Treat Me, Not My Age

TREAT ME, NOT MY AGE

A Doctor's Guide to Getting the Best Care
as You or a Loved One Gets Older

MARK LACHS, MD, MPH

Professor of Medicine, Weill Cornell Medical College
Director of Geriatrics, New York-Presbyterian Healthcare System

VIKING

VIKING
Published by the Penguin Group
Penguin Group (USA) Inc., 375 Hudson Street, New York, New York 10014, U.S.A. • Penguin Group (Canada), 90 Eglinton Avenue East, Suite 700, Toronto, Ontario, Canada M4P 2Y3 (a division of Pearson Penguin Canada Inc.) • Penguin Books Ltd, 80 Strand, London WC2R 0RL, England • Penguin Ireland, 25 St. Stephen's Green, Dublin 2, Ireland (a division of Penguin Books Ltd) • Penguin Books Australia Ltd, 250 Camberwell Road, Camberwell, Victoria 3124, Australia (a division of Pearson Australia Group Pty Ltd) • Penguin Books India Pvt Ltd, 11 Community Centre, Panchsheel Park, New Delhi—110 017, India • Penguin Group (NZ), 67 Apollo Drive, Rosedale, North Shore 0632, New Zealand (a division of Pearson New Zealand Ltd) • Penguin Books (South Africa) (Pty) Ltd, 24 Sturdee Avenue, Rosebank, Johannesburg 2196, South Africa

Penguin Books Ltd, Registered Offices: 80 Strand, London WC2R 0RL, England

First published in 2010 by Viking Penguin, a member of Penguin Group (USA) Inc.

10 9 8 7 6 5 4 3 2 1

Grateful acknowledgment is made for permission to use the following copyrighted works:

Selection by Robert N. Butler, MD. Used by permission of Robert N. Butler, MD. • Excerpt from *How to Live to Be 100—Or More* by George Burns (Putnam, 1983). By permission of InkWell Management. • Excerpt from *Halloween* by Jerry Seinfeld. By permission of Little, Brown and Company. • Cartoon by Mike Twohy. Copyright © Mike Twohy / The New Yorker Collection / www.cartoonbank.com. By permission of The Cartoon Bank. • Selection by Rodney Dangerfield. By permission of Joan Dangerfield. Excerpt from *You're Only Old Once!* by Dr. Seuss. Copyright TM & copyright © by Dr. Seuss Enterprises, L.P. 1986. Used by permission of Random House, Inc. • Selection by Brian Regan. By permission of Brian Regan. • Selection by Tom Cotter. By permission of Tom Cotter. • Selections from *Annals of Internal Medicine*: "Comparison of Yoga, Exercise, and Education for the Treatment of Chronic Low Back Pain" (December 20, 2005, vol. 143); "Glucosamine Sulfate to Treat Hip Osteoarthritis" (February 19, 2008, vol. 148); "The Relationship between Green Tea Intake and Type 2 Diabetes in Japanese Adults" (April 18, 2006, vol. 144); and "Adding Acupuncture to Physical Therapy and Anti-Inflammatory Drugs in the Treatment of Knee Osteoarthritis" (July 4, 2006, vol. 145). By permission of the American College of Physicians.

Author's Note
The views expressed in this book are not the views of the NewYork-Presbyterian Healthcare System or Weill Cornell Medical College.

Publisher's Note
Neither the publisher nor the author is engaged in rendering professional advice or services to the individual reader. The ideas, procedures, and suggestions contained in this book are not intended as a substitute for consulting with your physician. All matters regarding your health require medical supervision. Neither the author nor the publisher shall be liable or responsible for any loss or damage allegedly arising from any information or suggestion in this book.

LIBRARY OF CONGRESS CATALOGING-IN-PUBLICATION DATA
Lachs, Mark.
Treat me, not my age : a doctor's guide to getting the best care as you or a loved one gets older / Mark Lachs.
p. ; cm.
Includes bibliographical references and index.
ISBN 978-0-670-02210-6
1. Aging. 2. Ageism. 3. Geriatrics. I. Title.
[DNLM: 1. Aging—psychology. 2. Geriatrics. 3. Aged. 4. Attitude. WT 100 L138t 2010]
QP86.L335 2010
612.6'7—dc22
2010017487

Printed in the United States of America

For Susan, Joshua, David, and Lauren

ACKNOWLEDGMENTS

The buzzword in aging medicine and research these days is *interdisciplinary*. That applies to these acknowledgments, because the people who have helped me with this book were recruited—willingly and unwillingly—from all quarters of my personal and professional orbit. Gathered in a room they would constitute truly odd bedfellows, but I like to think that it now "all makes sense" given the topics tackled in this book, and how I've tried to present them: one part science, one part social work, and one part stand-up.

I have featured the research of several eminent scientists and clinicians who work in the field of gerontology. Their work is critical to the future of our aging nation. Without fanfare they toil endlessly in areas of scientific inquiry that no one else wants to (or has the superb scientific taste to pursue). Some of their personal and professional quests are featured in the book; several have provided useful edits and ideas—Sharon Inouye, Eric Coleman, and Sean Morrison to name a few. Others are mentioned in passing or perhaps inadvertently left out altogether; I apologize in advance to these colleagues. Many other geriatricians and gerontologists have reviewed chapters, sections, or permitted interviews to fortify the manuscript and help me develop the ideas. David Reuben at UCLA has been a constant source of advice and counsel throughout my career, as has Dr. Robert Butler, who coined the term *ageism*. My dear friend Karl Pillemer at Cornell University in Ithaca read the manuscript with both an academic and populist eye; David Pomeranz from the

Hebrew Home for the Aged provided assistance with the section on housing and long-term care, as did Eric Tyson for the chapters involving aging and money. The chapters on older people in the emergency department were ably fortified by Doctors Michael Stern and Carolyn Hullick. Dan Fish and Neil Cutler were generous with their time and ideas in the area of elder law and financial gerontology. While the citation and acknowledgment of these colleagues should in no way be construed as an endorsement of this book or my ideas, I am grateful that so many of the positions I have taken seem to resonate with the aging community.

Patients, families, and friends have contributed terabytes of useful information. I'm tempted to say you know who you are, but the truth is, I hope you don't. Although virtually every patient and family member I approached were delighted to tell their tales, I've gone to great lengths to "anonymize" them by amalgamating stories and changing names, diseases, genders (except the guy with prostate problems), locations, and some clinical details where warranted. So if you know who you are, I apologize to you, too.

I'm also indebted to my work family: The Division of Geriatric Medicine and Gerontology at Weill Cornell Medical College—New York–Presbyterian Hospital. To mention a few of them would be a profound injustice to the rest; every single one of them—physicians, nurses, social workers, support staff, administrators—has taught me something about aging. But I must mention one: my co-chief Ron Adelman, a constant source of encouragement, counsel, knowledge, and friendship.

The senior brass here has also made visionary investments in aging that should serve as an example for other academic medical centers. At the Medical College Dean Tony Gotto has understood and supported geriatrics from day one of his advent. My chairman Andy Schafer and his predecessor Ralph Nachman have listened to my ideas about geriatrics (and my intermittent whining) and given me sage advice about when to battle for my faculty or older constituency (usually battling with me or for me). At New York–Presbyterian Hospital, Herb Pardes, Steve Corwin, and Laura Forese have been similarly supportive, understanding that a great hospital needs a great aging program. I'll simply summarize by saying that I work in one of the finest medical centers in the country, if not the world.

Then there are the mentors who have had considerable influence on my choice of geriatrics and my style of doctoring, teaching, and researching. Towering among them is the late Alvan Feinstein. No one could meld mathematics, Camus, and Myron Cohen like Alvan; he taught me that disparate ideas and people could occupy the same paragraph or PowerPoint presentation and be a thrilling thing of exceptional beauty. The intellectual influence of others from my Yale days are also always with me: Leo Cooney, Ralph Horwitz, and Mary Tinetti are among those who have helped shaped my career.

Various foundations and organizations have been relentless in supporting aging research (including my own), policy, and services. The American Federation for Aging Research (led by Stephanie Lederman), The Hartford Foundation (led by Corrine Rieder), The Starr Foundation (led by Florence Davis), and The Commonwealth Fund (led by Karen Davis) are wonderful examples. The Atlantic Philanthropies has also had an unwavering commitment to geriatrics internationally. Locally, Julio Urbina and Lauren Weisenfeld of the Fan Fox and Leslie R. Samuels Foundation have been the "angel investors" in improving the lives of older New Yorkers. Sid Stahl at NIA has been my scientific program officer for over a decade, and I'm indebted to him not only for his wise counsel, but also for permitting the sabbatical that launched this excursion.

Our work in the division has also been championed and supported by some amazing ambassadors and their families, many of whom constitute our longevity council. In no particular order they include Paula and Ira Resnick (who did some fine editing), Teri Mendelson, Carol Einiger, Ellen Marram, Dana Stone, Cynthia Manocherian, Hilary Koota, and Daniella Lipper. Our extended family also includes Margot Adams as well as Steven and David Silbermann and their families.

There are a few great friends without whom this book would have never happened. I'm deeply indebted to Susan Burden and William Goldman (my rabbi in the writing process), not only for their encouragement, but for introducing me to my literary agent, Janis Donnaud and Peter Gethers. Wendy Wolf and Kevin Doughten at Viking Penguin have also put up with the schedule and penmanship of a full-time-geriatrician-trying-to-be-part-time-author with extraordinary patience. My old friend Mitch Blutt provided well-timed encouragement as well as edits, as did Kelly DeKeyser and *Seinfeld*-writer-turned-medical-student buddy Andy Robin. And on the friends list I would be remiss in not including Scott Brody and Jason Sebell at Camp Kenwood Evergreen; I crafted a good deal of this book sitting under shady trees in Wilmot, New Hampshire, during my stints as camp doctor in the company of good friends and good times.

But in the end it was my family that really made this book possible. My wife, Susan, was the first to read each and every chapter, opining thoughtfully like the avid reader she is. Writing this book infringed on some precious quality time with my kids, Lauren, David, and Joshua, who were already enduring their father's hectic schedule. They never complained. On the contrary, they often expressed pride in the undertaking in the face of grumpiness. God's greatest gift to me has been this outfit, and I could never thank them enough. A big shout-out and much love to all of you!

February 2010

CONTENTS

Acknowledgments   vii

1   Introduction   I

2   "You're a What?"   12
       Understanding How Geriatricians Think About Aging

3   The Biology of Aging   26
       An Embarrassment of Riches That You Were
       Never Supposed to Need

4   A Geriatrician's Perspective on Ageism   42
       It's Not Just Grandpa Who's Being Put Out to Pasture

5   Do No Harm, but for God's Sake, Do Something!   52

6   Cookbook Medicine   65
       A Recipe for Disaster at Any Age

7   Bedside Matters   78
       Do You Have an Aging-Friendly Primary Care Doctor?

8   How Many Specialists Does It Take to
       Screw in a Lightbulb (or Screw You Up)?   105

9   Care Transitions as We Get Older   116
       Cracks You Didn't Even Know You Could Fall Through

10 No Place for Sick People   131
   Hospitals as We Get Older

11 You Could Become Geriatric Just Waiting   156
   How to Emerge from the Emergency Room Unscathed

12 In Search of an Honorable Discharge   173

13 Maybe You're Not the Problem   192
   Disability Caused by Places and Not People (or Their Diseases)

14 Homes Away from Home as We Age   203

15 Medications as We Age   224

16 Complementary and Alternative Medicine,
   Vitamins, and Supplements   235
   Who Do You Believe?

17 Money and Aging   257

18 Financial Gerontology   275
   The Good, the Bad, and the Phony

19 It Ain't Over Till It's Over
   (and Sometimes Not Even Then)   294
   A Geriatrician Talks about Death and Dying

20 Staying in Control   319
   Making and Encouraging Good Choices as We Age

21 It's Never Too Late...   350

   Appendix   361
   Notes   371
   Index   379

Treat Me, Not My Age

Chapter 1

Introduction

Morris says to his doctor, "My right knee hurts."
"How old are you now, Morris?" asks the doctor.
"I'm 101," he replies.
"Well, what do you expect at your age?"
Morris pauses for a second, then rises in anger.
"The problem with that, Doc, is that my left knee is also 101, and it
   doesn't hurt at all!"

—Robert N. Butler, MD,
founding director, National Institute on Aging;
president, International Longevity Center

I wrote this book at the urging of many of my patients and their families who face a recurring conundrum that I suspect is probably familiar to you, too. Again and again I see patients of all ages—highly intelligent people—who are trying to reconcile two powerful forces that seem to be growing in ferocity with each passing day.

On the one hand, whether they're sick, well, or somewhere in between, they have a general awareness of scientific breakthroughs in aging, and they wonder whether they or their loved ones are fully availing themselves of that science. They may have read about a procedure, a supplement, a lifestyle change, or another nonmedical intervention (like mental exercises or calorie restriction) in the *New York Times* and wonder whether they should believe it, adopt it, or approach their primary care doc about it. But they may also have a nagging sense of insecurity about their longstanding trusted source of medical advice—the family doctor—especially if he or she has already started to write off their "aging concerns," like the man with the bum knee in the opening parable. They're smart and wary of folly but would hate to miss an important train that's about to leave the station without them. In short, they'd like to responsibly consider some health-promoting strategies as they age but don't want to learn that this year's darling supplement is next year's radon. It makes me think of the doctors of the future in Woody Allen's *Sleeper* who marvel that late-twentieth-century physicians had not discovered the health benefits of cigarettes and chocolate cake.

On the other hand, these patients have what my teenage daughter would describe as the "TMI" (too much information) problem. They are bombarded daily with emphatic pitches from the television, the Internet, health newsletters, radio shows, and the guy with a nearby locker at the health club (maybe even a physician) who outlines in explicit detail the steps they should be taking right now to extend life, run marathons, improve the performance or size of various body parts, or return mental acuity to undergraduate levels. And then there are the friends, colleagues, kids, or parents who subscribe to their own particular notions, potions, or life plans (or the gurus who espouse them) with the rapture of a televangelist. Modern medicine (the medicine *you* are getting *now*) has missed the boat entirely, they seem to say. That's tough to stomach if you've been led to believe you've been taking good care of yourself in partnership with your doctor, but it's especially jarring if you've been struggling with a chronic illness that you've been working hard to understand. Suddenly you're told you've been going about it all wrong. You think you've been responsible, only to learn that you've been duped by the system.

Where is the balance? How does one even begin to find and digest all the information that relates to getting older in a responsible way? What is important and what is noise? And even if you have the skill set to filter out the best information, how do you possibly find the time?

Oh, and I'm not done yet. There's an even lower floor to this house of cards, with a greater impact, that you probably haven't even considered, one that we folks in aging worry about all the time. Even if you could identify the "right" things to do or not to do to your body, there's unsettling news about the medical and social systems within which you make those decisions and try to implement them: These systems, which are meant to help you, are in fact failing you. It's clear from where I sit as a gerontologist that there's a new underclass in town. If you are over fifty, all you need to do is look in the mirror to find the newest object of American bigotry. We baby boomers and our parents no longer lead the way in the American processional. Now perceived as a drain on all kinds of resources in this youth-obsessed society, we have become the new scapegoats on the block.

Notice I said "underclass." I did not say "minority." We're not talking about a modest-sized constituency here. No, it's a growing tidal wave of older adults who—after years of poking fun at friends and colleagues with "over the hill" birthday cards, Viagra jokes, and jibes about Botox vacations—have survived and multiplied to become the target of their own discrimination.

Why as a physician am I so interested in this topic? Because we're not just talking about hurt feelings, nor is this simply about blood pressure, cholesterol, and mammograms. I hope to convince you that the factors that influence how well we age are related not only to personal health but also to the systems that claim to promote it. Over the past twenty-five years I've worked at some of the most respected medical institutions in our country and witnessed care received by my patients, my family, and myself at places great and small. I've been taught by some really smart and committed people and have reciprocated by training thousands of medical students and residents in internal medicine and geriatrics. And here's what I've learned: "Ageism" in American medicine and society is a matter of life and death, as dangerous as any incorrectly prescribed medication or slipped scalpel.

If that's not worrisome enough, there's another observation that should concern you. You don't have to be *that old* to experience this phenomenon. In the same way that people don't become "old" overnight when they hit some arbitrary retirement age, ageism in medicine sneaks up on patients long before they meet me for their first "geriatric" physical. It's a subtle process, one that begins as people enter their sixties, their fifties, and even their forties (which, in my business, is the neonatal unit). The comparison to infancy is not just a joke. In the same way that seemingly small errors or oversights in pediatric health care, such as poor nutrition or missed vaccinations, can produce preventable but lifelong misery, the improper care and feeding of baby boomers can lead to "later life" disabilities that could spell the difference between living independently and having a nursing home as your last address.

But here's the good news: You have more control than you think you do. You can live longer *and* live better, and many of the keys to this involve not only what care you receive but how you receive it. There are steps you can take to make sure you don't become the victim of the kind of medical and societal bigotry I'm talking about, and I'm just the guy to lay it out for you because I've seen it all: Older adults and their families undertreated, overtreated, or even untreated. Physical and psychological complaints that may be treatable but are dismissed by busy doctors with a fatalism that can send patients the subtle but poisonous message to go home and give up. Patients and families left in the dark. Institutions that were built—culturally, operationally, and architecturally—for twenty-somethings but are caring mostly for boomers and their parents in a bizarre medical mismatch that can be downright dangerous.

While I'm willing to take heat from colleagues and skewer the health-care system about many of the problems faced by people who are getting older, I'm only willing to do it up to a point. Patients and their families also bear substantial responsibility in perpetuating this "status quo." Adult children complain to me endlessly about their parents' bashfulness about "bothering the doctor" even when potentially serious symptoms arise. For God's sake, we're talking about your health here, not some body work your car needs! Or perhaps out of some misplaced sense of loyalty you might be unwilling to consider changing doctors even though he or she is not returning phone calls or taking your concerns seriously. Or maybe you've given up on Western medicine entirely, instead spending your hard-earned money on heavily marketed anti-aging or alternative medical products without any clear proof of the effectiveness of these treatments or understanding of how they might interact with any traditional stuff you're taking. So, no, I'm not letting you off the hook either.

What's in This Book—and What's Not

This book is about taking charge of your health and health care—or that of a parent or loved one you may be worrying about—but from a very specific vantage point: the "long view" unique to an internist-geriatrician who cares for those of us who are "young" or who have already hit seventy, eighty, or ninety; those of us who realize we are getting there; or those who are just beginning to understand and accept that it's where life's journey will ultimately (and hopefully) take us.

Sure, the book is about health, but it's even more about how systems and environments collide with our aging bodies to influence health. It also contains more than twenty-five years' worth of "insider" tips, tricks, and knowledge that I've collected while caring for thousands of patients and their families as well as immersing myself in the literature of my profession (to which I've also contributed). It makes use of invaluable insights and ideas gleaned from colleagues and, most important, from patients and their families. I'm constantly sharing these with other patients and families, and this book enables me to share them with you.

Now more than ever, it's important that you learn how to fish rather than just letting me spoon-feed you some geriatric paella. If you're looking for how much selenium to take this morning, exactly which tai chi class you should enroll in to prevent falling, or which company you should get your long-term care insurance from, you've come to the wrong guy. Those sands shift under our feet from day to day. That's why there are few truly enduring health books: Diet and exercise crazes come and go, supplements go in and out of favor, and every few years there's a new skin-care guru. But if I can explain to you what we know about aging and how the systems—medical and nonmedical—work and don't work as we get older, you'll be positioned to make the best decisions no matter what comes down the pike. It reminds me a bit of a very popular (and enduring) book about pregnancy that remained relevant to my wife over a decade of pregnancies because it provided expectant mothers with *an education about the science of pregnancy* (a part of the aging continuum, by the way) rather than simply spouting preferred yoga positions or specific vitamins for the gravid.

In the next chapter, I'll explain what I do, because it's the basis for understanding both how our needs change as we age and what "rules of the road" geriatricians use to look at patients as they age. You'll gain insight into how geriatricians think—it's vastly different from how most physicians are trained to think—and it will help you enormously as you consider the medical problems that you or a parent are confronting. I'll explain how medical and nonmedical needs begin to meld as people age. Even with the best medical care, you can still get sick as a dog when the nonmedical pieces of the equation are ignored, as is the tendency in most rushed modern health-care settings these days.

In chapter 4, I'll talk about medical ageism: not only why the health-care system is profoundly broken for older people but *how* it's broken. This is not some esoteric exercise in medical sociology and history. Rather, you need to understand where the medical quicksand is as you get older (everywhere, basically) and what it looks like in each health-care environment. Here and throughout the book, I will use patients' stories and cite very important (and sometimes unsettling) medical literature on how and why physicians often miss common problems associated with aging. It's a bit like the "pathophysiology" course taken by second-year medical students, in which they learn exactly how the body breaks down during specific illnesses, only I'll also break down how systems fail in these situations. This is critical, because if you don't understand the disease in detail, you can't devise a treatment.

Then I get even more specific. I'll talk about doctors. I'll tell you how physicians pick *their* physicians. I'll teach you how to assess the quality of a physician as you get older, not only with respect to technical ability, but also with regard to communication skills. You should be interested in the latter not only because it's nice to like your doctor (which, by the way, is usually but not always a key factor) but also because research is starting to suggest that a better bedside manner and communications skills are associated not only with greater satisfaction with medical care but also with better outcomes in some situations. If your doctor can't talk to you—and listen to you—there's a greater likelihood that you or your parent will be incorrectly diagnosed (and, along the way, sent for a series of expensive, useless, and potentially dangerous tests). I'll explain how you can tell if your doctor is a gem and whether you should hold on to him or her for dear life, and also when you should consider firing an underperforming medical man or woman.

I'll also talk about the other people who work in health care. As medicine becomes more hurried and expensive, much of the care that was previously delivered by physicians and nurses is being rendered by a slew of other folks with confusing degrees and abbreviations after their names. They are crucial players but still receive short shrift in a medical and lay world that remains doctor-centric. For example, I believe that for some chronic conditions and situations, physicians may be the *wrong day-to-day health-care provider*; you might be better served by a nurse practitioner or a physician's assistant ("physician extenders," as they're sometimes belittlingly called). I can't tell you how many times some of my misguided patients have recoiled at this idea, preferring to see a high-end cardiologist for a ten-minute monthly visit rather than having weekly or nearly daily interactions with a dedicated nurse practitioner who may have twenty years' more experience than the doctor. I'll tell you how to find the best one for the specific need you have. I see the same biases with health-care professionals in other settings as well. For example, I've seen patients obsess endlessly about which surgeon to choose for a complicated cardiac procedure but then give no thought whatsoever to the quality of the home health attendant who will be providing continuous and daily hands-on care to help them recover over the next month.

And then when I'm done with the health-care *people*, I'll talk in detail about the health-care *places*. I'll explain why, when it comes to older adults, the hospital can be a bad place for sick people. Folks young and old can get sick in the hospital apart from whatever brought them there in the first place. As frightening as that sounds, there are scientifically based interventions you can use to minimize this risk, and I'll go through them in detail.

I'll also discuss the places where people finish their recovery—at home, at rehabilitation facilities, and in nursing homes, which are no longer just the last stop on the train but increasingly a waypoint on the convalescence journey. Many people don't realize that, no matter what your age, there's a high likelihood that if you'll have a long recovery after a hospitalization and you're not well enough to go home, you'll wind up receiving "subacute care" in a nursing home. You may have gone to great lengths to pick your hospital, but how can you assess the quality of a nursing home that will complete the critical part of your recovery? Do you have any say as to which facility the hospital sends you to? What happens if you think you can go directly home to avoid such a place, but your doctor disagrees?

I'm also well aware that the decision many of us face for ourselves or our parents when it comes to a nursing home or an assisted-living facility involves more than just a brief stay. Sometimes we have to choose such a facility as a permanent address. As a geriatrician I've helped many families struggling to decide what type of facility to choose—nursing home, assisted-living facility, "life care" community—and I've also helped them decide between facilities of the same type. Not only are families in the midst of a medical crisis in a poor position to assess these places, usually physicians are, too. I'm amazed at how often families will ask a primary care or other doctor to choose or recommend a facility, when research suggests that most physicians never set foot in any long-term-care facility, except perhaps to visit their own grandparents! In fact, most physicians do not understand the differences among the various types of facilities or how each is paid for. But you will after reading this book. Finding a place to stay doesn't have to be a gloomy process if tackled with the right preemptive energy.

Other chapters deal with common issues I encounter in my practice in people of all ages. For example, I believe there are some alternative medicine treatments that are worth adopting and others you shouldn't waste your money on; I'll explain how, as a geriatrician, I help patients sort that out. Although it's not a cheery topic, I'll talk about advance directives, living wills, and health-care proxies in plain, easy-to-understand language; the "legalese" that's been injected into that topic has frozen many people into inaction and, as a result, caused unnecessary suffering not only for patients but also for their families as they stand by powerlessly without clear direction.

I'll talk about work and how retirement, at least for some people, can be one of the most stressful experiences in American life and can greatly impact physical and emotional health. I'll walk you through the decision to work, retire, or volunteer at every step of the way. And I'll talk about money. As the song goes: *it changes everything.* I don't care how much or how little wealth you or a parent has accumulated over a lifetime: you can burn through it quickly in the modern health-care world. Should it be spent on your care to modestly improve quality of life or left to squabbling adult kids? You don't seriously think that those playground sibling rivalries died when the kids left the nest, do you? No, they tend to resurface with a vengeance when Mom or Dad gets sick, and I'll advise you about how to approach these issues.

And if you're reading this book because of concerns for someone other than yourself, let me clarify something else. When I say "taking charge" of health, I'm well aware of how loaded the phrase is if we're talking about a parent or spouse. We hear so much about the role reversal that comes with caring for an aging parent, and let me give it to you straight—as a geriatrician I won't be a party to it. By "taking charge," I don't mean infantilizing or demeaning someone you care about by making him or her the child without a voice in this process. Geriatricians are very mindful of family dynamics—understanding them is part of our training after internal medicine. I like to believe this is one of the things that distinguishes us from other primary care docs. (One of my colleagues likes to say that part of the fun of training in our field is realizing that all families are screwed up, and that geriatrics enables you to figure out where your own clan ranks on the scoreboard.) I've been doing this a long time, and I assure you that in most cases getting your parent to accept the help he or she needs can be done in such a way that he or she runs the show to the greatest extent practical. Rob an older person of his or her dignity, and you're ruining quality of life, not enhancing it.

Throughout the book I'll cite relevant medical and sociological literature, not to drown you with detail but because it's interesting and I'd like you to understand the scientific basis for my assertions. An appendix at the back and an associated Web site (www .treatmenotmyage.com) can give you more detail or the "primary data" if you're interested.

One last thing: To introduce the ideas that I talk about in each chapter, I've chosen to reference snippets from popular culture—a memorable piece of stand-up comedy or one-liner, a cartoon, or a proverb or quotation. I don't care if you chuckle or not, because I'm going someplace else with these ditties: I'm trying to get you to think, reflect, maybe even wince a little at how we've come to view aging, as someone who's dedicated his career to preserving the health and dignity of people as they get older. As a mentor in medical school used to tell me, the harder a joke makes you laugh, the more important and serious the message is that it's conveying. I think the little story that began this chapter is emblematic of that: An older man whose symptoms are simply dismissed until his punch line shows us his intellectual strength and his courage while simultaneously lambasting his ageist doc.

One of the most dangerous ideas in American culture and medicine these days is that *aging is a disease.* How absurd! Aging is a part of the normal human development that begins in the womb. What's next? Is childhood a disease? To frame aging as a disease is to deny the idea itself—more or less the thrust of almost every popular book written about aging today. Yes, there are conditions that are more common as we age, but aging itself is not a disease. When we begin to believe that it is, we embark on a quest for a holy-grail cure that distracts us from addressing treatable needs in a way that can truly improve quality of life. Make no mistake: This is a book about gaining control as we get older, not surrendering it to people, places, ideas, or systems that are either anachronistic or just plain wrong about what it means to get older in these amazing times.

I'm not suggesting that anyone "go gentle into that good night"; my message is overwhelmingly one of hope. And I'm delighted that you've chosen to take a real and substantive journey with me.

Chapter 2

"You're a What?"

Understanding How Geriatricians Think About Aging

There's an old saying: "Life begins at forty."
That's silly—life begins every morning when you wake up.

—George Burns

My mother-in-law remains crestfallen. Although I graduated from medical school nearly twenty-five years ago, she still believes that her daughter endured my 110-hour workweek and meager intern compensation only to end up married to a social worker (a badge I wear proudly, by the way). To her way of thinking, the family should have gotten a surgeon or at least a cardiologist. She hasn't actually said it, but deep down I've always had this sinking suspicion that she believes I could have been a contender.

The questions usually surface at the end of Thanksgiving dinner:

"You have an office, right?"

"Do you use a stethoscope?"

"Can you prescribe medicine, or is that only the doctors who operate?"

"You're a *real doctor*, right? Not like a PhD. I'm only asking because one of the ladies I play canasta with wanted to know."

Since I'm well versed in reassuring her, permit me to do it again here; it lays the groundwork nicely for the crash course I'm about to give you, in the next chapter, about what we know about human longevity, the biology of aging, and how you can use that knowledge to your advantage.

I am a *geriatrician*—a physician who provides care to older people and support to their families in the same way that a pediatrician serves children and their families. But I'm also an *internist*—a physician who completed three years of internal-medicine training after medical school—studying the complex inner workings of the body and the nonsurgical treatment of diseases many adults acquire over the course of a lifetime (for example, high blood pressure, diabetes, arthritis). After completing training in internal medicine (our specialty), most practitioners of geriatrics (our subspecialty) spend an additional year or two learning our craft, as other internal-medicine graduates might select additional training in one of the other subspecialties of internal medicine that you're probably more familiar with, such as cardiology, gastroenterology, endocrinology, or oncology. The training content of geriatric medicine is vastly different from that of any of those subspecialties (and altogether different from training in any other area of medicine, really).

A *gerontologist* is generally someone who does research in the area of aging. But because aging can be defined broadly, there are researchers from a wide range of fields—economics, biology, housing, transportation, psychology—who call themselves gerontologists. Some gerontologists aren't physicians but provide direct clinical service exclusively to older people (such as a psychologist who might choose to work with older people exclusively).

Invariably, after I give my geriatrician-versus-gerontologist spiel and folks understand that I'm a "real" doctor, they ask a series of predictable questions. "How old do I have to be to see you?" or "How old is geriatric?" usually comes first. This is, in fact, the central metaphysical question in geriatrics, and since metaphysics contends that the universe is relative, I'll provide a relative answer: It depends.

Let me explain. Needing a geriatrician is partially about age but mostly about function. In my practice I have ninety-year-olds who are going to work on a daily basis, and providing care for them is very much like doctoring a fifty-year-old. But visit just about any nursing home in America and you'll find fifty- and sixty-year-olds who have been rendered impaired by diseases like multiple sclerosis or stroke, and caring for them is very similar to caring for frail ninety-year-olds. So there's really no age at which you become geriatric. If you're young or old and have many chronic diseases and functional problems, geriatricians are probably for you, but we're also delighted to see older patients who are doing well and are trying to avoid frailty. As one of my patients in her early sixties likes to say, "How old is geriatric? The older I get, the older it gets!"

Another question I'm frequently asked is whether I'm a primary care physician (like the doctor you see for your annual physical or when you have a cold) or a consultant (like the doc you see for a one- or two-shot deal when you have a specific problem, like an orthopedist for a broken bone or a bad shoulder). Answer: both. Most geriatricians provide primary care to older adults and see them annually or more frequently as the need arises, but we're also called on by patients, families, and other doctors to help with specific problems and questions like the following:

- Is my memory loss normal for my age?
- Am I taking too many medicines?
- Why is my mom falling?
- Is my hospitalized patient confused from medications, or is it another problem?
- Can Dad *really* live alone safely without help, or am I just being overprotective?

And finally, while we're dispensing with questions I'm most frequently asked, let me also deal with the ever-present, morbid end-of-life question: "Doc, it must be tough dealing with only dying patients. How do you do it?"

Well, first of all, the only people I know who are not dying, at whatever speed, are already dead.

Do I deal with end-of-life issues in my practice? Sure. But I prefer to frame it another way: While I certainly have expertise in hospice and palliative care, I am much more interested in *how people live* during the last years of their life on this planet, however long or short those years are. I have absolutely no interest in extending life expectancy to the extent that people are living and breathing but unable to do the things that mean the most to them. Those nursing homes with a smattering of prematurely disabled fifty-year-olds that I just told you about? Far more common are tenants aged eighty, ninety, and beyond, who have very limited quality of life. I would argue that the "life extension" these people have experienced—a good deal of it a result of technology—is as big a failure of medicine as any forty-year-old dying of breast cancer or fifty-year-old perishing from a heart attack.

As the Talmudic scholar Ben Azai said, "every man has his time." So for me, the question is not if or even when but, really, "how." My goal for patients is that when they leave the planet (believe it or not, not optional, a truth that has been lost on many Americans—see chapter 19), they do so enjoying the things they love most—family, golf, painting, theater, sex—ideally up until the very last minute possible. John Kennedy said it best in a special address to Congress in 1963, unbelievably prescient for its time:[1]

This increase in the life span and in the number of our senior citizens presents this Nation with increased opportunities: the opportunity to draw upon their skill and sagacity—and the opportunity to provide the respect and recognition they have earned. It is not enough for a great nation merely to have added new years to life—our objective must also be to add new life to those years.

Now that I have dispensed with my Thanksgiving soliloquy, it's time to get down to business.

At the core of it, two things separate geriatrics from all other forms of medical practice. The first is our emphasis on function, rather than on diagnoses or labels that people have accumulated over the course of their lifetime; and the second is our insistence on considering how factors that would seem outside the "traditional" purview of medicine have an impact on that function and on the patient and family. Let me talk about each of these factors individually so you can begin to understand the way we're taught and how we think.

Geriatrics Rule #1:
I Don't Really Care What They've Told You You Have

Several times a year I serve as the "hospitalist" for older patients who get admitted to my hospital. Typically I have not been the primary care physician for these people; they either enter the hospital through the emergency department or get transferred to the geriatric floor when problems arise that would be better handled by a team with our skill set rather than by the team on the floor to which they were initially admitted. While they're at my wonderful institution, I am the physician responsible for all aspects of their care, including the oversight provided by some superb eager-beaver residents I'm trying to convert to geriatrics. Each morning these young docs tell me about the new "cases" (I hate that word) that came in the night before, whereupon I'll try to impart some wisdom that will both help the patient get better and (I hope) offer some teaching pearls to these doctors-to-be.

One morning recently the medical residents presented the case of an eighty-four-year-old man who had come for a relatively simple procedure on his bladder. Besides bladder cancer, he had an extensive medical history that included prostate problems, heart disease, emphysema, a prior stroke, and a colon cancer that had been removed recently. Unfortunately, his procedure had been complicated by pneumonia, which landed him on our geriatric service. What was supposed to be a one- or two-night stay in the hospital had evolved into a three-week excursion, despite everyone's best efforts to help him.

The resident dutifully reported the long list of diseases that the man had experienced over his lifetime before this one had reared its head, followed by a list of at least a dozen medications the poor fellow was taking, those he came with and those that had become necessary during his stay. As I took notes my hand cramped from the litany of diagnoses, as well as the long list of medications being poured into him (the cost of which could have rivaled the entire pharmaceuticals budget of several small developing nations).

I studied the faces of the new medical students who had just joined my service as they listened and could see the mental image they were gathering of this poor man we were about to see. Maybe a bedridden man cared for at home by round-the-clock nurses? Perhaps a resident of the local nursing home who was wheeled to various meals and bingo games—if he had enough marbles to participate?

I said to the resident, "John, you've done a nice job of providing a detailed medical history about this fella, but you haven't told me anything at all about his functional ability, either now or before he was admitted to the hospital. Can he walk? Does he feed himself? Was he going to work before all this happened? Who does he live with? Can he take medicines by himself? What's his vision like? Does he wear glasses? Could he hear what you were saying to him when you examined him, and if he could, do you think that he could understand it?"

There was a long pause. The resident had, by all modern medical educational criteria, performed magnificently. He had dutifully explicated all the medical problems the man had acquired over a lifetime, detailed his medication list and allergies, and provided a family history going back three generations that any genealogist would be in awe of. But he could not tell me if this guy lived in a nursing home or ran a multinational corporation.

I work at a renowned teaching hospital (New York-Presbyterian Healthcare System) and its affiliated medical school (Weill Cornell Medical College), and if ever there was a "teachable moment," this was it. When we went to the bedside to examine the patient, I found a delightful man who motioned to me urgently. I thought he was having some kind of medical crisis. It was indeed a crisis, but more of a recreational one:

"Doctor! I need a ten-letter word that could be used to describe an honest drug dealer and begins with an *a*," he said.

"*Apothecary*," I replied.

He thanked me because my assistance permitted him to continue uninterrupted his twenty-two-year streak of completing the Sunday crossword puzzle every week. He said he loved doing it so much he even had his office fax it to him when he was in Europe on business trips.

Not a doddering nursing home resident.

That same morning, the team had admitted another patient for pneumonia as well. This seventy-nine-year-old lady had had absolutely no medical problems whatsoever and had taken not a single medicine until she had a major stroke six months earlier. She was volunteering at a museum as a docent five days a week and writing a book about orchids when she suffered this life-changing event, which left her unable to speak, walk, or care for herself. She was living in a nursing home when she was transferred to our hospital for treatment of the pneumonia.

What a compelling juxtaposition. Two patients of nearly the same age. One with a single medical problem—stroke—who was completely bed bound and without any meaningful quality of life. The other riddled with medical "labels"—heart disease, a prior stroke, prostate disease, bladder and colon cancer—who was functioning much as he had in his fifties—with complete independence.

Are you getting the picture here? Something is not quite right with the way modern medicine has taught doctors to think about patients. The medical words physicians use to describe maladies simply do not speak to the quality of life experienced by patients; there is all too often a complete disconnect between the two.

What geriatricians bring to this party is an emphasis on function rather than on labels. Yes, I'm an internist, and I know how to adjust insulin, prescribe blood pressure medicines, and read EKGs—it's all part of what I do, and I'm pretty darn good at it. But I'm much more interested in how various medical problems interact to produce the living, breathing patient sitting on the examining table across from me, and how it enables or disables him from doing whatever it is he wants to do. Why else would he come to see me?

I'm also a bit more interested and schooled in a bunch of areas that the average family doc might not be. I know a bit more about teeth—real ones and fake ones. I'm not a shrink, but I've had intensive training in psychiatry and psychology, since problems of depression and memory often complicate the care of older people (and because for a certain generation of patients, seeing a psychiatrist is stigmatizing and absolutely out of the question, so I'm "it"). I know more about podiatry than your average doc. I can teach a patient how to use a cane properly, and although I don't own a hearing aid, I know how to adjust one.

Geriatrics Rule #2:
I Don't Just Want You for Your Body

There are a few exceptions, but "traditional" medical care is primarily interested in how and why you got sick based solely on the body you bring to the doctor's office. What's trotted into the examining room is basically what's going to get assessed as the basis for your care. We geriatricians think bigger than that in a way that flies in the face of many trends in modern biomedical science.

If you haven't noticed recently, medicine has become more and more *reductionist*. It increasingly distills the human being down to the smallest parts studiable, based on the available science of the day. My father graduated from medical school in the 1950s, when the study of *organs* (hearts, livers, kidneys) was all the rage. By the 1960s, the *cells* that made up those organs were the science du jour. In the 1970s, cells came to seem gargantuan, and scientists embarked on the study of *organelles*—the parts of cells that could be visualized by high-powered microscopes, such as nuclei, chromosomes, and mitochondria. By the 1980s, you didn't really need a microscope much anymore, because by then we were down to the molecules that made up the organelles. Since the 1990s, we've drilled down to the individual atoms, and soon the subatomic particles that make up the molecules!

And don't be deceived into thinking that this "Honey I Shrunk the Patient" campaign is limited to laboratory scientists. No. Right there with those guys, at every medical school in the country, are the nonresearch doctors who have their own version of parse-the-patient. The tendency in American medicine toward specialization over the past fifty years is a very closely related phenomenon. There's typically one guy for each organ, and very often organ guy A has little interest in organ B or C, even if it's just next door.

The good news about this "fantastic voyage" of science is that remarkable discoveries have been made that will someday soon lead to treatments and even cures for some of the worst human afflictions. And as for supersubspecialists, I concede that some areas of clinical medicine are so complex and quickly changing that there's just no way to keep up-to-date on everything about organs A through Z; you pretty much have to limit yourself to just a few letters. At my medical school and hospital, I work alongside some of the most brilliant scientists and specialists of the day. I'm in awe of their intellect, drive, and tireless devotion to improving the human condition, both in the laboratory and at the bedside, and I ask for their help all the time.

But in my humble opinion as a geriatrician, there's also bad news in this trend toward specialization and microscience. I believe it has produced a kind of "molecular bigotry" in both science and clinical practice. Many of these breakthroughs at the molecular level have yet to have clinical relevance for my patients who are struggling to maintain independence or thinking about a nursing home in the here and now. On the research side, it has created a prejudice against researchers who are doing science involving anything bigger than quarks (and god forbid we should actually study the human being attached to all those subatomic particles). But there are many research questions not involving molecules that need to be answered to help patients, and they need to be answered quickly. My father had Alzheimer's disease, and I'm in my fifties—what should I be doing? What kinds of exercises might prevent my mom from falling? Should an eighty-five-year-old patient with slightly elevated cholesterol get treated if she's had no cardiovascular problems whatsoever? Should all eighty-year-old women still get annual mammograms? How can I tell if my eighty-eight-year-old patient should still be driving? If only the mitochondria could speak . . .

Enter the geriatrician, the antidote to reductionist medicine, whether it comes to research or the art of doctoring. Not only do we reassemble all those molecules, cells, and organs back into a living, breathing human being, we go much further. We're interested in your environment, for example. I care if your home is reasonably well lit, especially if you've taken some falls. I need to know if your insurance will cover the physical therapy I've suggested. If you've recently lost a job, a friend, or, god forbid, a child, I must hear about it, because it may well influence your ability to properly take the medication I've prescribed. If you're living with the kind of overwhelming stress and psychosocial problems that makes simply surviving the day difficult, taking your daily blood pressure pill may not be on the top of your priority list. These might be important things for me to know.

And it gets even broader than your "immediate" environment. I can also tell you how to get Meals on Wheels deliveries and what Medicare will and won't pay for if your mom or dad is coming home from the hospital. I know the support groups that can help you deal with a devastating diagnosis, or the good adult day care center for Mom that also has great child care for your kid. I know the difference between a rehabilitation facility, a nursing home, an assisted living facility, and a life-care community, and I can make a much better recommendation than most local docs about which one is best for you or Mom (because I've actually been to them to see patients, rather than simply read the promotional materials they sent over). And by the way, don't think that these places are just for Mom and Dad—there's a good chance that in the future you'll be spending some recuperation time in one instead of a hospital if you get sick, as hospitals begin to accept only the sickest patients with the most extensive (and expensive) medical needs. I'll talk about the confusing nomenclature used to classify these "homes away from home" and what goes on in them later.

Now at this point you might reasonably be asking: Why in the world would a highly trained internist be farting around with things like senior centers, Meals on Wheels, the treatment of loneliness, and family dynamics?

The answer is rather Machiavellian but ultimately rooted in the science of gerontology: Study after study has shown that you can get as sick as a dog from social consternation, and that this kind of *tsuris*, as my grandmother would call it (the Yiddish is loosely translated as "unspeakable troubles"), can produce as much medical illness as any bona fide medical condition. The most famous of these research studies you probably have heard of, although perhaps not by name: The Alameda County Study.[2] Conducted in the late 1970s, this study looked at how surviving spouses fared after bereavement; you can guess the results, I'm sure. Even after statistically adjusting for preexisting diseases and conditions, researchers found that older adults who lost a spouse were at increased risk of dying in the subsequent year. Since that landmark research, a bevy of studies have spoken to the influence of social or "nonmedical" factors both on survival generally and on how people recover from specific illnesses. Some examples:

- A Yale study conducted in the 1990s demonstrated that, among men who sustained a heart attack, having good emotional support was an independent predictor of survival, even after controlling for how severely and how much of their hearts were injured in the attack.[3]
- In a Duke study of nearly four thousand older adults, those who regularly attended religious services at least once a week had a better survival rate a decade later than those who attended less frequently.[4]

- In a nine-year study of nearly seven thousand older adults, those who lacked community and social ties were more likely to die during the study period than those who had extensive contacts with their community and friends. Men were nearly three times as likely to die when socially isolated; women's risk was doubled.[5]

- In a European study of patients who had undergone invasive cardiovascular procedures (such as inserting stents) to treat narrowing of their coronary arteries, patients were asked how they perceived their general health after the procedure, independent of any physician assessment of their well-being. One year later, those who had reported their health to be good were two to three times more likely to be alive than those who rated their health less favorably.[6] This finding remained true even after considering the subjects' actual postoperative health as measured by medical professionals.

- In a study of women with newly diagnosed breast cancer, those who were socially isolated had a 66 percent increased risk of dying from the disease when compared to those with more extensive social networks. The researchers postulated that while poor social networks could limit access to care, such women also enjoyed less direct assistance and caregiving from friends, relatives, and children.[7]

I suspect you're getting the big picture here. As we age, medical problems and social problems become inextricably intertwined and interrelated. Medical illness can cause social difficulties, and social difficulties profoundly affect both the development of illness in the first place and/or the ability to weather an illness successfully. Whether the paramedics find you on the ground from a heart rhythm disturbance or from dehydration caused by your unwillingness to drink fluids after losing a loved one, you're sick and you're going to the hospital. If in the course of providing traditional medical care for you I prescribe a drug so expensive that you can't afford groceries and you become sick from malnourishment, I haven't really accomplished very much. The ability to show up for the physical therapy that I've suggested can be derailed by problems at home, such as poverty, family violence, or the mental illness of another family member. But most physicians would never know of these environmental circumstances from a fifteen-minute office visit. I have to if I am to do my job correctly.

Now, to be fair, this medical-social conspiracy theory we geriatricians cling to isn't just for older people. Dealing with medical illness at any age is going to be compounded by accompanying nonmedical grief. Weathering breast cancer when you're in the midst of a divorce is harder than when you have a supportive spouse. Having a heart attack is bad, but it's really bad if it happens the same week you lose your job (and I don't just mean affording the cardiac care you'll need). Think managing diabetes is tough? Try testing your blood sugar and dosing your insulin while you're worrying about a child with drug addiction or newly diagnosed schizophrenia. But what is it about getting older that makes the medical-social interplay so much more critical? Shouldn't medicine be attentive to interacting problems in people of all ages?

Answer: Of course it should. But as we get older, concurrent medical and social assaults begin to take a bigger toll and have a higher probability of resulting in demonstrable quality-of-life declines. Why? Because we begin to deplete some of the "extra capacity" we had when we were younger that enabled us to shoulder these problems without getting discombobulated. Medical and social stresses that would have elicited nary a burp from us as a twenty-five-year-old can produce gargantuan problems as we approach fifty. When stressed, "young folks" can "dig down" and tap into an extra capacity that takes many medical and social forms: wider coronary arteries to tolerate the rapid pulse that comes with a fever; a bigger social network to pitch in when a spouse is sick; better upper-body strength to use crutches when a leg is broken.

Geriatricians call that extra capacity *physiologic reserve*; it's important that you understand it, because it serves as the basis for many of the life-enhancing interventions I will describe in later chapters. And the best way I can help you to understand physiologic reserve is to offer a brief and interesting immersion course in how the biology of aging has collided with startling increases in longevity for the first time in the history of the human race.

Why as we age does every sports injury seem to last longer? When we get out of bed, why does every bone seem to creak louder? And why is every hangover tougher? For answers to this and other existential boomer questions, read on.

Chapter 3

The Biology of Aging

An Embarrassment of Riches That You Were Never Supposed to Need

*At the end of Halloween I was able to fill a punch bowl so full of candy
that the top of it would be curved. It was like a planet.
Next morning I'd wake up, feel fantastic. And that's when I realized,
when you're a kid you don't need a costume, you are Superman.*

—Jerry Seinfeld

Allow me to succinctly summarize a good deal of the first year of medical school for you (and save you a substantial tuition tab): The good lord was very generous when he or she put us together. Not only did we get too many of the organs we need to thrive, survive, and procreate (kidneys, eyes, ovaries, testicles, and so on); within those organs there is also an enormous amount of redundancy. For example, you probably know that you can survive perfectly fine with a single kidney; it's what makes kidney transplantation from a living donor possible—the donor experiences no ill health effects from offering a sibling this remarkable gift.

Have you ever asked yourself how this could be? How could removing an entire vital organ have absolutely no effect—and, in fact, produce no abnormality in the blood test physicians routinely use to measure kidney function? The answer is physiologic reserve, the extra capacity that was given to us in each kidney at birth. Even if you have two kidneys throughout a long and happy eighty-five-year lifetime, and even if you never develop kidney disease of any type, you can still lose up to 90 percent of the kidney function you had as a child and never experience any symptoms whatsoever related to kidney function failure. That extra capacity is what enables you to give away a kidney and suffer no ill effects.

And I'm not just talking kidneys. At birth we're given billions of brain cells we'll never use. A female fetus has millions of eggs in her ovaries, yet over her reproductive years she'll ovulate only several hundred of them and only a few will be fertilized. There are countless examples of how our bodies have been endowed with excess capacity, a bounty that until recently we'd never lived even remotely long enough to plunder.

In the following figure, I've demonstrated these ideas pictorially. Let me walk you carefully through this graph, because it conveys some important ideas. The vertical axis shows muscular strength, and the horizontal axis shows time—advancing age in years. The shaded bar shows how muscle strength declines over a hypothetical

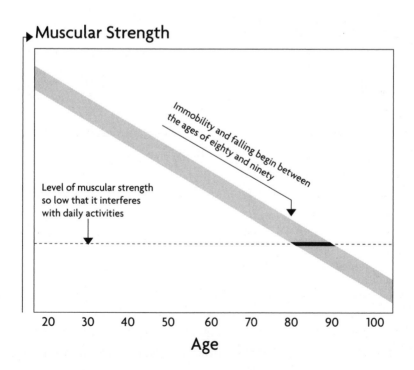

one-hundred-year lifetime, even in the absence of muscular disease. I've added what I call the "dreaded dashed line" to indicate the level of muscle strength at which people actually begin to experience symptoms from muscle weakness—falling, trouble rising from a chair, or perhaps getting into or out of a bathtub without difficulty.

You need to take away a few things from this little graph that say a lot about the biology of getting older. The first is obvious: over the course of a (hopefully) long lifetime, we begin to lose muscular strength.* Seems depressing, I know. But bear with me and look more carefully. Because we have so much extra capacity at birth, the bar does not cross the dreaded dashed line (the point at which we're actually incapacitated from muscle weakness) until between the age of eighty and ninety—pretty late in life. This is a good news/bad news story. Long before many of us would ever become completely immobile, something else—perhaps cancer, perhaps a heart attack—will do us in. In short, we'll never live nearly long enough to experience muscle frailty.

Note also that the bar is wide. This reflects the fact that we're all different at birth, when we start this journey. Some of us inherit a marathon runner's thighs or a yogi's flexibility, regardless of whether or not we later decide to jog daily or do Pilates. Despite what you may think or have been told, we now believe that, for most people, genetics contributes a smaller proportion to healthy aging than we once thought (a factor over which we have less influence), and the wide line creates a range of years (eighty to ninety in this example) over which we might experience mobility problems.

---

* If you're a body builder or an exercise physiologist, you may recognize that I've simplified the graph slightly for the purpose of illustration. For most of us, peak muscular strength does indeed occur between ages twenty and thirty, but this can vary considerably by muscle group (e.g., biceps versus hamstrings). Furthermore, the decline that occurs over a lifetime may or may not be a smooth regular one for all muscle groups. For example, in many people, grip strength can peak as late as age thirty-five, and then remain relatively stable for a few decades before beginning a more steady decline.

Another important point made by the diagram: There is no one, absolute point of failure. The loss of reserve occurs throughout our lifetime, but age is imperceptible or barely perceptible to most people before, say, forty because they never experience symptoms. Unless you run marathons in your twenties, thirties, and forties and assiduously keep track of your times on a spreadsheet, or you're a NASA astronaut who has his or her muscle strength measured in an exercise physiology laboratory every year as part of a scientific experiment, you'd probably not know that you were losing some capacity, because you'd never have a need for it in the course of your daily life. Very few of us have our fastball clocked with a radar gun each spring to see if we'll have our contract renewed or be released as a free agent. It's simply not an issue in remaining healthy and functioning (and employed).

One final point about the graph: I made the vertical axis muscular strength and the dashed line the level of muscle strength at which you develop immobility, but I could have picked any physiologic parameter to make my point. I could have made the vertical axis brain cells and the dashed line the point when you begin to miss appointments. Or I could have picked manual dexterity, and the dreaded dashed line could have been when you can no longer dress yourself or brush your teeth. My point is that this phenomenon occurs in many bodily systems.

When Worlds Collide: "Physiologic Reserve, Meet Unprecedented Longevity"

Now reconsider the previous graph in the context of how life expectancy has changed over the past few thousand years of human development. You've certainly heard about the unprecedented longevity humans have started to enjoy recently. But perhaps you don't realize how recent a phenomenon this is. As the following graph shows,[1] until the mid-1800s, average life expectancy remained pretty much the same for thousands of years, hovering in the midtwenties.

So if you happened to be born before 1800, odds are you'd never

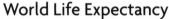

World Life Expectancy

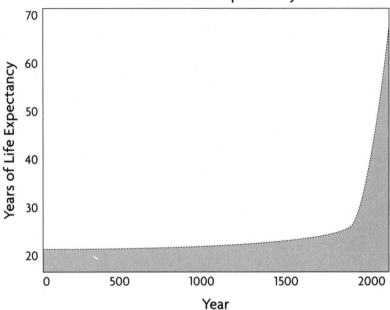

even come close to living long enough to need your physiologic reserve. Long before you would lose enough muscle mass to make you bed-bound, you would more likely than not have perished in some other way. As a hunter-gatherer in preagricultural societies you might have been skewered by a wild boar, a hazard rarely encountered during modern-day foraging at the supermarket. As a citizen of the Roman Empire you might have died from something as routine as appendicitis. In medieval Europe you could have been a victim of smallpox—a disease that has now been essentially eliminated from the planet. If you were a Renaissance-era woman in childbirth, and the baby you were carrying was too big to be delivered vaginally, a C-section was a roll of the dice—gruesome and perilous, performed without anesthesia, transfusions, or modern surgical instruments. But whatever your mode of exodus, you were very unlikely to become geriatric. You'd never even come close to needing a medieval walker or an American Revolution–era hearing aid. In fact, a fifty-year-old was probably viewed as "long in the tooth" throughout much of world history.

The first boon in longevity—raising life expectancy from the twenties to the forties between about 1800 and 1900—had little to do with medicine and more to do with toilets. People began to catch on that having drinking water near sewage was probably not a good idea, and it was sanitation—the arrival of sewers and the widespread availability of cleaner water—that greatly reduced the spread of infectious diseases that had taken the lives of so many people.

But only in the last hundred years or so have things really started to get interesting. Life expectancy at birth has increased from the forties to the late seventies. In fact, a baby born at my hospital this morning will have a median life expectancy of about eighty years (a bit more if she's a girl). And that's a *median*. Half of the babies born today will live longer.

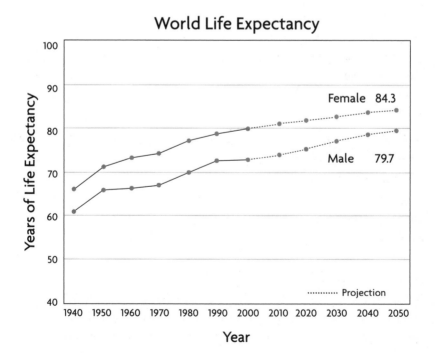

These more recent advances in longevity did not come from better sanitation; they came from modern medicine. Colon cancers that would have felled many are now detected through colonoscopy before they become fatal. Blockages of coronary arteries that were untreatable only a few decades ago can be propped open with medical rigatoni. Death in childbirth is an exceedingly uncommon event in modern medicine because of advanced surgical techniques, ultrasound, antibiotics, and transfusions.

Now think about how this newfound longevity affects my earlier muscle-strength graph. Today millions of people have survived long enough to keep a date with immobility and the dreaded dashed line. Aging muscles survive long enough to produce noticeable symptoms. In short, that physiologic reserve that we never even remotely needed as a citizen of ancient Rome or as a medieval castle dweller has become something many of us rely upon simply to function.

As I said earlier, I chose "muscular strength" for the vertical axis of my first graph and "level of strength when you begin to get immobile" as the dreaded dashed line to demonstrate the interplay between aging and real-world mobility problems, but I could have chosen nearly any organ or function. For example, the vertical axis could have been "reaction time," and the dashed line could have been the level at which you can no longer drive a car safely. Or I could have picked "bone density" and made the dashed line the level at which you begin to develop hip or spinal fractures from evolving osteoporosis. Even in the absence of disease, these changes are advancing simultaneously in several different organ systems within an individual. We've also discovered that, for reasons we don't understand, different rates of decline can be seen in different physiologic systems in the same person. For example, an eighty-year-old may have the kidney function (and reserve) of a ninety-year-old but the reaction time of a sixty-five-year-old.

As you'll learn shortly, this becomes critically important as we near impairment, because the interaction of these different organs and systems enables us to carry out our daily lives; human activity (like walking or cooking) is never the exclusive product of one organ or physiologic system. Preparing a meal, for example, involves the muscle strength to stand, the manual dexterity to stir, and the visual and cognitive abilities to read an instruction label. If one physiologic ability we need to cook declines out of proportion to another, it may be possible to call upon strengths in other systems to maintain or restore function. For example, one of my patients, a former professional chef with relatively mild Alzheimer's disease, had memory loss severe enough that he became completely disorganized in the kitchen; he was unable to find the utensils, cups, and plates needed to prepare and present a simple meal. He became flustered and stopped puttering around the kitchen altogether, which led to a profound depression and life-threatening weight loss. His loving and creative daughter got the great idea of labeling every drawer and cabinet to indicate where he could find each item. That worked for a while until his reading ability began to plummet from a combination of cataracts and his dementia-related cognitive inability to process the written word. The problem was ultimately solved when, instead of labels, his daughter put pictures of items (a cup, a plate) on the cabinet doors. The scheme worked flawlessly—he was back tooling around the kitchen and gaining weight in no time, because his *visual-processing skills* remained strong despite declining *language-processing skills*. Parents of children with learning disabilities will recognize these strategies, which are frequently employed to build on a child's cognitive strengths so as to compensate for areas of relative weakness.

Sure, I've chosen an example of someone living with significant impairment to make my case, but such clever interventions can play a role long before people develop disability.

Age-Related Disability Is Not Like the Weather: There *Is* Something You Can Do About It

So I've depressed you, you say? I know what you're thinking: Killjoy Dr. Lachs has just rattled off a litany of bodily processes that will inevitably decline. Am I to simply sit back and watch myself slide down the disability bar over time only to collide with the dreaded dashed line, winding up immobile, incontinent, and feeble?

Not so fast, my friend! Here the science of gerontology has some good news: The graph can be tweaked to your advantage—or disadvantage—by a variety of interventions, many of which are known to you and many of which are not. And it often doesn't matter whether you're fifty or ninety when you start tweaking, nor does it take dramatic interventions to change the slope of that line just enough to delay your date with the margins of physiologic reserve—you just need to get started. Doing so will let you increase the probability of leaving the planet in any way you'd like—whatever "turns your gears," as one of my patients likes to say—as opposed to spending your later years bed-bound at home or in a nursing home. My plan does not begin or end with a supplement or an exercycle. Getting age-appropriate medical care (and avoiding ageism in your or a parent's interaction with the health-care system) is part of this strategy.

In introducing this book, I told you that the embers of disability start glowing long before you're handed a walker. Next, I've modified my first graph to depict how midlife decisions have an impact on late-life functional ability. Specifically, I've shown how the decline bar gets modified ever so slightly—for better or worse—based on the lifestyle choices you make at forty-five, fifty-five, or any year for that matter, and how even small changes in slope can produce dramatic late-life differences in disability.

Let's look at how two hypothetical lifestyle decisions, made years before immobility in later life, change the path of the curve, and what the "downstream" implications are.

Let's say that at age forty-five you fall into some not so great habits, like becoming a "couch potato." Maybe you had a foot injury that put an end to your weekend racquetball ritual, but it also dramatically limited your daily walking and general strength and fitness, and you didn't seek medical attention. Or maybe you did seek

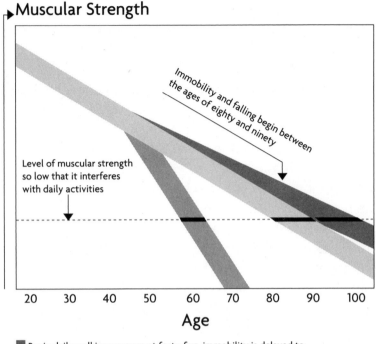

Muscular Strength

Immobility and falling begin between the ages of eighty and ninety

Level of muscular strength so low that it interferes with daily activities

Age

20   30   40   50   60   70   80   90   100

■ Begin daily walking program at forty-five, immobility is delayed to between ninety and one hundred

■ Become a couch potato at age forty-five, immobility begins between sixty and seventy

medical attention and your doc blew it off, as mine once did. Or maybe your kids finished Little League, your coaching gig ended, and there simply isn't the same impetus to be physically active. "No big deal," you say to yourself. You're a young guy, right? Certainly you're deserving of a brief couch potato phase after all the heavy lifting you did. What could this decision have to do with how you spend your silver years?

Actually, the implications are huge! By changing the curve ever so slightly downward (the left bar in the graph), you've now hastened your appointment with disability. You've moved up the time line in such a way that your immobility becomes life altering somewhere between the ages of sixty and seventy, rather than between eighty and ninety. This doesn't necessarily mean you've shortened your life, but it does vastly increase the odds that whatever time you have remaining will be spent confined to a bed or a wheelchair, or with profound mobility problems, such as frequent falling.

Now the good news: This effect works in the other direction, too. In the same way that nudging the slope of that bar slightly downward can accelerate your appointment with a wheelchair, the bar can also be nudged to become more flat, so that this day is forestalled—with any luck, long enough so you can depart this mortal coil without ever experiencing severe disability. Of course, all things come to an end, but the idea is to "go out on a high note"—making love at home, for example, rather than making pottery in the nursing home.

And another point: Even the smallest of interventions—such as walking to maintain or slow the decline of muscle mass—can produce substantial benefits "downstream," because the slope of the line doesn't have to be changed that much to significantly delay your date with disability. It's a bit like sailing a ship that's heading toward an iceberg directly in front of you but still far off in the distance: A 1 percent course correction, if made reasonably early, can avert disaster completely.

This should be an especially empowering truth for the oldest readers: You don't have to begin these kinds of reservoir-building activities in your forties to derive benefit. In fact, it's never too late for a course correction, even if your ship is dangerously close to the iceberg already. The best evidence and testament to this idea is illustrated by several studies over the past decade involving weight training for older women at risk for falling and fracturing, or people who have actually fallen and broken a hip already (in other words, people who are already flirting with the dreaded dashed line). These studies typically split the subjects into one of two treatment groups.[2] The first got customary hip-fracture care after repair—a course of physical therapy in the hospital or the rehab unit of a nursing home—then were sent home to fend for themselves. The second group, however, after finishing their "standard" rehabilitation, got to go to the gym, using the same body building machines you might find in a swanky health club. We had one of these studies at Cornell a few years back,[3] and I tell you this was quite a sight: adorable grandmas pumping iron as muscle-bound personal trainer types shouted boxing-ring expletives of encouragement to motivate them to grind out the last rep.

But whatever ribbing investigators got about putting these little old ladies through basic training dissipated when the results were published. In general, women who participated in these programs had decreased rates of falling, refracturing, and osteoporosis. What is even more remarkable about these studies is that we're not talking about pumping that much iron here—a few pounds in most cases, but with multiple repetitions.[4]

How could this be, you say? Very simple. Just look at the next graph. As I said, these women live right at the dreaded dashed line (in actuality, they probably crossed it already). But even a tiny improvement in muscle strength can make their curve ever so slightly flatter; now they reside decidedly above that danger line, and their mobility is restored enough that they can walk more safely using just a small amount of their newfound muscle strength. Their date with wheelchairs and walkers has been delayed, perhaps by a few years. Not by much, you say? A few years can be over half the life expectancy of an eighty-eight-year-old, who can now spend that life as a productive community dweller.

If you're not experiencing symptoms like a dramatic broken hip, it's often less motivating to take on and sustain a program of regular exercise to avoid disability that seems so far off in the distance. This is why, in my experience, many younger people stink at sustaining interventions intended to improve their medical or emotional health unless they experience some immediate return on their investment, such as rapid weight loss or a dramatic improvement in physique. If the results aren't immediate, they can't fathom what later benefit

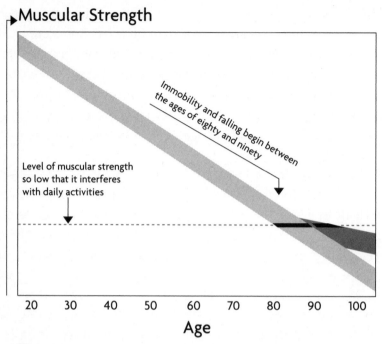

Muscular Strength

Immobility and falling begin between the ages of eighty and ninety

Level of muscular strength so low that it interferes with daily activities

Age

20   30   40   50   60   70   80   90   100

■ Weight training started at age eighty after hip fracture; immobility was forestalled by a few years, or a substantial proportion of remaining life expectancy

they might possibly derive. Perhaps our somewhat eggheaded excursion has convinced you that there is real and lasting benefit even if you don't drop four dress sizes overnight.

No Need to "Swing for the Fences"

Whatever your age, modest efforts to shift the line are always desirable. Think about the amount of muscle strength that had to be added to "rescue" the older hip-fracture patients from traversing the dreaded dashed line. It was not extraordinary. The researchers were not looking to create geriatric "Miss Universe" contestants. They simply wanted to improve muscle strength to the extent that it would impact daily functioning—and it did.

That's another extremely important difference in the way geriatricians think about treating patients of all ages: Complete eradication of disease is often not possible, and therefore a cure is not necessarily the goal of therapy. Minor interventions that may seem trivial can lead to dramatic improvements in quality of life.

Why, then, has medicine not embraced these low-tech, approaches to improving the health of older people and people who are getting old? I have some ideas about that.

Having participated in the training of thousands of medical students, I can tell you that most students do not enter the first year with that mind-set. They've come to cure, and they've been taught to "throw the book" at medical problems toward that end or else not bother trying. This tendency in American medical education is one of the factors that produces overtreatment or undertreatment of people of all ages, a phenomenon I'll describe later in this book.

But for the purpose of this discussion, let's dig deeper. I believe there's a larger organizational reason for this physician "cure crusade," which derives from more "institutional" sources: I think these young physicians, like the public at large, have been bamboozled by what I would call the overselling of medicine. Competing hospitals, HMOs, and insurers in every major city in this country try to outdo one another with claims of miraculous care, always rendered with the greatest dignity and affection. You've seen these beautifully crafted advertisements that tug on your heartstrings, featuring perhaps a pregnant ingénue with a heart defect or a teenager with leukemia. Invariably these lucky people have been cured of their afflictions, often with minimally invasive interventions.

Certainly these are wonderful stories, and I'm proud to work at an institution that's proffered many of them. But they also lead medical students to enter the system imagining that they, too, will be the laser- or catheter-wielding physician who metes out stunning technologies for the betterment of humanity. When it comes time to actually practice medicine, however, they find a situation altogether different. Instead of twentysomethings with one rare but curable disease, they find eightysomethings with many common chronic diseases that aren't curable. As a geriatrician, I deal with a lot of that: arthritis, narrowed heart arteries, diabetes, hearing loss, usually occurring together in the same patient. I rarely "cure" anybody, except maybe someone who has a urinary infection or bronchitis heaped upon a long list of medical diagnoses and conditions. By age seventy-five, Americans have developed, on average, two or three chronic conditions. Someone has to manage them and work to minimize their impact on day-to-day quality of life. If you've hit fifty, more likely than not, you've already started to accumulate them. My job is to make sure that patients have the highest possible quality of life given their chronic conditions, which may be inevitable, no matter how excellent their medical care has been or how well they've taken care of themselves.

That goal does not require cure! Technology and health-care overpromising have obscured this point, but it makes perfect sense if you stop to think about it: A patient with arthritis, young or old, whose pain medication dosage can be reduced from four times daily to four times a week is not "cured" but *is* dramatically improved. A seventy-year-old with urinary difficulty whose geriatrician's interventions decrease the number of "accidents" from three a week to three a month is an immensely grateful patient, even though he is not "cured." Wouldn't you be interested in meeting a doctor who could provide this kind of help in your daily life even if he couldn't "cure" you?

One final observation here: A hundred years ago, this is what docs did, and they did it pretty well within the limits of that era, maybe because there were no alternatives. A patient came from the shop or the farm or the factory with a problem: It hurts here. I can't walk. I'm having trouble breathing. The human suffering was before the doctor, without corporate or technological distractions. He was forced to address these problems with his eyes, ears, hands, and ingenuity. Patients' expectations had not been whipped into a frenzy by marketing campaigns; patients understood that *healing* need not be synonymous with *cure*. No test or scan could relieve the physician from "the laying on of hands" or from (gasp!) the obligation to actually talk to a patient. To this day, I maintain, these are essential parts of the process of doctoring. How ironic that the modern forces that have allegedly improved the quality of medicine may be the same ones responsible for robbing it of its humanity and jeopardizing our ability to care for an aging society.

Chapter 4

A Geriatrician's Perspective on Ageism

It's Not Just Grandpa Who's Being Put Out to Pasture

"If there are younger women in the store, the salesperson makes a beeline straight to them. It's like I'm not even in the room. I'm not even sixty yet!"

"I don't really want a face-lift; I'm only fifty-five. But I work in a business where everybody is young, and I feel like people just aren't taking me seriously anymore. I'm worried that I might lose my job. My mind and ideas are better than ever, and maybe if I look younger, people will listen to what I have to say again."

"My kids are well meaning, but they meddle in my social life, living situation, and personal finances as if I'm a blithering idiot. I've got my marbles, and I'm still the parent, damn it!"

"I'm eighty, and my doctor still insists that I get a colonoscopy every five years, as I have done since I was fifty-five. It's just not that easy for me to do anymore. I've never had a single abnormal finding, and I have no symptoms or family history of colon cancer. But when I asked him if I could stop, he wouldn't even discuss it with me."

"The man at the ticket counter shouted, 'HOW MANY TICKETS AND TO WHAT SHOW?' I was mortified. I'm seventy, but my hearing is fine."

"The pharmacist filled the prescription and went over the directions with me as if I was in kindergarten. It seemed like the whole store was watching. It was completely humiliating."

"After I finally found an orthopedist who would accept Medicare, I sat in his waiting room for over an hour, watching thirtysomethings with ski injuries and better health insurance come and go. When I finally saw him, he spent a grand total of three minutes with my bum knee and me. He said, 'What do you expect at your age?' I told him I finished a marathon last year, then stormed out."

"The oncologist said that the treatment for my breast cancer was a cocktail of various chemotherapies that was likely to make me too sick for my grandson's wedding next month. I've lived a long and good life, and that wedding means more to me than anything else on this planet, so I don't think I'd want treatment like that under any circumstances. But his only response was 'This is the proper treatment for your kind of breast cancer.'"

Discrimination against older people? Old news. What's noteworthy is how early in life people are starting to experience it, and the many new and different forms it's taking. Getting spoken to as if you're not following, perhaps because you have some gray or thinning hair? Having trouble getting the salesperson's attention at the Gap? Got the queasy feeling that those thirtysomethings didn't have to wait as long as you did for the primo table at that new restaurant? Does the doc seem to be examining you a bit more quickly these days, perhaps eager to move on to the next victim? I hear it every day; the stories above are all true and were told to me by patients.

Now imagine you heard those patient confessionals again but with a slightly different twist. What if I were to replace the patients' ages in the vignettes (which appears to be the source of their consternation in all these situations) with another immutable attribute like their skin color, gender, or sexual orientation? At the beginning of the twenty-first century in America, how long would a restaurant or boutique remain open whose staff seats or serves white people first? What medical society would defend an orthopedist who spends thirty minutes with each straight patient and two minutes with each gay patient even though they have the same medical problem? And how would you feel if people assumed that you could not hear, think clearly, or understand directions because of your gender? No, none of this bizarre behavior would survive in broad daylight. But it's all gone now, right?

Well, not *all* of it. Get ready, boomer: You're the new scapegoat on the block. Whether you came into this world—black or white, ugly or attractive, native or immigrant—and no matter what you did for the first fifty or so years while you were here—got rich, got poor, got educated, got incarcerated, got famous, stayed obscure—sheer longevity makes you the newest low man on the totem pole, maybe for the first time in your life. The best solace I can offer is that you're in good and huge company. The bad news is that being old in America today puts you at high risk not only for a bruised ego but also for a bruised body. This is not simply because bodies tend to break down more frequently as people get older. It's also because the health-care system that's supposed to serve us breaks down, too, and in some pretty remarkable ways. But before I talk about ageism in health care (which can kill you), allow me to talk a little bit about ageism in society generally (which may make you wish someone would). And I'll use a true story that just happens to have taken place in a hospital.

A physician colleague of mine (I'll call him Phil) likes to tell the story of how he first got exposed to ageism in medical care. We did our residencies in different hospitals, and from time to time we would call each other up to commiserate, compare notes, whatever. After being on call one night, he phoned me, rather shell-shocked, to tell me this chilling story, which has stayed with me:

I was a new intern rotating through the veterans' hospital when I got a call from the resident in the emergency room to come admit a patient to the medical service. "I've got an old GOMER* down here with your name on him, Phil," he told me over the house telephone.

So it was not without trepidation that I got out of bed in the on-call room and made my way down to the ER at three in the morning. I had just gotten to lie down after what had been an abysmal and exhausting evening of emergencies, and I was not in a good mood. I had all kinds of fantasies about what I would find. A schizophrenic trying to spit on me? An alcoholic with the shakes? An addict in heroin withdrawal? Maybe a homeless patient covered with lice?

This resident was one whom I respected. He was thorough with patients and communicated with families well. He had a large fund of knowledge and always seemed to make a great diagnosis when everyone else had missed it. He'd seen a lot, so I figured that whatever he was calling in would not be a day at the beach.

When I arrived, I grabbed the chart and made my way over to the patient's bay. I drew the curtain and found a lovely but frightened old man, delirious and breathless from a bout of emphysema. He could barely speak because of his huffing and puffing but managed to eek out "Help me, Doctor!" His wrists were restrained to prevent him from pulling out his intravenous lines. He was confused, probably because his lungs could not get enough oxygen into his blood. Through all the indignity, I could tell from the look on his face that he could not have been happier to see me—a doctor finally willing to help him.

Most troubling about meeting this new patient was not his complex medical illnesses—I knew how to treat those. No, it was the piece of masking tape that had been stuck to this poor man's

---

* GOMER is a derisive acronym (stands for "get out of my emergency room") used by some interns for patients who were not especially fun to take care of—unappreciative drug users, assaultive patients with psychosis, malingerers—and quite often older adults who were frustrating to communicate with if they were confused, hard of hearing, or generally just too slow in getting their story out.

head. The resident whom I so respected had placed it there and written "Phil" on it.

He was, quite literally, a patient with my name on him.

When I heard this story, I went numb. Such odious bigotry from "the healing profession"? As an undergraduate I read Dr. Robert Butler's 1976 Pulitzer Prize–winning tour de force, *Why Survive?*;[1] this book coined the term *ageism* and predicted the medical, social, and political landscape we see before us today with regard to aging. But frankly, as a very young man I was skeptical of ageism's pervasiveness and had not experienced its ugly depths up close. Later, as a medical student, I'd certainly seen physicians refer to older people pejoratively, sometimes even when they were in earshot (implicit justification: The patient was too deaf or impaired to perceive the affront). But Phil's story described an act of discrimination that was willful, blatant, and hideous. To add insult to injury, after the patient's confusion had lifted, Phil discovered that the man was a decorated World War II veteran who had fought in some of the most dangerous battles in the European theater.

As I drove home from work that night I thought about Phil's patient. I had to pull my car to the side of the road to digest the enormity of it: This man's youthful courage and sacrifice had been met in his later years with ingratitude and indignity!

How eagerly our nation devours the fruits of our youthful labor. But after our fertility has peaked, after our children have been raised, after our country has been defended, and after our general heavy lifting for the common good is finished, what sentiment survives? Somehow we transition from main event to sideshow or, worse, an embarrassment that should be hidden out of sight or ridiculed. We're underemployed at work despite loyalty to the company and the capacity to contribute. Underserviced at the sales counter despite an appetite to buy and the capacity to spend. Underutilized as a family resource despite the need to be needed and the ability to mentor.

And in health care, we can wind up undertreated or overtreated, despite having the greatest chance of being helped (or harmed) by the newest dazzling technology medicine has to offer. I've seen physicians deliberate more intensely over what to have for breakfast than over whether to prescribe a medication to an older patient.

Ageism in Medicine:
Too Much, Too Little, but Not Necessarily Too Late

There are many different definitions of *ageism*, but for the purpose of this book, I'll define it as systematic discrimination against older people due to their age, such that they are denied opportunities, potential or real, on the basis of that discrimination. My patient who got the cold shoulder from the salesclerk when younger patrons entered the establishment is a good example, as is the patient who waited hours for the orthopedist and then got a two-minute "drive-by" for his bad knee while other (younger) patients came and went. Discrimination like this and its consequences may be very familiar to you, like having a taxi pass you by only to stop at the next corner to pick up a passenger of a different color, or seeing an incompetent coworker get promoted over a competent one because of gender. But when we're talking about medical ageism, this definition doesn't fully pass muster, because (a) you don't have to be that old to experience it, and (b) it doesn't necessarily result in denial of an opportunity—paradoxically, it may actually result in too *many* medical opportunities.

You've heard the saying that "youth is wasted on the young." As a geriatrician taking the long view, I'd say that it's pretty accurate, but it doesn't fully apply to ageism in medicine. Age-inappropriate care at any age is ageist care, like when your gynecologist recommends a hysterectomy because he assumes you're done having kids, or when, without hearing you out, your orthopedist reminds you that you're no spring chicken and advises against a tendon repair that would enable you to play your favorite sport. In fact, if you've experienced rotten medical care as a forty- or fifty-year-old, it's quite possible that such care has some or all of its roots in ageism, subtle or otherwise, even though you may have summarized it as generically "bad." This is because you've not been conditioned to think about it in terms of aging. For example, all other things being equal, who do you think is more likely to receive an attentive evaluation of possible appendicitis in an emergency room, a fifty-five-year-old housewife or a twenty-one-year-old fashion model?

The excessive medical opportunities brought about by medical ageism can lead to all kinds of health-care misadventures. Examples include the woman who was given a one-size-fits-all approach to her breast cancer despite her deeply held convictions and preferences, or the man who was ignored when he dared to challenge the screening dogma of a regular colonoscopy (gasp!) because he could barely tolerate it and was fully prepared to accept the remote possibility of a missed colon cancer.

In the next chapter, I'll deal with the problems of misdiagnosis and missed diagnosis (they're different), and how and why these problems start when we're young and escalate as we get older. In chapter 6, I'll deal with the perils of overtreatment, its causes and origins, and why it's especially a problem for younger aging folks. I'll also talk about how and why we boomers, often sticklers for customer service and bang-for-the-buck results, haven't helped matters in bringing these sensibilities to our health care and the health care of our parents.

———

Several years ago, when John Glenn was shot into space at the age of seventy-six, many of us marveled at his achievement. I watched on television, but a group of my gerontology colleagues went to view the launch at the Kennedy Space Center; they told me that grown men and women of a certain age literally weeped with joy when the space shuttle pierced the cloudless blue sky on that beautiful morning. We were all sure that a great man, a hero of our youth, had just permanently shattered the stereotype of older adults as feeble and frail, with nothing to contribute to society. And he did it in a way that could not have been more dramatic. Older adults would never again be portrayed in the same way, we believed. On television, for example, older people are often shown as forgetful, decrepit, or asexual or simply as laughable props meant to embellish a story line inhabited by younger actors. But the former senator's exploits were to change all that—I was certain of it.

I could not have been more wrong. The next day, several political cartoons appeared in the newspapers, among them this one:

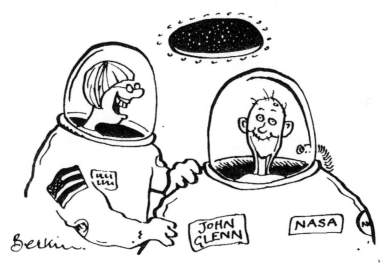

"We'll go for a nice space walk later on."

Other cartoons showed Glenn taking a space walk with a walker, asking mission control for laxatives, and generally acting the way older people are often portrayed—insultingly—in the media and popular culture. What should have been heralded as one of the greatest events in the history of gerontology and human development was being belittled by a substantial proportion of the media. But what was even more curious to me was the public's willingness to stand by and acquiesce to this frankly prejudiced viewpoint. When Glenn orbited the earth at the height of the cold war in 1961, President Kennedy pronounced, "Godspeed, John Glenn." Now, forty years later, an icon of the cold war, the very human emblem of American drive and ingenuity, was being welcomed home as a doddering nursing home resident.

My mind immediately drifted back to a book on the history of racism in America that I read as an undergraduate. It included a discussion of racist political cartoons from the late nineteenth and early twentieth centuries. These now unfathomable illustrations appeared in many of the most mainstream publications of the day, just as the disparaging cartoons of John Glenn's shuttle mission had appeared in some of the most respected national newspapers.

I suspect that your gut reaction to a racist political cartoon from the turn of the last century is like mine. It's how I react when I see newsreel footage of the civil rights movement that boomers grew up with, images indelibly seared into our consciousness: However left or right our political leaning, most of us cringe. Lunch counters marked "whites only." Students sprayed with water cannons as they appeared for their first day of classes. Religious leaders publicly uttering some of the most intolerant racial epithets imaginable.

And so we cringe. But then an unsettling emotion begins to percolate. It's hard to describe at first: one part bewilderment, one part outrage. How, we wonder, could so many sit idly by and acquiesce to bigotry that now seems so clearly outrageous? Why weren't there more brave and clearheaded souls willing to stand up and say: This is wrong. How did an entire community collectively come to regard this as okay? In short, what exactly was everybody thinking? And then, of course, what would I have done?

As someone who has devoted much of my life and my entire professional career to the medical, emotional, and social health of older people, I believe deep in my heart that the opportunity to bravely stand up and speak about a deafening social injustice is presenting itself again for Americans of a certain age. And while a highly calibrated moral compass would be a nice motivator to get you onto this bus, you don't necessarily need one. Enlightened self-interest will suffice. We're the new pariahs (or we're about to be), and we've got tons of company. We just don't matter as much as we used to. Not in courtship. Not in commerce. Not at work. And certainly not in health care.

Fifty or a hundred years from now, will our great-great-grand-children cringe at those derisive depictions of John Glenn as they leaf through old newspapers and periodicals at a tag sale? Or will they still see older people as worthless and disposable vestiges with little to contribute to society? And what happens as they approach their own "middle years" and realize that they have become what they have feared for most of their adult lives: old?

Your mission, should you decide to accept it, is to make sure that medical ageism doesn't undermine your medical care and your health, through undertreatment, overtreatment, or no treatment.

But there are some big problems in trying to do that. Unlike Goldilocks in the fairy tale, you're at a disadvantage. She knew exactly what she was looking for; an arbiter of her own taste. She could tell for herself when the bed, the porridge, and the bath were just right. But as you're about to learn, that's often not the case when you're trying to get health care in an aging America. You often can't know what you need, and even if you could, you probably wouldn't know how much or how little to buy. And to make matters even more complicated, there are many purveyors of porridge out there who are trying to decide for you just how hot or cold yours should be, and not all of them have your best interest at heart.

I can't turn you into a geriatrician, but I can help you figure out on your own when things are just right.

Chapter 5

Do No Harm, but for God's Sake, Do Something!

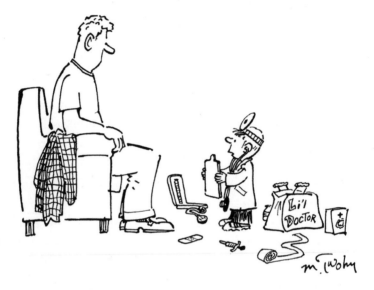

"Because of your age, I'm going to recommend doing nothing."

What geriatrician could argue with one of the central rules doctors are supposed to adopt early in their training: *primum non nocere*—first, do no harm? We've seen too many older people injured by injudiciously prescribed medications, aggressive testing, or ill-advised surgical approaches. On the other hand, there are many medical problems we experience as we age that merit aggressive intervention; far too often a strange combination of ageism and "do no harm" are used to justify, implicitly or explicitly, a posture of sitting idly by while Rome burns. There are some patients, even very old ones, for whom a "full-court press" is very appropriate. Let me tell you about two of them.

The first was a lovely ninety-year-old man (I'll call him JB), who worked every day importing olive oil from his native Italy. His wife of sixty years had passed away a decade ago, and his response was to throw himself even more feverishly into his highly successful business. Every day he woke at the crack of dawn to go to work, and he delighted in sharing the business and his knowledge with his children and grandchildren who worked with him. The last year had been a particularly good one for him because a beloved great-granddaughter had spent her college summer working in the business and he took great pleasure in her company and energy.

Over the course of a week, he had developed progressively worsening chest pain and breathlessness. These symptoms were exacerbated by exertion. Any third-year medical student, even a bad one, would have immediately recognized these symptoms as classic angina pectoris—pain from the heart caused by narrowing of the blood vessels that serve it. The pain is prompted by activity because when we exert ourselves, the heart has to pump more forcefully to handle the increased demands of exercising muscles and other organs. The pain stops when exertion stops, because the supply of available blood and the tissues' need for oxygen become balanced again. In most cases the heart does not suffer irreversible damage, but when angina persists for a long period of time—say, ten minutes or more—the heart muscle can die. In layman's terms, the patient suffers a heart attack. If the condition is diagnosed before the death of heart tissue, it is eminently treatable using a variety of interventions ranging from medications to stents (essentially rigatoni inserted into the arteries in a procedure to prop the blood vessel open after it is scraped clean) to bypass surgery, a major surgical procedure in which the narrowed arteries are "jumped," or bypassed, using veins from the leg. You may recall that former president Bill Clinton had both (and at my hospital, parenthetically). In short, there are many options.

But when this otherwise robust man went to see his physician of thirty years and explained his symptoms, his doctor gave him nitroglycerin to place under the tongue when the episodes occurred (not unreasonable *temporary* therapy to treat the symptoms, mind you) and told him (because he was "old" and probably could not tolerate more aggressive therapy) to go home and just put up with it. JB received no electrocardiogram. No stress test. And certainly no cardiac catheterization, wherein dye is squirted into the arteries to determine the nature and extent of the narrowings.

When my patients with angina get upset at being given a new cardiac diagnosis, I often tell them to be grateful for their angina. After they look at me quizzically, I explain that about 25 percent of patients with narrowing of the coronary arteries experience no angina—the first indication that they have heart disease of this type is a huge heart attack or even sudden death. "Be grateful that you had symptoms that caused you to come see me," I tell them.

But JB subsequently was not so fortunate. After his doctors ignored his anginal symptoms, he had an enormous heart attack, and after that he became totally disabled. His heart could no longer pump blood, and fluid backed up into his lungs. His legs became swollen. He could not walk. He was short of breath twenty-four hours a day and required oxygen.

I met JB when he was admitted to a nursing home from the hospital after his heart attack; he was simply too sick to live at home independently anymore. At first glance, he looked like he had been in the nursing home for the past ten years. He was in a wheelchair and gaunt, with his head drooped in a sleepy kind of surrender. His swollen legs looked like tree trunks. He was so short of breath he could barely finish sentences. Medical paraphernalia—an oxygen tank, IV tubing, and so on—was always nearby or in tow. I simply assumed that he had been this debilitated for years.

How ageist of me.

As he began to tell the story of his life before the heart attack, I simply couldn't believe what I was hearing. Only two months ago he had been working a fifty-hour week! He had planned to spend the fall taking his great-granddaughter to Italy to show her the vineyards and olive trees. He went to the opera nearly every night he could get home from work early enough. He was becoming romantically involved with a new flame in her seventies, and they were starting to become sexually intimate.

But when I pieced together the medical records from the previous two or three months, I became furious. His cardiograms from before the heart attack were better than my own, and I was in my thirties at the time. All his laboratory tests were completely normal. But the imaging studies of his heart done after the heart attack showed a muscle that barely quivered. It had been damaged irrevocably, and no one was going to transplant a new heart into a ninety-year-old. He was going to die soon, and what time he had left was going to stink—he would be breathless, swollen, uncomfortable, and quite understandably depressed. But the worst part was, this did not have to happen!

What I did next was something I've never done before in this context: I called his old doctor, the one who had dropped the ball so egregiously. Let me clarify: Sure, I call patients' former docs all the time to get vital information that might aid in treatment, old lab results, whatever. But even though I might have justified it to myself as a part of providing holistic and comprehensive care to JB, calling this guy would add absolutely nothing to helping the patient; that ship had already sailed. Nothing the doctor could say would change my management of JB in any way. No, this was more of a fact-finding mission. I was angry and wanted to understand how a magnificent man like this could get dropped on his head so flippantly.

I guess I was really hoping not to like the doctor. But the truth is, he couldn't have been sweeter. He came to the phone right away, despite having an officeful of patients. Oh, yes, he said, he knew the patient. Lovely old man, cared for him for years, his late wife, too. Makes olive oil. Had a heart attack? Gee, that's too bad. In fact, I saw him in the office with chest pain a few months back. Thought it was probably angina. Didn't think at ninety he'd want or be able to tolerate a stress test or angiogram. Didn't really lay it out for him, either—thought it might upset him.

I guess I should be grateful for the doctor's candor. He made his thought processes completely transparent for me. JB was ninety, and the doc didn't think he would want or could tolerate a cardiac evaluation. Didn't want to upset him. Didn't offer it to him. Didn't discuss it with him, either. Just gave him some pills, no instructions.

If this physician did not think his patient could tolerate a cardiac evaluation, I wish he could have seen how poorly he was tolerating dying of congestive heart failure in a nursing home.

JB's physician made several common errors in the course of caring for him, but the most serious one was *rationing his health care on the basis of age and not on the basis of his functional ability or his preferences.* As I often say, if you've seen one ninety-year-old, then you've seen one ninety-year-old—they're all different. JB was more like many fifty-five-year-olds in my practice—working hard, interacting with family and friends, sexually active—than the ninety-year-old patient his doc had in mind. JB should have been offered intensive evaluation and treatment, even the most aggressive treatment for coronary artery disease, because he had so much to lose, even from the smallest heart attack. A forty-year-old who loses a little bit of pumping activity in the heart will likely go on without much of a change in daily functioning. But for a ninety-year-old with fewer reserves, it could be the difference between living at home or being in the nursing home for the rest of a short life.

Notice I said he should have been "offered" an intensive cardiac evaluation and treatment. I've cared for many patients who have been presented with such an option and who have then, after getting all the facts, vehemently refused. But that was their decision to make. In JB's case the options were never even presented. He trusted his doctor but was denied the opportunity for complete treatment. Even if the treatment came down to aggressive cardiac bypass surgery, it was his choice to either give it a shot or risk subsequent illness and disability, not his doctor's choice.

Nota bene: I struggled for weeks as to whether I should tell JB (and his more medically sophisticated children and grandchildren) about my impressions of the care he'd received. This struggle was not born of some lofty Hippocratic loyalty or some physician's code of silence; it was just that there was little to be done about it now, and I did not want to heap any psychological suffering on top of his physical ailments. Eventually I worked up the courage and gumption to say something, because I felt he deserved to know. I approached him with reserve: "I spoke with your old doctor, Joe," I ventured cautiously. His face brightened for the first time in weeks: "The most wonderful doctor in the world!" he replied. "The best you could find!" "How great that he would call you to check up on me." I said nothing more about it.

This story reflects the most common form of medical ageism: picking up a medical record, noting a date of birth, and assuming that the patient you're about to see is like every other ninety-year-old you've met, with the same goals and values—then using this assumption as a justification for doing nothing or next to nothing, often without eliciting any input from the patient directly. It's as if the physician's approach to JB was ordained before he walked into the examining room.

Misdiagnosis versus Missed Diagnosis

As egregious as this treatment (or nontreatment) may sound, I'm willing to give JB's doc a good deal of credit for making an accurate diagnosis, because this often fails to happen as patients get older. Many elderly patients like JB are diagnosed incorrectly (or misdiagnosed)—for instance, ascribing the chest pain to a muscle injury in the chest wall rather than the heart, perhaps because the doctor does not spend enough time to find out that the pain comes with exertion and subsides with rest. No, in JB's case the doc made the right diagnosis and gave the right medication; he just wasn't aggressive enough in evaluating the condition and treating it.

Contrast this with an even more common problem as we age, what I would call a *missed* diagnosis: when a significant problem goes completely unrecognized. In fact, a sizable body of scientific research shows that many conditions common in older people (depression, pain, sleep disturbance, confusion, hearing loss, visual impairment, incontinence, memory loss, falling, mobility problems) are never detected by physicians, even when there's a long-standing doctor-patient relationship. In these studies, research staff is placed in the waiting room of the doctor's office; after the patient visit the researchers do a focused assessment to determine whether patients have problems like major depression or memory loss. These results are then directly compared to what the doctor just noted in the exam room. Dozens of studies show that physicians miss many of these problems in a typical office visit.

How is this possible? The reasons are endless, and many are rooted in ageism. One physician might rationalize that a little urine leaking as we age is normal and not consider it a problem. Another may simply not have time and decide not to ask about these common problems—patients are rarely falling or tearful during an office visit, so why go looking for trouble? The way medical students are trained to examine patients—looking at their eyes with an ophthalmoscope rather than making them read a prescription bottle to determine if they have functional vision, for example—is a vestige of a time when older people were uncommon patients in medical practice. And what if a physician actually does do a good, careful job? God forbid you actually uncover an older patient who's depressed during the course of a physical examination—that's going to take some time to evaluate, and there's a waiting room full of patients out there! When grown children bring a parent to the doctor, they may do all or most of the talking; the physician is often delighted to remain silent (no need to talk to the patient, who is slow to get his story out). Patients also play a role in this ageist dance; when they come to see me, they are often on their "best behavior" and deny or try to hide problems with function because they fear I'll send them to a nursing home rather than try to help them (an ageist view, too).

Furthermore, these oversights are not limited to the doctor's office. In one remarkable study, physicians were interviewed after they left the hospital room of patients they had examined. They were asked, "Does your patient have a urinary catheter?" Fully 38 percent of physicians were completely unaware that their patients (whom they had been seeing daily) had a catheter in their bladder draining to an external collecting bag![1]

I also believe that ageism is an occupational hazard in medicine, because society is ageist and we doctors are mortal members of that society (notwithstanding the beliefs of a few surgical egos I have encountered over the years). My division at the hospital once ran a wonderful volunteer program in which medical students accompanied older adults to appointments with physicians in the community. I always instructed the students before they went to resist the temptation to identify themselves as medical students. I wanted them to see these docs warts and all, not on their best behavior because they knew they were being observed by a future colleague. Usually these community physicians were wonderful, but sometimes the stories the students would bring back were dispiriting. Many of the older people they accompanied were socially isolated, and this monthly visit to the physician was an important ritual, a highlight of their calendar. Often they would carefully prepare long lists of questions and dress up proudly for the occasion as if it were a major social event. But in many instances, the doctors didn't treat these appointments with the same importance. For patients to prepare in this way and then be asked to wait for an hour, only to get dismissed after three minutes with the doctor (questions still in hand, mostly unanswered) was demoralizing. But I felt that the students needed to see that.

Finding the Medical Sweet Spot as We Get Older

Now let me tell you about a patient whose experience is in stark contrast to JB's. Mrs. J was diagnosed with breast cancer at age eighty-four when a "heads-up" primary care doc felt a lump in her right breast. A biopsy confirmed the diagnosis as well as the fact that the tumor had spread to lymph nodes under her arm. The "standard" treatment should have been fairly intensive chemotherapy, followed up with local radiation therapy to "mop up" any tumor that the chemo might have missed, but the oncologist at her community hospital actively dissuaded Mrs. J from getting this therapy, citing primarily her "old age" as a mitigating factor in choosing not to pursue overly aggressive treatment. You're no spring chicken, he told her. That's a common refrain patients hear from doctors as justification for being told to go home and do nothing.

The problem with this plan was that Mrs. J was biologically more like a sixty-year-old than an eighty-four-year-old. She swam half a mile every day, volunteered as a mentor at the local youth center, and had no significant "comorbidity" (other diseases that would make cancer treatment especially onerous). In fact, the only problem she had was very minor hearing loss in both ears and some modest arthritis in her left knee. Her son was a friend and called me for advice. I suggested she see—brace yourself for this—a "geriatric oncologist."

When my dad graduated from medical school in the 1950s, much of the chemotherapy and other cancer treatments that were administered (there were very few, and they were pretty feeble) were given by internal-medicine doctors. But in the 1960s and 70s, as cancer research enjoyed explosive growth, the field of oncology (a subspecialty of medicine) was born. By the time I made it to medical school in the 1980s, oncology was a relatively new but established and full-fledged specialty of internal medicine. Trainees who finished internal medicine could do a couple of years of additional training and be qualified to treat all kinds of cancer with drugs and other therapies that required special expertise. I suspect that Mrs. J's oncologist trained in this paradigm and probably took fine care of his patients.

Fast-forward some twenty-five-plus years, and oncology is undergoing a rather remarkable transformation, dividing into ever more subspecialties. In my institution, for example, there are oncologists who treat only lung cancer or only breast cancer in the same way that there are cardiologists who treat only rhythm disturbances or congestive heart failure. In the case of Mrs. J, a referral to a geriatric oncologist with special expertise in breast cancer led to an entirely different recommendation. Because of her relatively "youthful" biology and lack of other complicating diseases, the oncologist explained to her that there was much quality of life to be lost in simply ignoring or undertreating her breast cancer and suggested that a more aggressive route be pursued. He skillfully calculated her anticipated life expectancy based not on her age but on her real physiology and devised a treatment plan that balanced the greatest chance of success with the potential for life-altering side effects.

The lady who was "too old for chemotherapy" tolerated the treatment better than many forty-five-year-olds I knew and remained free of any detectable cancer some five years later.

Not Just for Grandma

So maybe you're a forty-, fifty-, or sixtysomething and believe that these stories have no particular relevance for you.

Well, you're dead wrong. I picked these stories of undertreatment and appropriate treatment in older people not only to demonstrate medical ageism but also because I wanted you to see the immediate effects of decisive, age-appropriate medical care versus complete inaction—disease-free survival and high quality of life for Mrs. J, on the one hand, and extreme disability for JB on the other. But you really don't have to be *that old* to experience medical ageism, and furthermore, you may not even realize you've experienced it, because the consequences and benefits are so far downstream in your future. To demonstrate that point, I'll describe one final patient: me.

In my forties, I fell and broke a toe and quibbled with the local "doc-in-the-box" at an urgent-care center about the need for an X-ray. "Why bother?" he argued. "You're just going to buddy-tape it to the toe next to it, whether it's broken or not." I protested again. Pause. And then, out it came: "Dr. Lachs, it's not like you're a teenager trying to get a spot on the Olympic snowboard team."

No, I'm no teenager. But come to my practice and I'll introduce you to a bunch of nice older people who fall several times a year and live in terror of a hip fracture. Many of them fall because, among other things, they neglected (or their doctor neglected) these kinds of "trivial" issues a couple of decades earlier. Why see a podiatrist for that corn or hammertoe? Men don't look at my feet anymore; why bother with a pedicure? My feet hurt, but I doubt the doctor could do anything about it, so I'll just stop walking to work and take a bus. Bad idea. The embers of disability occur decades before they give you a walker.

And if you don't have a foot fetish, I could give you endless other examples from my own practice that extend well north of your feet. How about mild midlife depression after your kids flee the nest for college (for some, I believe, a low-grade form of bereavement) that leaves you trudging through the day but choosing not to "bother the doctor"? Or, worse, you tell the doctor, and he chalks it up to "overprotective parenting" or some such situational nonsense without any further evaluation or serious consideration of treatment.

For one such patient of mine, this initial "midlife crisis" was never dealt with and set in motion a series of progressively more severe depressive episodes over the subsequent thirty years, from which he has never really recovered. He's absolutely miserable, to the point where we had serious discussions about electroconvulsive therapy when no medication seemed to work (it's safe and can work wonders, by the way; it just got a bad rap from the movies, and one in particular). I was curious as to why his problem didn't get nipped in the bud when it first started, in the 1970s—even back then we had highly effective treatments for mild forms of depression, treatments that might have aborted all the difficulty that was to follow. "Why didn't you tell your doc at the time, Fred?" I asked him. "You might have avoided three decades of misery." The reason: His doctor was another practitioner of age discrimination in health care. "I did tell him, Mark," Fred recounted. "He told me the best treatment for my midlife crisis was to go out and buy a sports car."

Look, there are things that happen to some of us as we get older that we simply have no control over. We may be bereaved. We might have a stroke or a heart attack despite meticulous monitoring of cholesterol and blood pressure. We might suffer surprising and devastating financial reversals. The disabilities that may or may not result from these often random events are cards we are dealt and simply must play. We have no choice. But there is another source of disability—what some gerontologists call "excess disability"—over which you can have influence. And nothing drives geriatricians nuts like disability that didn't have to happen.

Not every bad card we get is dealt by fate; some are dealt by our health-care system's actions and inactions (or *our* passive acceptance of them, as described in some of the stories above). These cards, like those in a game of draw poker, are ones you can put back in the deck to try to get a better hand. The key is recognizing when you've been dealt a bad hand and having the gumption to do something about it. That is what this book is about.

Often it's precisely the cards you can put back that produce the worst excess disability, sometimes by themselves but more frequently in concert with the cards that you're stuck with. We wind up suffering from decisions—bad treatment decisions, bad lifestyle decisions, bad environmental decisions, to name a few. And while some of those decisions are made after you're old, they frequently get made when you're in middle age or younger, long before you realize the down-the-road impact they're going to have. These decisions take many forms: "playing through" a weekend sports injury that's not improving after several weeks; making your arthritis worse by choosing to live in a home with beautiful views but difficult-to-negotiate steps; letting your doctor dismiss physical, psychological or other symptoms that he perceives as trivial because "you're no longer a teenager."

As you travel through your forties, fifties, and sixties, you begin to accumulate these health-care experiences and navigate the choices they place before you. Although they may seem transient or even trivial at the time, few are truly without consequences in the long run. They get recorded on a kind of aging ledger. Think of it as a geriatric profit and loss statement that profoundly influences what you'll look like a decade or two down the road. Furthermore, these accumulated experiences and the impact they have begin to interact in potentially worrisome ways with the stuff you can't change. A small stroke at eighty that produces mild walking difficulties is terrible, but add an undertreated foot injury from twenty years earlier, and now you're never walking again. Losing a spouse at seventy is awful under the best of circumstances; but if you come to that experience especially poorly prepared (like my patient who wasn't properly treated for his empty-nesting bereavement), you may never function meaningfully in the world again. As I said, excess disability drives geriatricians nuts, especially when it's avoidable.

The famous serenity prayer says: *God grant me the serenity to accept the things I cannot change, the courage to change the things I can, and the wisdom to know the difference.* As a geriatrician, I'll modify that a bit: *God give me the wisdom to recognize whether my doctor is really listening to me when he ascribes my medical complaints to just getting old, and the courage to call him on it if I'm not sure, before I choose less aggressive treatment as a reasoned course of action as opposed to the ageist default.*

Sure, doctors should do no harm with their treatment, and think long and hard about tests, drugs, and surgeries they recommend to patients of any age. But inaction can be harmful, too, and physicians, patients, and their family members should constantly reevaluate the advisability of inaction.

Having covered the dangers of doing nothing, it's time to talk about that other equally perilous minefield: doing too much.

Chapter 6

Cookbook Medicine

A Recipe for Disaster at Any Age

An older man visits his physician for a routine physical.
"Before you can see the doctor, every patient must give a blood sample,
*   a urine sample, and a stool sample," demands the nurse.*
"Just take my underwear!" he says.

Earlier I told you about my sixtysomething patient—an absolute knockout—who would have dropped a bundle at the counter of a fancy clothing boutique but instead was abandoned by the sales clerk when a younger patron appeared. It's easy to understand how this kind of general discrimination could hurt your feelings. Nobody should be treated that way in the course of daily interaction, whether purchasing health care or a carton of milk. The problem, of course, is that ageism is not limited to the dairy aisle—it's everywhere.* But when it starts showing up in health

---

*Some of the most elegant studies on ageism in America have been conducted by Duke University sociologist Erdman Palmore, who has created a variety of survey tools, including "The Ageism Survey"; he's even published an *Encyclopedia of Ageism*, eds. E. Palmore, Laurence Branch, and Diana K. Harris (Binghamton, NY: Haworth Press, 2005). Dr. Palmore has been interviewing groups of older adults for some time, asking them about their personal experiences with societal ageism; the results are unsettling. Some examples: 43 percent of respondents said that on at least one occasion a physician immediately ascribed their ailment to old age; 69 percent said that someone had told a joke that "poked fun" at their age; 43 percent said they were told "you're too old for that" when pursuing new interests; 33 percent said that people assumed they did not hear well simply because of their age; and 31 percent said people assumed that they did not understand information provided to them.

care, there's yet another problem that's worse than bruised pride: getting too much care.

You must be thinking: Too *much* care? Is there such a thing? How could there be when there are millions of people in this country with no health insurance and with poor access to care? And even if it were happening to me, couldn't I put the brakes on it if I saw it coming?

First of all, yes, there is such a thing. And no, you can't always put the brakes on it, the way you might if you were buying just about any other product or service. Sure, while you might be influenced by a persuasive car salesman to upgrade to leather seats, the product you walk out of the store with—a car—is ultimately of your own choosing.

Not so in health care! The fact is, when you or your mom goes to the doctor with or without symptoms, *you often don't know what you need*. As a result, the physician is likely to decide for you, and it's precisely this peculiar situation that can combine with ageism to produce too much of a good thing.

Your next reasonable question might be: Isn't the treatment of most medical conditions similar and straightforward, assuming that you're correctly diagnosed? If I have appendicitis, I need to have my appendix taken out, right? My arthritic right hip will need to be replaced, won't it?

Very frequently, nothing could be further from the truth. A growing body of literature on this very idea demonstrates something that every physician knows deep in his or her heart but rarely articulates: Medicine is profoundly discretionary, and more often than not we just don't know what works best. Given a patient who appears to have a discrete and straightforward medical problem, ten physicians can take ten radically different approaches to diagnosis and treatment. What's even more disquieting about this literature is another dirty little secret about medicine: Some of the factors that determine how you get treated for a particular problem have nothing to do with your symptoms or other "clinical" parameters. Features like your gender, your race, your age (of course!), your health insurance, and even the number of doctors in your community appear to play a role in whether and how you're treated.

Some of the most famous examples of this phenomenon come from Dartmouth Medical School researcher Jack Wennberg, who was the first to scientifically study a phenomenon sometimes called *practice variation*. In an extraordinary series of studies that began in the 1980s, he looked at how frequently men in different communities throughout the United States got operations for benign prostate enlargement, a condition that can either be managed with a surgical procedure called a TURP (trans-urethral resection of the prostate), essentially a "Roto-Rooter" type of affair (sorry, male readers), or medications that in many cases postpone the need for surgery. Thus, the timing of when to do a TURP is discretionary— for most men there is no absolute right time to have it if they're still able to empty their bladder completely, however slowly. The choice of treatment depends more on individual patient factors, like how annoying he finds the symptoms (for example, how many times he needs to get up at night to pee, or how long he keeps his date waiting while he's in the powder room). But there also appear to be physician variables that influence the frequency of this operation. After controlling for factors like age, when researchers studied large geographic areas (there's no plausible reason to believe that rates of prostate enlargement should be different in different cities), variations in surgical rates had to be due in some degree to physician factors. The findings: If during the period of study you were a man with urinary difficulties, you were four times more likely to wind up in an operating room for the problem if you lived in Salt Lake City as opposed to New York.[1] Furthermore, one of the factors that correlated with high rates of the procedure was the number of surgeons in a town who perform it.

Is it disquieting for patients to learn that a significant predictor of the medical care you receive is which city you live in or which urologist you were referred to or picked from the yellow pages? Absolutely. But it's also disquieting for doctors, who'd like to believe that there's some science to the care we're rendering, and even more worrisome for the folks who have to pay for all this care (like the government, employers, and health insurers). I don't believe for a minute that the majority of physicians who sorted into the "quick to recommend surgery" group had anything other than their patient's best interest in mind when they decided a surgery was advisable. No, I think there are many factors responsible for this phenomenon, and a branch of medical science (most recently called comparative effectiveness research) is now trying to figure out why physicians vary so in their approach to the same medical problems. More important, comparative effectiveness researchers are trying to figure out which treatment doctors should select to produce the best and most cost efficient outcome based on what symptoms the patient is experiencing.

Cookbook Medicine Can Be Ageist Medicine at Any Age

Whatever the origin of practice variation, many doctors—including those who conduct comparative effectiveness research—have tried to rein it in. How? By trying to create, to the greatest extent possible, standard approaches to common medical problems. The aim is to make sure physicians move in lockstep when encountering specific symptoms in a variety of medical conditions.

This isn't really a bad idea; clinical guidelines can be a very good thing. Practice variation occurs for reasons beyond physicians having differing opinions and can lead to substandard care. In some cases, physicians are simply not up-to-date on the newest, most cost-effective and scientifically supported medications, tests, or screening strategies, either because they graduated from medical school decades ago or because they simply don't have time to keep up with the literature. I'm completely on board with approaching medical conditions in a uniform way, particularly when good data suggests what to do and especially when a good chunk of doctors aren't rendering modern medical care.

But when lockstep, uniform care for the masses becomes the

robotic norm in every patient interaction and for the evaluation and treatment of every symptom or condition, regardless of a patient's preferences, age, and living environment, I start to get queasy.

This trend has been called "cookbook" medicine,[2] and some of its tenets may sound familiar. You must have a screening colonoscopy every X years, even if you're eighty-five and have no personal or family history of colon cancer and you've had several negative screening studies in the past. You must always get a lipid-lowering drug for mildly elevated cholesterol levels, even if you've made it to eighty with no cardiac events, have no other risk factors for heart disease, have no family history of it, and hate taking medications. In situations like these, uniform approaches to medical care are ill advised. A doctor's time might be better spent explaining the pros and cons of a test or treatment—for example, why annual mammography for an eighty-two-year-old woman with many negative mammograms, no history of breast problems, and no family history of breast cancer might be overdoing it.

Yes, in the same way "babying the ball" (undertreatment) can lead to hellacious outcomes for patients, robotic approaches to patient care—at any age—can be equally ridiculous and just as traumatic for patients and families. To show you what I mean, I'll share two stories about overtreatment, one involving an older patient and the other a young one.

A few years back I got a call from an old buddy who asked me for some help with his mom, who was living in a nursing home. She had Alzheimer's disease and had been lovingly cared for by her family at home for almost a decade until it just became too difficult for them to provide the twenty-four-hour care she needed: She was essentially bed-bound and unable to communicate intelligibly; additionally, she often grew highly agitated at night and would scream out the way patients with dementia sometimes do. The family found what they thought was an outstanding nursing home. It had marble floors, beautiful chandeliers, and all the nice furnishings you'd want in such a facility. But after I heard the story that came next, I wished the nursing home had spent more money on medical care and nursing education than on fine china.

My friend was calling out of concern not for her Alzheimer's disease but for her diabetes, a problem from which she had suffered for more than twenty years. The physician and nurses caring for her at her well-appointed facility had become obsessed with her blood sugars and her insulin dosages. They would stick her finger four times a day to check it, causing her to holler out that someone was trying to kill her. They would change the dosages of her insulin nearly daily, sometimes administering several additional injections into her abdomen to respond to blood sugars that were slightly high; this too made her cry out. On several occasions her blood sugars became dangerously low because of overadministration of insulin; she then had to be given orange juice or candies to raise her blood sugar levels. The problem was that the Alzheimer's was causing her to lose her ability to eat and swallow; when candies or juice were stuffed in her mouth, she either choked or screamed out that they were trying to poison her. On two occasions when they could not get her sugars up, they had to call 911; the paramedics put a large IV into her to administer sugar water and then took her to the local ER, where she spent about eight hours—and predictably became more confused than ever.

With as much restraint as I could muster in my indignation, I told my friend that this was an insane situation. Yes, the doc was doing everything by the book. "Tight" control of diabetes is a very desirable thing—most studies show it slows or prevents complications that can occur years down the road, including vision loss, kidney disease, and nerve problems. But my friend's mother was a bed-bound patient with dementia whose ultimate functional prognosis was poor. What were they trying to prevent? Dialysis a decade from now? Diabetic eye damage in the future? She had stopped reading four years ago because her brain could not process the signals produced by reading written words. Why were they torturing this poor lady with injections and finger sticks that would have absolutely no bearing on the quality of her life other than to ruin what little quality she had left? She may have been paranoid from her dementia, but she was not entirely wrong when she claimed they were trying to kill her. Their robotic devotion to a strategy of care that would be great for a forty-year-old was just terrible given her specific situation. It was a complete disconnect.

My friend asked if I would speak to her doctor. This led to another instructive interaction, one that was in many ways the mirror opposite of the conversation with JB's physician that I described in the last chapter.

This guy was a baby doctor. By that I mean he had probably finished his residency in the past two hours (it's the new guy in the medical practice who usually has to cover the nursing home), and it wouldn't surprise me if he had graduated at the top of his class. He had clearly read and dutifully digested every textbook ever handed to him but managed to have not a single inquisitive bone in his body, as far as I could tell.

I felt like I was talking to a machine. Was I not aware of the American Diabetes Association's guidelines on diabetic control? (Yes, I teach that stuff at an Ivy League medical school and tell residents to apply it assiduously to patients who could benefit from it.) Wasn't I familiar with the complications of diabetes? (Please! I'm an internist!) Why would one not want to be aggressive in such a patient?

When I calmly explained that it might be more realistic for him to widen his idea of "reasonable" blood sugar control in the context of this patient, he listened but seemed unimpressed. I suggested that a more appropriate goal for patient and family, who were also being driven nuts watching this absurd circumstance (calls from the nursing home at two in the morning every time her sugar bottomed out or skyrocketed) would be to define a sugar range that made sense—not so low that the patient needed to be schlepped to the hospital each time she had a life-threatening "insulin reaction" (complete or partial loss of consciousness from low blood sugar), but not so high that she became dehydrated and comatose from diabetic coma. That, I felt, was all he really needed to worry about in a patient like this. He could dispense with the four-times-a-day finger sticks or even just test her urine for sugar to avoid that trauma altogether. The doc was cordial but wanted no part of it. "The guidelines say . . . ," he went on.

While JB's physician rationed health care on the basis of age, this doctor's approach was ageist in a different way: He was providing care on the basis of no rationale whatsoever. He was a student of what I call the "One Size Fits All" approach, which can be incredibly dangerous for young and old alike.

There's no shortage of blood tests that I can order for a patient of any age. The list of X-rays, scans, MRIs, and other imaging studies at my disposal is nearly endless. Furthermore, Medicare or private insurers will pay for most of these little excursions. Combine this profusion of diagnostics with the reasonable expectation of most patients—that the doctor will do something about their problems—and you can understand why people feel disappointed if all they get is a lecture about holding off.

But here's my side of things: In explaining to a patient why a drug they saw on TV last night is not for him, or why a screening test her sister had might be great for the sister's situation but age-inappropriate for my patient, I am trying to provide a kind of care that is increasingly unavailable as medicine becomes more regimented. I *am* doing something, but I'm up against some powerful forces that want me to do something different. I can't tell you how many times I've gone through this exercise with patients—explaining why a particular test posed more harm than risk, or recommending against an elective procedure or a new medication, only to find that after weeks of obsessing, the patient found another physician who was willing to countermand me and offer the opinion the patient wanted. Many times I was right and the patient suffered a cascade of subsequent complications. Sometimes I was wrong and the patient sailed through the procedure with nary a peep, leaving them understandably irritated at my conservatism. I can accept being wrong; medicine is a humbling business. What I have more trouble with is how quickly patients can be shepherded into treatment decisions in the course of a single office visit with a new doctor, when I have had the benefit of the long view of their medical care and their ability to tolerate medicines and surgeries.

Now, this story makes it pretty clear how a physician could "overtreat" a frail older person because of a lack of "gero-sensitivity" and by adopting a cookbook approach. But how does a robust forty-five- or fifty-five-year-old get overtreated? And what does age discrimination have to do with that? Does it really happen?

It happens all the time. Just as with eighty-year-olds, sweeping generalizations are made about us "younger" people in our forties, fifties, and sixties on the basis of age, helped along by ugly and unfair boomer stereotypes that come from the media. Depending on whom you read, we're the self-absorbed consumers of the earth's resources; many in the next generation believe they'll be left to clean up our mess. Those who preceded us like to remind us we've been coddled and can't possibly appreciate what true struggle, which they endured, really means. And most of the cable television channels I surf appear to be directed at an audience that is obsessed with customer service, ready to part with money for any item that can relieve any form of inconvenience. We're in control of our destinies. We want to be waited on. We want the best of everything including health care.

So what solutions are being offered to quell our self-indulgent anxiety about not having every last possible health-care option at our fingertips? Ironically, in an attempt to escape cookbook medicine and get personalized care, what many of us are being sold is nothing more than cookbook medicine on steroids. The ads tell the story: Virtual body scans marketed directly to you, no matter what your medical history is and because your doctor, with his medieval exam, misses all kinds of terrible diseases (You haven't even met my doctor, I mutter to myself). Commercials market vitamin and supplement cocktails, now directed not only at general well-being but at specific organs while failing to provide high-quality evidence of effectiveness (You've never met my prostate, either, but my doctor has, and I'd like him to worry about my "prostate health," thank you).

If you're an inquisitive baby boomer intent on getting to the bottom of a medical concern or you're just seeking the best preventative health care, your high-speed Internet connection and your health insurance can be as dangerous as they are valuable. Just scratch the surface and you'll be offered all manner of screenings, comprehensive preventative health examinations, and supplements from folks who have no knowledge of your medical history. Make no mistake about it: You've been targeted on the basis of your age, your demographic, and your wallet. And if you take the bait, there's a very good chance that at some point you'll get what you wished for—and then some.

One story—involving a physician, no less—was reported in the *New York Times* several years back.[3] When "virtual colonoscopy" became available, this doctor decided to avail himself of the new technology rather than submit to the usual invasive procedure, which many people find so unappealing. The good news: His colon was just fine. The bad news: When they put you in the scanner, they don't just look at your colon. The scan showed that the patient had smallish cysts on his kidneys and liver and nodules in his lungs, common incidental findings that usually don't reflect anything nefarious. But the cat was out of the bag, and the patient was understandably anxious. Rather than simply follow the lesions with serial scans to see if they got bigger, the doctor-patient had his liver and kidney nodules biopsied via needles—not a full surgery but not a day at the beach, either. Checking the lung nodules, however, required a bigger procedure, which collapsed his lungs.

The biopsies were negative. The nodules were probably scar tissue from an old fungal infection. But it took the doctor months to recover, and all the procedures cost him (get ready) $47,000—thanks to a "health promotion" activity that was marketed to an age-specific segment of society hungry for information, anxious about health, and eager and willing to spend.

A nasty story for sure. Fortunately, the patient was a younger man, not an elderly person who might well have been permanently injured by such an unnecessary medical excursion. Remember that "geriatric ledger" I told you about, the accumulated conditions we accrue and the tests we endure over a medical lifetime by fate, inaction, or choice? This undertaking turned out to be a substantial withdrawal. What if twenty-five years from now this patient gets what would have been simple pneumonia or another lung problem and needs to call upon the lung reserve that was squandered here? A disease that could be treated with a few days of oral antibiotics at home might wind up being a more serious medical extravaganza. And what's so frustrating is that the lung reserve was squandered needlessly on a medical wild goose chase. As I said, nothing drives geriatricians nuts like avoidable excess disability, especially when it's caused by ill-advised collisions with the health-care system.

Contrast this story with that of another patient of mine, age seventy-six, whose senior housing community had an outbreak of influenza a few years ago. The housing administration ordered that every patient on the affected floor be seen by a doctor and receive a chest X-ray. My patient had only some mild cold symptoms and no abnormal breath sounds when I listened to her chest with my stethoscope, so an X-ray seemed nuts. But her ability to stay in her apartment hinged on my complying with the bureaucrats, so I indulged them. I could have kicked myself for doing it, but it was easier to order the test than to argue with them.

Her chest X-ray revealed a small lung nodule that could have been a very early lung cancer but was more likely benign. The only way to know for sure would be to do a biopsy of her lung. I could have predicted her reaction to this news: "I want no part of it!" she said. "You doctors with your crazy tests, all you do is look for trouble!"

She had a point. And the truth is that I was somewhat relieved; I had no stomach for talking her into this, because frankly, I wasn't sure whether the procedure was such a good idea myself.

Her high-powered daughter, on the other hand, had very strong ideas about the whole affair. She was a "doer" and would have been delighted to see the procedure done right then and there in the office. "Mom, when you have something that could be cancer, it needs to come out, period!" she argued. "And right away! Why are you playing with fire?"

Her mother countered that the "fire" here wasn't the nodule in her lung but the needle in the radiologist's hand. The daughter looked to me for backup, but I wasn't biting. After I (a) explained to the mother the small but real possibility that this could be cancer; (b) pointed out that, if it was, a major subsequent surgery would be the only real opportunity for cure; and (c) described both the needle biopsy and what that would entail, I was convinced she had all the info she needed to make her own decision.

And then she spoke: "Mark, if this was supposed to convince me, you've done it," she declared. "I'm more convinced than ever that there's no way in hell I'm doing this. I'll roll the dice."

She rolled and she won. A decade later the nodule in her chest had grown slightly. (I'm still not sure to this day what it was: Possibly it was cancer—some older people coexist with theirs very well.) She sallied along with no symptoms whatsoever. Every time I saw her after this heated exchange, she delighted in reminding me, and more pointedly her daughter, of who was right (her) and who was wrong (everybody else) in this medical decision-making exercise. It became our running joke, a "testimony to my incompetence," she would say with a wink. But the truth is that she sidestepped cookbook medicine with nominal help from me, and not only did she live to tell about it—she lived well. And as they say, living well (especially while sticking it to your doctor and meddling daughter) is the best revenge.

I hope I've convinced you that the boomer-driven pilgrimage for ever more health-care whistles and bells can be viewed as

a variant of ageism with huge potential for unintended consequences. But who could blame some of us for seeking it out? In
America, we've been conditioned to believe that more is better.
Supersize that meal. Get more horsepower for your SUV. How
about a suite instead of that standard room at the Marriott? I hear
it from well-meaning but naïve spouses and adult children all the
time: "I want Mom to have the best care possible. Do everything
you can!"

The problem is that, as we age, more can be more, more can
be the same, or more can actually be less. Well-meaning patients,
families, and doctors who reflexively forge ahead with medical tests
and treatments run the risk of violating the "do no harm" edict
through doing too much. It's a form of unintentional killing with
kindness.

We geriatricians have a saying: "Doing" is easy; it's knowing when
"not to do" that portrays geriatric medicine at its finest.

Chapter 7

Bedside Matters

Do You Have an Aging-Friendly Primary Care Doctor?

"You're a very sick man," said the doctor after my annual physical.
"I want a second opinion!" I demanded.
"Okay," he said. "You're also very ugly."

—Rodney Dangerfield

I'm sure you've heard about physician stereotypes or seen them portrayed on television. Pediatricians are cheerful. Heart surgeons are cowboys. Pathologists are introverted. Internists are brainy. So what about the doctors who choose to care for older people? What are they like, and why did they make that choice?

I can only speak for myself, but my story is a common one among geriatricians. Most will tell you about an older adult who had a significant influence on their lives. In my case it was my grandfather. He spent a good portion of his last few years helping to raise me in his home. His daughter, my mother, was an only child, and looking back, I think he lavished attention on me that he would have given to a son, had he been blessed with one. And at the time, I desperately needed it. I remember having friends over in elementary school who thought my father-figure-in-residence was old, but if my grandfather's state of mind and body could be described as old, tell me where I can sign up. This guy was larger than life—an amateur boxer, attorney, Scrabble god, stand-up comedian. I remember being seven and unable to keep up with him on the two-wheeler he had just taught me to ride. When he became sick and ultimately died, the loss was unfathomable to me as a ten-year-old. It was as if I had lost a father twice.

It would be disingenuous to say I signed on for a medical career as an immediate outgrowth of that formative experience. Over time I've come to see geriatrics as a way of honoring that which is steady, venerated, and reliable, and my grandfather was all these things. It's also an unusual marriage of science and art, of hunch and data, and of function and form. We geriatricians embrace the long and holistic view, not only of our patients but of history and the value of "old" things. We're willing to use technology, but we're also interested in the patient story; we see geriatrics as the perfect marriage of the medical and social sciences with the humanities. And we delight in being able to play a meaningful role not only in patients' health but also in their lives. Yes, we're a self-selected bunch who like people. We also like what we do for a living. In fact, at a time of extraordinary cynicism among physicians, geriatricians have the highest job satisfaction of any specialty in medicine.[1]

I believe that many of the qualities found in an enduring relationship with a grandparent (for those of us lucky enough to experience it) can be found in a great doctor-patient relationship, too. Most of us want a physician who is knowledgeable about our families, work, and life but not so immersed in our minute-to-minute struggles that he or she can't step back and provide perspective. We'd like a health educator who can offer sincere advice in our best interest but nonjudgmentally. And it's great to have a reliable source of wisdom and counsel who ages with us. Unfortunately, there are strong headwinds that blow against this kind of doctor-patient relationship these days.

But we're all getting old, and we all need a doctor. So in this chapter I'll provide a strategy for evaluating the kind of primary care you're getting as it relates to aging. I'll give you some perspective on what's reasonable to expect from a doctor's visit and what's not. I'll provide advice on how to make the most of what is becoming increasingly limited time with your physician. If you believe the relationship you have with your doc is suffering to the extent that you're thinking about ending it, I've got some thoughts about that, too. (Not so fast, my friend!) But if it turns out that you indeed have irreconcilable differences, I can offer some advice on how to find your next doctor. Finally, I'll describe other models of medical practice that you might not know about and may want to consider if nothing seems to meet your needs.

The Most Important Quality in a Primary Care Physician vis-à-vis Aging

Here's the question I'm most frequently asked about finding a doctor who can provide good care for an aging parent or an adult child: Dr. Lachs, if you had to pick one attribute or quality to look for in a primary care physician who'll care for you or your aging parent, what would it be? Superb diagnostic abilities? Exemplary physical examination skills? Superior technical prowess, such as in interpreting blood tests or an EKG? Or would it be exceptional bedside manners, and empathy?

My answer: None of the above.

Assuming that all the docs I get to pick from have a basic level of medical competence and a decent fund of knowledge, the most desirable attribute I would seek in a physician caring for a patient with "aging issues" or "aging concerns" would be a mild obsessive-compulsive disorder.

Let me explain.

You know that book about not sweating the small stuff? When it comes to aging, that's an incredibly bad idea. I want a doc who sweats everything: every pill I take, every consultant he sends me to, every test result that comes back, every symptom I experience, no matter how trivial I believe it might be. I want a guy who tosses and turns at night as to why he prescribed Tylenol versus Advil for the knee pain I told him about earlier that day. I want a gal who goes and looks at my chest X-ray herself because she doesn't trust the radiologist's written report.

I'll put it even more bluntly: Given the choice between the

valedictorian of the medical school and the guy who graduated in the middle of his class who dots every *i* and crosses every *t*, I'll take the second fella nearly every time, especially as a primary care physician. (There are exceptions based on your psychological makeup and preferences, as well as the diseases or conditions you have, but they are few and far between; I'll get to that issue later.)

Why this seemingly strange choice? It might already be obvious to you from my previous diatribes. Internal medicine generally, and geriatric medicine specifically, is detail work. As I've described, as we get older, big and often permanent life-altering problems can arise from neglected medical and social issues, even those that may seem trivial when they come up. I believe ageism is at the core of many of these oversights, but there are other factors as well. One is great insurance reimbursement for docs who do procedures and little reward for those who take the time to think. Another is a subspecialty culture that divides care among many doctors with no single captain of the ship. The uncoordinated care that results from the latter may seem cutting-edge when viewed through the narrow prism of the specialist, but it can be outright dangerous. When too many doctors start messin' around with your care and your medicine, you're asking for trouble. And as we get older, we tend to get more and more doctors, particularly in this subspecialty-oriented culture, where one hand often doesn't know what the other one is doing.

And here's the real rub: I believe that never in the history of American medicine have conditions been less conducive to the "compulsive" style of doctoring that I'm encouraging and that an aging population needs. The average primary care physician in the United States can have more than two thousand patients in his practice. It's not uncommon for a family doctor to see thirty or more "customers" a day as outpatients. The demands of managed care often pressure docs to spend eight or ten minutes with "the ear" or "the foot" that's acting up on a particular day, but there's (usually) an entire person attached to the body part when it's brought to the office. While subspecialized care might be fine for an eighteen-year-old with a sprained knee, it's a recipe for disaster in an eighty-year-old whose "chief complaint" (the reason he came to the doctor) is infrequently so neat and tidy. Very few of my patients come to see me with just one problem, and when they do, it's rarely so straightforward that I can let my guard down to focus solely on that one organ or anatomic area. Tempting as it may be at times to do so, geriatricians cannot declare other body parts off-limits when patients come to them for a particular problem. A rash could be from an infection or from a medication the dentist prescribed. Belly pain could be anything from an upset stomach or life-threatening diverticulitis to depression. A patient may be falling from cataracts, medications, arthritis, or a combination of all three. Try figuring that out in eight minutes.

So what happens when doctors try (or are forced) to deal with these problems of aging in a younger man's world? Lack of attention to detail. Shortcuts. Carelessness that's unintentional, but carelessness just the same. And in many cases, medical error. If I were to write a book about the process of care experienced by many older people in the United States, I might paraphrase the title of another popular book about physician practice: *How Doctors Don't Think*.

Scary stuff, but here's the good news: Armed with a little forethought about your interpersonal style and preferences, and informed by what I'll tell you about the art of doctoring, you can make some more intelligent choices about your medical care. The first step involves a bit of medical self-reflection.

How Do You Want to Be Doctored?

I'm a big believer in bedside manner, but I'm an even bigger believer in what I'd call "doctor-patient fit"—particularly as we get older. Most patients I speak to tell me that if their relationship with a doctor isn't right (or is even simply average), less "healing" gets done, no matter how technically skilled the physician is. Data are starting to bear this out. Studies now suggest that patients' adherence to all kinds of medical advice might be influenced not only by whether physicians actually deliver the appropriate message but also by *how* they deliver it and whether their communication and cultural styles are compatible with their patients'. And this isn't limited to suggestions involving lifestyle choices, such as when your finger-wagging doc admonishes you to lose weight or stop smoking. Stylistic nuances and compatibilities may someday be shown to influence whether or not you'll actually get a screening colonoscopy or take medication as prescribed.

By doctor-patient fit, I mean individualized expectations and preferences with respect to getting doctored. If we're talking about your parents or your spouse, then I mean *their* expectations and preferences, not yours. If you have no faith in Mom or Dad's physician and haven't been shy about making your feelings known, your strategy is probably not helping anyone. In my experience, the more you impugn the ability of your loved one's physician, the deeper he will dig his heels in around that issue, and nothing will get solved. Most patients remain fiercely loyal to their physician, even in the face of some underwhelming doctoring. When you try to point that out, it's often experienced as a personal affront, like critiquing Mom's taste in music or booing Dad's beloved baseball team. You're going to have to join that team, not battle it, if you're going to make any progress.

But when it comes to your own care, you'd be smart to ask yourself (and answer honestly) a few questions about what it is you want in a physician, because if there ever was an area in which "one size fits all" doesn't apply, this is it.

Perhaps you've been led to believe that all patients should want a doc with great bedside manners or directness, or perhaps a communicator. In my experience, nothing could be further from the truth. Different people want different things from their physician, as they have individual preferences for everything else, from clothes to foods to mates. Why should something this personal (choosing the person you get naked in front of and presumably reveal details you'd tell no one else) be an exception?

Some folks (and many doctors themselves fall into this category) couldn't care less about interpersonal abilities; they want technical prowess, period. (As one of my surgeon buddies likes to say, "I've come to be doctored, not mothered.") Some patients want big communicators—they need to know every potential cause of their symptom and every option to treat it. Others simply hate it when the doctor provides too many gory details—"TMI." "Just tell me which medication to take, how much to take, and when to take it," one of my patients likes to rant. "I don't want to go to medical school, I just want to get better."

I, on the other hand, never got over "second-year medical student's disease." It's a strange condition that sets in during the pathology course typically given in year two of medical school, when the student experiences every disease he's learning about. (I still seem to have a stubborn brain tumor that comes and goes.) As a result, I like a communicator who's willing to patiently entertain my paranoid medical mind and then reassure me thoughtfully. Most of my colleagues (of the doctoring-not-mothering ilk) see no need for this. Which type of patient are you?

It's important to know, because you have choices! Whether you're accompanying Mom to her doctor or dealing with your own, there are some ageist land mines that need to be avoided in the doctor-patient discourse. Light has been shed on this issue by several elegant studies of interactions between doctors and older patients conducted by my co-chief of geriatric medicine, Dr. Ronald Adelman, at Weill Cornell.[2] He and collaborators throughout the United States audiotaped doctor-patient encounters (with patient consent, of course), and some rather dramatic findings emerged, including some troubling patterns of doctoring. I'd strongly suggest that you be on the lookout for the following problems with a doctor in the course of procuring care. If you spot one, you can redirect the physician gently or find another if he or she is incorrigible.

- **Talking down:** You may notice you or your mom being addressed with patronizing colloquialisms ("sweetie," "honey") that certainly wouldn't fly with younger patients. I'm not saying that this is necessarily inappropriate in every case (I've had a few patients call me by such endearments on occasion; a ton of folks I care for seem to see me as a surrogate child or grand-child), but the assumption of informality and intimacy in a new doctor-patient relationship strikes me as inappropriate.

- **Ignoring the patient:** This happens most frequently when a patient is accompanied to the medical visit by someone else, no matter how well-meaning the third party is. Audiotapes of these so-called "triadic encounters" reveal that doctors often talk about patients as if they're not in the room or are so impaired they can't fathom what's going on. One patient who had this experience said she felt "as if I were a pet brought by my owner to the veterinarian." When you come with your spouse or parent to my office, I understand that it's because you want to help him or her articulate symptoms more clearly to me; or because when Mom gets home, she can't produce even a scrap of detail about what happened at her doctor's appointment, and that's frustrating. But don't forget who the patient is here, and don't let the doctor forget, either. This is indeed an occupational hazard in geriatrics; I often find myself having to redirect eye contact and dis-course toward the patient when a third party is present, no matter how probing and appropriate questions from the "third wheel" might be. Older patients have rights, too. Be aware of physicians who don't acknowledge them, and gently ask the doc to speak directly to the person being cared for, whether it's your husband or you.
- **Interrupting:** This happens with patients of all ages but especially oldsters. There's evidence to suggest that most patients get interrupted and/or waylaid by the doctor within the first minute of articulating their "chief complaint." You're especially at risk for this if your thoughts are not well orga-nized before you get to the doctor; shortly, I'll show you some tricks to minimize this danger.

- **Dismissive of complaints:** As patients age, physicians increasingly tend to minimize their problems and attribute them to just getting old. As I've discussed, this can have disastrous consequences. I'll say it again: Aging is not a disease. There are diseases that become more common as people age, but attributing all symptoms in older persons—tiredness, aches and pains, memory loss—to advancing age is intellectually lazy. Any physician who practices this way is eventually going to miss a significant treatable condition. Any worrisome symptom should be evaluated before you and your doctor decide you're "just going to live with it."

- **Quick to refer, test, or prescribe:** Another way some doctors deal with patients who take up too much time is to quickly write a prescription or send them for a test or to another doctor. (Patients love prescriptions; many feel as if they really haven't been to the doctor unless they leave with one.) It takes a lot of time for me to give you a careful physical exam and then explain why I am confident you don't have a brain tumor, but it takes almost none to send you for an MRI of your head. The problem is, as you'll see in a subsequent chapter, tests and medications are a mixed blessing as we get older. And while seeing a specialist might seem like a good idea, there's almost always a cost to parsing out body parts to subspecialists or ordering tests to get patients on their way.

I have even heard physicians describe a variety of "tricks" they use to keep the line moving. It made me queasy and embarrassed for our profession. One bragged to me that he kept no chairs (other than his own) in his consultation room; older people simply did not have the physical endurance to stand long enough to ask questions. One patient recently told me that her physician brought a discussion to an abrupt end because the patient's insurer "did not pay me enough money." While I'm certainly sympathetic to the underfunding of care for older people (it's the reason many physicians are leaving Medicare), the doc should have kept that comment to himself.

The Age-Appropriate Doctor's Appointment: Making the Most of It

Since the forces that have led to "the incredible shrinking office visit" are unlikely to end soon, and since we're all getting older and need the best care we can get, the question is: What's a boomer to do?

Answer: Plan accordingly. You wouldn't go to your accountant, your lawyer, or even your hairdresser without a sense of what you wanted from the transaction; why would you be any less prepared for a visit to the doctor? Here are some tips to help you get the most out of what is increasingly likely to be a time-pressured encounter. Underlying every piece of advice is a simple edict: *Get organized.* The visit will be more productive for you and more efficient for your physician.

Articulate your chief complaint. The cornerstone of med students' training is the "chief complaint"—the reason you sought medical attention ("It hurts here" or "I have a cough"). But as we age, chief complaints often become nebulous or difficult to put your finger on. If you can't tick off specific symptoms, note whatever functional problems you're having, for example, "I can't put on my overcoat" or "I keep losing things." If you don't have a chief complaint (perhaps you're here for an annual physical and everything is hunky-dory), that's fine, too. Say that.

Organize your thoughts before the doctor visit. Geriatricians (and all primary care docs, for that matter) don't have scalpels. The tool of our trade is what we call the medical history—understanding your story is the key to making an accurate diagnosis. So think about what's troubling you in some detail before coming to the doctor to tell your story. For example, if you have pain, when did it start? What makes it worse? Is there anything that makes it better—perhaps position, ice, or Tylenol? Does it move or radiate anywhere? Providing as much accurate detail as you can about what's troubling you will likely lead to a better outcome. You're not a doctor, and you're not going to be able to anticipate all the questions you'll be asked, but a good doc should leave no nit unpicked in probing you about specific symptoms. If you are accompanying a loved one who typically "clams up" during a doctor visit, I'd interview him or her beforehand to practice responding—maybe try a little role playing, with you starring as the doctor.

Prioritize your complaints. Many patients I see have a laundry list of issues that they find overwhelming. Believe me, it can be overwhelming for us, too, as we do our best to help you with ten problems in the fifteen minutes the system may have allotted us. (You can see why meds get dispensed and specialists are invoked indiscriminately.) The expression "Rome wasn't built in a day" applies in this case. You need to be practical. If you wind up spending only a minute or two of your precious office-visit time on each of a smorgasbord of issues, none of them will get solved. My suggestion: a top-three list. I encourage new patients to do this: I might say something like "I see from your list, Mrs. Smith, that a number of things are bothering you. If you were forced to pick the top three things I could most help with, what would they be?" Or I might provide orientation myself: "Today I'm going to focus on the arthritis pain you've been calling about, and if we have time, I'll explain the results of the cholesterol tests you had when you were here last visit. Does that sound reasonable?" Everybody's happier when expectations are managed.

List all "interval events." By this, I mean major things that have happened to you since you last saw your doctor. Examples include hospitalizations, surgeries, bad infections, a trip to the ER for a cut, or visits with other doctors, who may have offered advice or changed your medications. Big life events count, too: a divorce, the birth of a grandchild, loss of a job, unusual financial reversals—if you feel comfortable discussing these. As I said earlier, the medical and social components of our lives become more inextricably linked as we age and conspire to influence health. Basic rule of thumb: If you're not sure if something constitutes a significant event, then include it.

Bring a list of your medications. The list should be up-to-date and complete, including dosages and frequencies. (Even better, bring the medicines themselves in a bag.) Know beforehand what you're running out of so you can ask for any renewals you might need or take care of after the visit by phone or with office staff so your time with the doctor is not usurped by an administrative task. One of the biggest areas of medical error with patients of any age is what medical quality experts call *medication reconciliation* (see chapter 15 on medications). In older people, this is especially critical, because medications can interact with one another; more important, they can interact with or have unexpected effects on the chronic conditions you have (so-called drug-disease interactions).

Get a specific follow-up plan. At the end of the visit, you should leave with several "action items" that need to be followed up on. These could be blood tests or X-rays, a referral to another doc, or a change of medication. Go over with your doctor what's going to happen and when once you walk out the door. Example: "So I'm going to get an MRI of my head for these headaches. Will you be calling me with the results even if they're normal, or should I call you?" Or: "So I start taking the medication for my knee arthritis tomorrow. When should I come back to see you to assess whether or not it's been effective?" Or: "Will you be calling Dr. Jones, the lung doctor, to explain why you're sending me?" Again, getting the follow-up plan clear and setting expectations goes a long way toward avoiding miscommunication and trouble down the road.

Get the doctor to be transparent. If you bought this book, I assume that you're pretty darn intelligent (and have good taste to boot). That being the case, there's something seriously wrong if you walk out of the doctor's office without understanding what he's trying to tell you. If it's because he's using medical jargon, remind him kindly that you're not a doctor (assuming that's true) and you need it in lay terms. If you're anxious about something specific, let the doctor know that. Perhaps he can list the things he believes might be causing your symptom, and you'll be relieved to learn that mad cow disease, swine flu, or the Ebola virus is not at the top of his list, though it might be on the top of yours. If after making this request several times it still feels like you're at the Tower of Babel, then you might need to start looking for another doctor.

Finding a "Gero-Friendly" Doctor

Now that I've suggested that there might be a perfect Marcus Welby for every aging patient on the planet, you might be asking, "How do I find one of these guys? That's a superb question for which, sadly, there aren't always great answers. But here's some help.

There are very few geriatricians; at last count via our professional organization, the American Geriatrics Society (visit them at www.americangeriatricssociety.org or their foundation's Web site that includes a physician referral link at http://www.healthinaging.org/public_education/physician_referral.php), there were about eight thousand of us in the United States to care for 30 million people over the age of sixty-five.[3] You don't have to be a demographer to realize that this presents a pretty shocking supply and demand problem. Not only are there not enough of us, but at the rate we're minting new geriatricians (and losing old ones to retirement) in comparison to how the population over age sixty-five (and eighty-five especially) is growing, *there will simply never be enough of us.* So you'll need to do some sophisticated sleuthing to find a bona fide geriatrician (or a physician who is sensitive to the needs of older people) near where you live.

By far, the best place to find a geriatrician is at an academic medical center—a hospital with a medical school on or near its campus. For example, I teach at Cornell's Medical School (the Weill Cornell Medical College), and our major teaching hospital, New York–Presbyterian Hospital, is literally attached to the school. Call the hospital or the associated medical school and ask to be connected to the geriatrics division. Typically it resides within a department of internal medicine (as I mentioned earlier, most geriatricians are internists before they become geriatricians); in some cases it is located within a department of family practice, since this is a recognized pathway to geriatric board certification.

If there is no local medical school, you can try a couple of things. One is to find the nearest medical school and contact its department of internal medicine or family medicine to see if it recently graduated any geriatricians in your area. There are other places to look that you probably haven't thought about. You might be pleasantly surprised to learn that the Veterans Health Administration has been at the vanguard of training geriatricians and creating innovative clinical programs to care for its aging constituency. If you're a veteran, call them. If you're a member of an HMO or other managed-care plan, inquire with them; you might think that HMOs would have absolutely no interest in providing this kind of care, but that is not always the case. Motivated by recent financial incentives created by the government, many HMOs are beginning to reenter the senior market. To do that well, they have to make sure that their older members are kept well and high-functioning— frail patients are expensive patients. Sure, that costs money, but not as much as not doing it. Remember, under managed care the costs of many tests and hospitalizations are borne by the insurer to various degrees. Minimizing these costs requires geriatricians, who know how to manage older patients or create systems of care for them; or at the very least, gero-friendly primary care providers, who can keep older people healthy and out of the hospital. Some HMOs are beginning to incorporate geriatricians or geriatric-type practices into their offerings.

Finally, your community hospital may have some kind of geriatric program. Even in the face of relatively poor medical economics (which should, I hope, improve under health-care reform), these are beginning to spring up as the growing number of older Americans makes it simply impossible for any credible health institution to call itself enlightened if it doesn't offer something for older members of the community.

Another warning: Once you locate a program or a physician who fits the bill, you are very likely to encounter a long waiting list. No matter how long it is, I would advise you to get on it. Very few of the patients I see have issues so acute that they need to see me immediately. The problems that I typically encounter in geriatrics are serious but more smoldering than emergent.

A community-advocacy point here: If you can find no geriatric program in your community, at your local hospital, or in your local health system (or find one that does only research, not patient care), and you are in a position of influence, I would holler about it to the powers that be. In this day and age, such an oversight is a travesty.

Walks Like a Duck

What happens if you simply cannot identify someone with geriatric credentials in your immediate environment? Should you travel substantial distances to receive specialized care? That depends.

About five years ago, a spry sixty-five-year-old man came to my office seeking a new primary care physician. He had seen a lecture I gave at a local community center about geriatric medicine and decided this was for him. He'd passed the "magical" sixty-five milestone (an insane and arbitrary demarcation for what's old, if you ask me) and decided, unbeknownst to his long-standing internist, that it was time to seek me out. In fact, one of his major anxieties in coming to me was offending his doc, with whom he had a fine relationship extending back two decades. His substantially younger wife was under this doc's care and would remain so after he transitioned to me, he explained.

One of the other interesting things about my business is that you get to learn a lot about how other people practice medicine. Patients who have made it to sixty-five or older invariably come with at least some medical history (more often than not, a ton of it). I probably spend as much time reviewing old office records, hospital admissions, tests, medication lists, and other medical novellas as I do examining various body parts. In reviewing this stuff, not infrequently I see some pretty questionable choices—tests and procedures that I would not have ordered that were, others I would have ordered that weren't, and even tests and procedures I didn't know were done anymore. I've seen prescriptions written for medications that should never be used for elderly patients (or many younger ones, for that matter) and obvious diagnoses missed. It can be a bit disconcerting.

But I also get to see some pretty great doctoring. That was the case with this man's internist. He was simply superb: detailed problem lists, cautious use of medications, sensible ordering of tests, completely up-to-date and appropriate screening tests and vaccinations, and to my delight, a variety of geriatric measures as well—memory testing, depression screening, even an evaluation of gait. (What primary care doctor has actually watched *you* walk?)

Though they're dwindling in number, there are still outstanding primary care physicians who provide excellent care to older people, essentially functioning as geriatricians but *without a portfolio*. I hope health-care reform will produce more of them, but the problem now is finding one. If you've stumbled onto one of these national treasures, stay put. If there's no wait to see him or her, that won't be the case for long, I guarantee you.

My advice to this gentleman was to count his blessings and stay connected to this wonderful doctor who had provided him with years of dedicated service. Not only was the doc gero-friendly, he had the long view of this patient's life course and family (having cared for several other family members). Such doctor-patient relationships in modern American medicine are increasingly rare and priceless.

Time to Find a New Doctor? Not So Fast!

Okay, so you're increasingly dissatisfied with the medical care you or your parent is receiving. Perhaps you're feeling ignored or rushed during "the incredible shrinking office visit." Maybe you had a test or biopsy done days or weeks ago and the doctor hasn't called you back, oblivious to the fact that you've been pacing the floor at night waiting for the results. Or maybe you tried to call your doc with an acute medical problem (a cough, a rash, a fever) and weren't even afforded the courtesy of a response.

Look, I'm not going to defend any of this. If I did, I'd lose credibility with you because, frankly, if these things occur on a regular basis, they're simply indefensible. And I'd be lying to you if I told you that the medical practice I work in hasn't screwed up customer service from time to time.

But before you pull up stakes and go shopping for a new primary care physician, let me educate you a bit about why the tenor of primary care medical practice has deteriorated over the past decade. I'm doing this for two reasons. First, if you're considering giving your doc a pink slip for unreasonable medical or customer service, you'll need an objective sense of what "reasonable" is in this day and age; I can provide that with a glimpse inside medical practice. Second, before you jump ship (often irreversibly), you'll need to make sure that what's out there is superior to the care you've been receiving, or you may discover that you've jumped from the frying pan into the fire. It's a bit like the classic Henny Youngman joke: When asked how his wife was, he famously replied, "Compared to what?"

If you've been in any business in your life that requires interaction with the public, you know that customers come in all shapes and sizes, and with all kinds of expectations. While I still harbor the fantasy that what I do is not a business and that my patients are not customers, there is without doubt a customer service element to medical care. And because logic often flies out the window when your health is at stake, customer expectations can be all over the map. For example, how would you rate (reasonable or unreasonable) the following medical encounters I've had with patients and their families over the past year or so? There are no right answers—it's a question of perspective:

- The daughter of an elderly patient who faxed me to say, "Call me at home tonight after 9 p.m. to discuss my mother's care."
- A patient who repeatedly phones the physician on call for me on weekends and holidays to renew her blood pressure medicines.
- A patient who doesn't call me at night with chest pain and shortness of breath because he doesn't want to disturb me.
- A patient who sustains a laceration while cutting bread in the middle of the night insists I meet him in the emergency department to explain his medical problems to the ER physician.

What's Reasonable? What's Not?

Having said all this, I'm willing to lay out some general principles about what you have the right to expect from a primary care physician and when you should be looking elsewhere.

Test results: For relatively routine tests, I have no objection to a physician's saying something like "If you don't hear from me, it means the blood tests I drew today are fine." But as the nature of the tests moves from routine to more unusual, or if they are performed to exclude a specific disease or problem, I don't buy it. For example, you shouldn't have to hunt down a physician to get the results—within a reasonable period of time—of a breast biopsy for a mass that was discovered on mammography, or the results of a CAT scan of the head that was done because you're having headaches. To avoid these potentially agonizing waiting games, *when the test is ordered, ask your physician how long it will take to get the results back and how you can obtain them.* Will he call you? Will you call him?

Physician telephone accessibility: In this day and age, unless you're in an unusual practice, I don't think it is reasonable to expect a physician to come to the phone immediately when you call, unless the problem you report seems urgent to his nurse or whoever takes the call. But I do believe that it's reasonable to expect a call back that day or that night, depending on the nature of your problem. (It's unreasonable to expect a call back in two minutes: This is not a hospital environment in which a surgeon is getting paged to the operating room to save a trauma victim.) If you believe that it's urgent, tell the person answering the phone that this is the case. If you're not sure, ask for the nurse. If you have a specific medical condition or conditions that occasionally flare up, next time you're with your doctor for a routine office visit, ask what kinds of problems constitute an emergency and when and how that should be conveyed when you call the office.

After office hours: I am a firm believer that if you're providing primary care to older adults, a health-care provider (not necessarily your physician) must be on call 24/7 for that practice. If your primary care doctor has an after-hours message on his answering machine that says something like "There's nobody here, nobody on call, so call back tomorrow" or "If this seems like an emergency, go to the nearest emergency room," I'd start trying to find another doctor. While telephone medicine is certainly imperfect, there are subtle nuances to figuring out what exactly is going on when a patient calls after hours. Perfunctorily sending an older patient to an ER for what could be a trivial problem could be more dangerous than the problem itself (more on that in chapter 11, where I'll teach you how to navigate the ER).

Waiting: When I'm the patient, I hate waiting for the doctor. When I'm the doctor, I hate keeping patients waiting (and get equally annoyed when patients are late). But the nature of this business is that there are emergencies from time to time, and you need to be tolerant of that. If chronic tardiness is a habitual problem with your doctor, you might want to first chat with the office staff about this before pulling the plug on the relationship.

Hospitalists: An increasing trend in health care is for patients admitted to the hospital to be treated by someone other than their primary care physician: It's simply too inefficient for physicians to leave an office full of patients to travel across town for the sake of one or two hospitalized patients. Additionally, hospital medicine has become an entirely different skill set, and many experts believe that you'd be better served by someone who practices it exclusively. If you have the expectation that your doc will come to see you in the hospital, you may be disappointed, so you need to discuss the doctor's policy *before* you're admitted. Personally, I have a bit of a problem with this arrangement, as do many geriatricians; there is no greater need for continuity of care than when an older person is admitted to the hospital. But there are strategies to minimize the potentially negative impact of being admitted to the hospital, which I'll describe in chapter 10.

Physician Extenders

Physician extender refers generally to two types of health-care professionals who can be of enormous value to older adults: nurse practitioners and physician's assistants. While I absolutely love nurse practitioners and physician's assistants (full disclosure: I married one), I absolutely hate the term *physician extender*; it sounds like some kind of Hamburger Helper you mix with an overextended doctor to create a care situation that's marginally better than an overwhelmed doc practicing alone.

The truth is, good nurse practitioners and physician's assistants are worth their weight in gold. When properly integrated into a medical practice, they can provide care that far exceeds anything you could get from a "customary" primary care doc (except perhaps for a "concierge" service, see page 101). In my division we employ several NPs and PAs, who work shoulder-to-shoulder with physicians in a variety of settings (office practice, inpatient practice, house call program, and so on). These folks are full-fledged faculty in every sense of the word, and I'm not at all ashamed to admit that a good deal of the geriatric medicine I've learned in my life has been taught to me not by stodgy professors with lofty academic titles but by these profoundly dedicated and talented individuals. In many ways they are in a better position to understand the problems of older people than anyone else in medicine.

Why? Because these folks live at the nexus of the clinical practice of medicine and a broken health-care system they must skillfully navigate every single day to advocate for patients. The thirty- or sixty-minute doctor (or nurse practitioner) visit is in many ways the easiest part of the patient encounter. What is invisible to many patients and families is the subsequent torrent of administrative and clinical follow-up activity that takes place behind the scenes, long after the patient has left the appointment and is home eating dinner. As an example, I'll tell you about a woman I saw recently.

Mrs. R is a terrific seventy-year-old who is a highly successful author. I've had the honor of caring for her for a few years. Well educated and well-to-do, she was sent to me by a friend of mine, because "he just wasn't impressed with her doctors." Despite their fancy Park Avenue addresses, neither was I after I reviewed her records. She had a litany of medical problems that were basically undertreated or ignored: arthritis of her knees that made her unstable, high blood pressure that was not adequately addressed, and intermittent weakness on one side of her body that I discovered was probably the result of an abnormal heart rhythm causing blood clots that were going to her brain. I aggressively treated her arthritis and put her on blood-thinning medications, and she did just great—walking again and getting out into the world.

Unfortunately, one month she forgot to take her blood-thinning medications and had a pretty serious stroke. She was admitted to a rehabilitation facility, where she recovered much of her speech and mobility. She was eventually discharged, and soon afterward I saw her in the office for the first time in months. She looked great. I did the usual geriatric doctor stuff—watched her walk, took her blood pressure, reviewed her functional abilities, and made some recommendations about her home-care environment. All in all, it was a wonderful forty-five-minute visit (for which Medicare probably paid me less than the price of a not-too-fancy haircut in New York City).

But after she left, the (uncompensated) fun began for my nurse practitioner and me. I kept a log of all the activity that grew from that visit:

- Her visiting nurse called, wanting to confirm her discharge medications as she was on an unusually high dose of cholesterol-lowering medication. I called the nursing home; they got those dosages from the hospital. So I called the hospital.
- The hospital had no information and could only refer me to the neurologist who had cared for her during her stay. So I called him.
- He indicated that the high dose of Lipitor was prescribed as a matter of protocol. I lowered the dose, mindful that the drugs can produce muscle weakness in older people when taken in doses that would be fine in younger folks.
- Her blood thinner required that a blood test be drawn twice weekly. Her cardiologist called: Would I be doing that or should he? And how will those lab results be forwarded to each of us, since we both needed to know if her blood was "thin enough"?

- The company that manages her Medicare drug benefit called. Would I be willing to substitute a generic version of one of her blood pressure medicines?
- Her son called, wanting a complete update of her condition over the past three months. He had been away.
- Not to be outdone, his sister from California called with precisely the same question. I went over everything again.
- While my patient was in the rehab center, she did not pay her bills, and her landlord began an eviction proceeding. Her neighbor called to see if I knew someone who could help her with this. I did. A local senior center had a retired lawyer who volunteered by helping to contest evictions such as this.
- That lawyer called me to ask if I would write a letter on behalf of my patient, indicating that she was "indisposed" with medical problems that precluded timely payment of her bills. I was delighted to do so.
- Later in the month he called again, thanking me for the letter and asking if I would testify downtown on my patient's behalf in housing court. I was less than delighted.

As you can see, the vast majority of Mrs. R's care occurred long after her office visit ended. Furthermore, much of that "detail work" I could not have handled myself—I had the assistance of an able nurse practitioner. Note also that less than 50 percent of what we had to do was "medical"; in her aftercare we were dealing with the legal system, insurance companies, and a devoted family who reasonably wanted information. We could have ignored or delegated many of these requests; that would not have been malpractice or below the standard of care. It would have saved our practice considerable time and expense. But it also had a very high likelihood of landing this lady back in the hospital, whereupon she might never have recovered enough ability to live independently again.

Yet almost every time I see a new patient, tell them about the way our practice works, and dutifully explain that very often they will be seeing a nurse practitioner for minor problems between scheduled appointments if I am traveling or at the hospital, they respond the same way: They want to see me, their doctor, not "a nurse." But just as reliably, as their relationship with our practice evolves, I soon find myself vying with my nurse practitioner for patient attention. The reason is obvious: Besides being as good for basic medical stuff as just about any primary care internist in New York City, nurse practitioners and physician's assistants often possess more of one specific resource than any of their physician counterparts: time. Why? At academic medical centers they may be supported by institutional funds or foundation grants, rather than patient billing, so they are not always beholden to the time pressures that physicians face to move on to the next patient. In environments where their wages are paid from patient billing, their substantially lower compensation in comparison to that of physicians enables them to spend more time with patients while still earning their keep. And as I hope I've convinced you, the practice of providing proper primary care to older adults (and their aging baby boomer children) is an intensely time-consuming activity.

So if you find yourself joining a practice that features physician extenders, don't regret; rather, rejoice. You've probably found an enlightened practice. You're likely to get far more quality time in such an environment and come to love your nurse practitioner or physician assistant as much as or more than your doctor.

Concierge Medicine

I'd be both remiss and out-of-date if I neglected to mention a trend that is becoming more and more popular and that addresses many or most of the shortfalls I've discussed in this chapter: concierge medicine. In this membership-based service, instead of caring for a census of up to several thousand patients in a regular practice, a physician may care for hundreds, or even fewer than one hundred—thus making possible much more hands-on involvement. Each "member" pays an annual fee or retainer in addition to the cost of each physician visit or interaction.

Concierge medicine comes in many shapes and sizes. At one extreme, there are practices that charge in excess of $10,000 annually for this service. In these cases, physicians typically have such a small number of patients that they may have no schedule—they are at your beck and call, coming to your home or wherever you happen to fall ill. In some cases physicians will even accompany you to a subspecialty visit to "interpret" the medical interaction.

In less intense versions of concierge practice, a smaller annual fee, say $1,000, is charged. For that amount, appointments are generally expedited (within a day), the physician (not the nurse) returns your call promptly, and care is coordinated with hospitals and subspecialists. (Gee, the more I think about it, the more it sounds like the way medicine used to be practiced. In fact, it sounds a lot like the way geriatricians approach patients, don't ya think?)

How do I feel about concierge practice as someone who has publicly and privately advocated for a system of national health insurance and universal access for all Americans? I'm absolutely fine with it. If you have the resources to join a practice like this— especially if you're not happy with the practice you're in—consider doing so (after performing some due diligence on the physicians involved and ideally speaking with patients who are in the practice). If you've taken away anything from this chapter, I hope it is the notion that the best medicine for people who are getting older is practiced compulsively; and a concierge model provides time for a physician to be detail-oriented and offer continuity across all the places you receive care and all the people you get it from. Good geriatric medicine is very much like concierge medicine, only at bargain-basement prices (thus the long lines). In my medical center's academic geriatric medicine practice, I like to believe that we practice an unusual brand of concierge medicine for both rich and poor. We can afford to do it without regard for the patient's ability to pay only through the generosity of a great hospital and medical school that believes in our mission and helps the practice, and through the philanthropy of a few patients who want to see that the good care they receive can be afforded to older people from all walks of life. I'm immensely proud of this "Robin Hood" arrangement; it's a bit like concierge medicine with "scholarships."

So, to repeat, if you have the resources to expend on concierge care, I would probably do it, especially if you are dealing with multiple chronic conditions that require coordination. As one of my former patients (a wealthy retiree who moved to another community and then joined such a practice) said to me, "Mark, what am I going to do with my money? Buy more art? My body is the most important thing I own!"

I understand the inequity of the "two-tier" system this creates. Concierge medicine offers the kind of care every older American who paid into the Medicare system over much of a lifetime should be receiving. And I'm aware that concierge medicine for the masses underwritten by philanthropy is not a widely sustainable model in areas where there is no wealthy community to "subsidize" the care of those who cannot afford to pay. But I'll end this chapter on an optimistic and prescriptive note, which is also an advertisement for my craft.

Want to rein in medical costs in the United States and improve the quality of care for all? Put primary care geriatricians in charge. I'm not kidding. The best physicians I know are quite often geriatricians, and they routinely are the least frequent test orderers, the least likely to request specialty consultations, and the last to hospitalize patients—not out of some financial pressure but out of good clinical judgment and concern for their patients. I'll again repeat one of our favorite geriatric aphorisms: "It's easy to *do*; it's knowing when *not* to do that makes a great geriatrician." That edict not only protects patients; it saves money. Similarly, my experience is that patients who have transitioned to concierge care—however it is financed—generally find themselves needing hospitalization and expensive services far less frequently than their "traditional" patient counterparts, who these days seem to get attention only when they become seriously ill. And seriously ill patients are expensive to treat.

I believe that an army of "high touch" but "low-tech" geriatricians could care for America at a fraction of the cost of the status quo, produce equivalent clinical outcomes, and engender enormous patient and family satisfaction in the process. Now, that's real doctoring.

Chapter 8

How Many Specialists Does It Take to Screw in a Lightbulb (or Screw You Up)?

Then, into the New Wing! We'll see Dr. Spreckles,
who does the Three F's—Footsies, Fungus, and Freckles.
And nextly we'll drop in on young Dr. Ginns,
our A and S Man who does Antrums and Shins.

—Theodore Geisel (Dr. Seuss), *You're Only Old Once*

In much of what I've so far set down here, I've been talking about the *primary care doctor*—the guy or gal you go to for an annual checkup but also when you have a new medical complaint—the person also known as your family doctor. While many of the pearls I've tried to impart about making your office visits more efficient work equally well with specialists (such as encouraging transparency and making a follow-up plan), the world of subspecialty medicine raises a separate series of issues for people who are aging.

Without a doubt, the explosive growth of specialty and subspecialty medicine has provided huge health and quality-of-life improvements for many, many Americans. It is in large part responsible for our "age wave"; many recipients of subspecialty care are alive today only because of highly trained doctors who could discover and remove their early colon cancers, or open their blocked heart arteries with stents to prevent a fatal heart attack. We also need specialists because there's simply too much medical knowledge these days to fit into one doctor's head or proverbial black bag. That was tough fifty years ago, when most docs were generalists; today it is impossible.

But as we get older, subspecialty medicine becomes yet another mixed blessing. Why? It's the "too-many-cooks" phenomenon. More doctors means more to keep track of. And with that comes more opportunities for miscommunication. Again I'll illustrate with a patient story.

Mr. V was one of my favorites. He was a real New York character. Often when he'd come for his checkup, he'd have the daily racing pages with him, and usually a tip for me on which horse to play. (Disclosure: I'm not a gambler, but one time one of his picks went by a pet name that I used for one of my kids, so I played it and it won.) If there were no winning horses, then he was usually good for a stock tip. (Those I avoided.)

Mr. V's only medical problems were osteoarthritis in one of his knees (the "wear-and-tear" kind) and lifelong bipolar disorder, which I had finally gotten under control using a small dose of psychiatric medication that we adjusted together very carefully. Previously this problem had caused profound difficulties in many of his relationships, but when he was treated, he was the sweetest guy you ever met. Whenever I looked at my schedule for the day and saw his name, I found myself smiling.

Then one day, unbeknownst to me, he sought out an orthopedist for right-hip pain. The orthopedist examined him, did some tests, and determined that he had bursitis (inflammation of a sac called the bursa that just overlies a joint). Without so much as reviewing the medical history of the patient, and without calling me, the orthopedist decided to give Mr. V a short course of prednisone, a form of steroids (not the ones abused in sports but the kind that lowers inflammation in the body). Mr. V was old school, a trusting sort, reverential of physicians (to a fault), and not one of those patients who needs all the information. He dutifully filled the prescription and began taking the prednisone.

Perhaps you've read about the side effects of steroids; the list is too long to print here, but it includes diabetes, osteoporosis, cataracts, fluid retention, weight gain, hypertension, and then some. One of the less common side effects is mania—a hyperactive state in which patients often become revved up and develop unusual ideas and behaviors.

With Mr. V's preexisting but controlled bipolar disorder, it only took a couple of days of high-dose prednisone to push him into a florid manic state. He became absolutely unhinged. He lost thousands of dollars at the track. He stopped all his other meds, which only worsened his mania. He wandered the streets. Ultimately we found that he had been admitted to the psychiatric floor of a community hospital through the emergency room when the police brought him in for disturbing the peace. All because of bursitis and a failure of the orthopedist to do a little due diligence. (By the way, this was an example of a drug-disease interaction, just as common as we age as a "drug-drug interaction" and very important to be on the lookout for. More on this later when we cover medications.)

I felt horrible about Mr. V's troubles, and I replayed his story in my mind. Was I responsible? I was, after all, his primary care physician. I tell all my patients to let me know when someone tries to start them on a new medication; I'm guessing about half actually call me to do this. Should I have been in contact with the orthopedist directly? How was I to know that Mr. V even sought him out? He worked at another hospital.

Mr. V's story is my issue, and I'm still smarting from it. But here's what you should take away from it as it applies to your situation: If you've got lots of doctors, there are many places where things can break down, and you need to adopt a Harry Truman approach. Ultimately the buck stops with you as the repository of all medical information. I'll be even blunter: If you want to find the best primary care provider for yourself in a world of specialty medicine, look in the mirror. You must be ultimately responsible for the flow of information from primary care doc to specialist and subspecialist* and vice versa. Toward that end, here are some practices to adopt as you navigate that world:

Don't assume that your medical information will travel with you from primary care physician to specialist. In fact, assume it will get lost. I hate to break it to you, but it is distinctly unusual for a primary care physician referring someone to a subspecialist for consultation to pick up the phone and explain exactly what's going on (if yours does, that's an indication you should be holding on to him). Oftentimes documents are sent physically or electronically, but very frequently that fails to happen in a timely manner. That leaves a busy subspecialist retaking a detailed history about what's going on directly from you (that's actually good; another set of eyes is always a good thing) but also trying to re-create your primary care doctor's thinking about what might be going on (not so good). My suggestion: Be your own courier. Ask for a copy of your physician's consultation request form (a note with a sentence or two that describes the reason for referral) so you can make sure the specialist sees it.

I'm not suggesting that extensive communication needs to occur between your doc and a specialist for all issues, including more trivial concerns (say, a new rash to be evaluated by a dermatologist or your regular screening colonoscopy by a gastroenterologist), but for unusual concerns (such as when a diagnosis needs to be nailed down) you should take responsibility.

---

*I've been a little lax in not distinguishing between specialist and subspecialist in these comments, in part because their definitions are always shifting. Not long ago most U.S. physicians were primary care doctors or general practitioners, and an internist or a pediatrician was considered a specialist. Now, as I discussed in chapter 2, most medical students become specialists (by doing a residency in internal medicine or pediatrics, for example) and then do subspecialty training in areas like oncology or gastroenterology (subspecialties of internal medicine). But stay tuned, because even these subspecialists are becoming yet more narrow in their practices, selecting a specific organ or disease area within their subspecialty (like a cardiologist specializing in heart rhythm disturbances or an oncologist specializing in breast cancer). I guess we'll need a new name for these folks soon (subsubspecialists?).

Make sure the specialist knows what medications you're taking and about your medical "greatest hits" list. In a subsequent chapter, I describe the basic "crib sheet" of medical information you should always be carrying with you. Show it to the specialist. Make sure he or she knows what you're taking and what conditions you have; any treatment he prescribes could conceivably interact with what you're already on, or with the diseases or conditions you have (the "drug-disease interactions" I mentioned above).

Make sure information from the specialist flows back to your primary care doc. In the same way that you have to make sure the specialist understands why you're seeing her, you need to make sure that whatever she did or discovered is conveyed back to your regular doctor. In nearly all cases, specialists send a letter to the doc indicating what they did or found (it's good manners and invites more business back). But sometimes busier docs don't do this, or the consultation letter is so delayed that it doesn't make it into your chart for weeks or months. This drives me nuts. (At my institution, we have an electronic medical record that makes this instantaneous—almost.) Ask the specialist when and how he will convey information to your doc. If you're due to see your physician very shortly and a dictation will be delayed, ask the specialist to call your doc or simply jot down on his prescription pad what his major findings were and what he thinks should be done about it.

Be your own medical records and radiology department. I'll never forget the time when, as a young intern at the Hospital of the University of Pennsylvania, I saw an elderly man in the emergency room with chest pain. He had an incredibly complicated cardiac history—bypass, valve replacements, heart attacks—with procedures done at several different Philadelphia hospitals over a span of twenty years. In trying to help him, I was still inexperienced and grew frustrated at how vague he was about much of his history. For example, when I asked him what meds he took ("a blue pill, a white pill, and another white pill that was not as round as the first white pill") and about his history ("heart stuff"), he eventually became frustrated with me and said, "I'm a patient here! It's in your records. Just go look it up!"

Now, look: Medical information technology has improved since my internship, and a lot of this stuff is indeed stored on computers. But you're making a huge mistake if you assume that it will be at your doc's fingertips every time you enter the health-care system—not to mention the fact that you may be traversing several health systems. Some hospitals don't have computerized records; most private docs still don't, despite the government's push to get them with the program. Then there are other lapses. Hospitals and clinics close and physicians move; who knows what happened to their documents (about you) after they pulled up stakes?

Whenever you have blood work or a test—especially anything nonroutine, such as a stress test or an MRI—get a copy for your own records (it's your body and your money). Many of my patients request copies of all the blood work I order, even the routine stuff. I also suggest that you keep copies (digital or physical) of X-rays, MRIs, and CT scans that have been done on you. Many people don't realize that those scans, which are often hidden in the bowels of the hospital, belong to you and not the institution. So get them, and get them soon! Hospitals are digitalizing their records and discarding older ones, which may not get archived. At New York–Presbyterian Hospital, we're creating a revolutionary Internet portal so patients can have direct access to many of their medical records.

Don't leave your health to the specialists; you still need a primary care physician. This is true for an overwhelming majority of patients, and the need becomes more urgent as we get older. I hope that this chapter and the preceding one have convinced you of that, not only for your own health but for that of our health-care system. Subspecialty care is all the rage; everybody wants to go to the doc who specializes in the body part that's bothering them. But you need a "traffic cop" through whom all information flows and all specialty care can be coordinated. If the example of Mr. V doesn't convince you of this, then I don't know what will.

Sure, most primary care physicians wince at the label *gatekeeper* (managed-care-speak for how we are supposed to regulate access to the system in response to financial constraints), but I'm not sure a gatekeeper is a bad thing for a patient of any age if there are dozens of different people who provide you with care, prescribe medicines that the others don't know about, and order tests that very often are duplicative. *Gatekeeper* is really an inadequate description. How about *orchestra conductor*, to reflect the art in all this science?

———

Above, I said the "overwhelming majority" of patients need a primary care doc; there is one exception. If a single chronic illness is the major obstacle in your life, it is not unreasonable to have an internal medicine subspecialist act as a specialist for that disease as well as a primary care doctor. An example might be a patient with lifelong rheumatoid arthritis who sees a rheumatologist often or someone with Crohn's disease who is under the regular care of a gastroenterologist. In these cases, the specialist may also choose to provide what amounts to primary care, and I applaud the attempt to keep all the work in-house. This is also a reasonable strategy, because patients with specific chronic diseases may develop additional or unusual primary care needs that a subspecialist would be more attuned to, such as the need to pay extra attention to osteoporosis prevention in a lupus patient who requires steroids (which thins the bones), or the increased risk of colon cancer in patients with colitis, a case in which more frequent screening becomes especially important.

Evaluating the Quality of Subspecialty Care: Science versus Service

I spent a good deal of time in the last chapter talking about the interpersonal skills of primary care doctors and the idea of doctor-patient fit. You might expect that I have the same advice about your relationships with the specialists and subspecialists who care for you. Not exactly.

Sure, it would be wonderful to have great chemistry not only with your primary care physician but with every doctor who comes in contact with each one of your body parts. Unfortunately, that's both statistically improbable and pragmatically undoable. It reminds me of the double-dating conundrum that all newlyweds face. Before we got married, my wife and I had a list of each other's friends whom, well, let's just say that we'd prefer not to spend an evening with—so we didn't. After we got hitched, the number of couples we both could tolerate for a full evening dropped precipitously—but we had to socialize periodically to preserve each other's friendships with old chums. Thus it is with subspecialists: Your primary care physician may refer you to a highly competent knee, GI, or headache guy who is clinically terrific but perhaps not your interpersonal cup of tea. Here you might have to suck it up a bit and endure, in the same way my wife puts up with an old fraternity buddy now and then lest we never get out of the house. Why? Well for one thing, most of your interactions with specialists should be brief and more limited than those with your primary care physician, so sacrificing quality for personality and customer service should be endurable unless you're seeing Dr. House. Second, and more important, specialty referral by physicians may not always be driven first by technical excellence. I found this out from one of my oldest medical buddies through a story about community practice in his town.

Fred was superbly trained in one of the medical subspecialties—as good as any physician in any top medical school in the country. He could have been a department chair had he decided to stay at a medical school. The two of us trained together and obsessed endlessly about where we would apply for jobs afterward; we were both offered the option of "staying on" as junior faculty members. I decided to accept the offer; he didn't and moved away to take a job as a specialist to be nearer to his aging parents. A year later he was coming to New York for a medical meeting and called me to meet for a drink. This was a good opportunity to compare notes on the "academic life" versus private practice. What were his colleagues like? Was the environment intellectually stimulating enough? How were the "top docs" chosen in the community where he was working? I'll never forget how he framed it for me.

It's the three A's, he said: availability, affability, and ability—and usually in that order.

He went on to explain that in his world, most docs were really good, but medical care had become profoundly time pressured and harried. He attributed this to declining reimbursement and the lack of other funds to support protected "academic time" (such as grants for teaching and research) that might be simply available in a medical school, time that could be used in those environments to fully "think through" a problem. As a result of this and other forces, the primary care physicians who called on him to consult on their patients were certainly interested in (and impressed with) his credentials and expected a basic level of competence, but what they wanted most was for him to see their patients right away. When they called asking for his help, he would begin suggesting what might be causing the symptoms described, but they really had no time or patience for it. With a waiting room full of folks, they just wanted him to see the patient. Quickly, please.

After just showing up, what docs in his community ranked next was affability. They wanted the specialist to be nice, or at least not mean. Patients complained if they didn't like their referrals, no matter how technically excellent a physician might be in the eyes of colleagues. "Table manners matter to my patients," a senior physician in town told him, trying to provide some well-intentioned but eye-opening mentorship. "You may be a great cook, but if they don't like you, you won't get invited to dinner."

This I could relate to. I can't tell you the number of times I have referred patients to highly regarded specialists at top medical schools who, in some cases, have clearly saved the patient's life with a great diagnosis or an innovative surgical procedure. What amazes me is how completely that "technical home run" can be obscured by a nasty bedside manner. I had one patient who was probably cured of a rare form of lymphoma by a brilliant oncologist who thought outside the box and saved this lady's life using a combination of therapies no one else considered. Here's what she remembered about the experience: He didn't look at her when he spoke, and he always kept her waiting. ("Please don't send me back there," she said.") As one of my former professors liked to joke, "You can cure their leukemia, but if they're still constipated, you've failed!"

And finally, there's ability. In the eyes of many patients, it's the least of the criteria. But that's not because they don't care; they care a lot. In all fairness, most lay folk have no technical basis for judging how good their doc really is. As a result, physician performance is often too heavily evaluated on the basis of the customer service experience—in both directions. Patients usually feel that if a physician is nice and/or engaging, he must be a good doc medically, and if he's a pill, vice versa. But one thing doesn't necessarily have anything to do with the other.

Let me be clear: I don't fault patients or families who critique physicians for poor customer service. It's a critically important part of getting or staying well and a key piece of patient satisfaction. But it's not the only piece. Yes, you may hate Dr. House's bedside manner, but I bet you'd be willing to give him some latitude if he could figure out what's wrong with you after everyone else has failed.

The Medical Home

Finally, my remarks about specialists and their relationship to primary care physicians would be incomplete if I didn't include something about a movement that's gaining momentum as America gets older and as its health-care system gets more complicated and closer to bankruptcy: the medical home.

Now endorsed by major specialty societies as well as the Association of American Medical Colleges (AAMC), the concept of the medical home is best explained by describing its exact opposite: medical homelessness, a state most of us share. I'm not talking about being uninsured, although certainly uninsured folks are at the greatest risk of medical homelessness. Wealthy or poor, black or white, young or old, you're medically homeless when no single person is coordinating your care or taking ultimate responsibility for its oversight.

The medical home need not be a location; in fact, it's more of a virtual place where all your care is coordinated. While there's no universally agreed upon definition of the medical home, I like the AAMC's description:

> The medical home is a concept or model of care delivery that includes an ongoing relationship between a provider and patient, around the clock access to medical consultation, respect for the patient/family's cultural and religious beliefs, and a comprehensive approach to care and coordination of care through providers and community services. . . . Every person should have access to a medical home—a person who serves as a trusted advisor and provider supported by a coordinated team—with whom they have a continuous relationship. The medical home promotes prevention; provides care for most problems and serves as the point of first-contact for that care; coordinates care with other providers and community resources when necessary; integrates care across the health system.[1]

Notice anything familiar? There may be no precise definition of the medical home, nor a precise definition of geriatric medicine, but the two sure sound similar. I'll squirrel out of providing my own definition by quoting Supreme Court Justice Potter Stewart, who was asked to define pornography in a famous 1964 obscenity trial: I can't define it, he said, but I know it when I see it.

Most of the troubling stories I tell in this book involve some variant of medical homelessness. Virtually all the good ones involve care coordination of specialists, facilities, and other providers, which could be described as a medical home with a geriatrician as the patriarch or matriarch. That's a pretty good arrangement for the future, since I believe a major risk factor for medical homelessness is accruing more and more subspecialists as we age. I'll describe why this is so in the next chapter.

Innkeeper, gatekeeper, call us whatever you like; it's far preferable to "six characters in search of an author," which is what much of medical care has become for older people these days. That's what happens as we interact with more and more doctors, with no single one flying the airplane.

Chapter 9

Care Transitions as We Get Older

Cracks You Didn't Even Know You Could Fall Through

A man goes to the doctor complaining about his sex life.
"Every day take one of these pills and jog ten miles," the doctor tells
*   him, "then call me back in a week to report on your progress."*
A week later the man calls back. "How is the medicine?" the doctor
*   asks.*
"Fine," the man says. "No side effects whatsoever."
"And is your sex life any better?" he inquires.
"I'm not sure," says the man. "I'm seventy miles from home!"

One of my most jarring experiences with medical miscommunication (or noncommunication) occurred when I was a resident in Philadelphia. In addition to long stints in the hospital as part of training, residents care for a panel of outpatients, serving as their primary care doc for the three years of residency. For me, this was one of the most rewarding aspects of residency; while I liked dramatically intervening for critically ill patients with heart attacks or unusual infections, I got a bigger kick out of prevention. I really enjoyed helping people change their lifestyles and risk factors to stay out of trouble in the first place.

And I loved the population we cared for in the residents' practice. The patients were by and large hardworking west Philadelphians, mostly African American, many of them poor or near poor, who were getting very attentive care from some really smart young doctors at one of the best medical centers in the world.

One of my favorite patients was a transit worker in his fifties who was a mess when I inherited him from the departing resident. (The only bad thing about having a resident as your doctor is you get a new one every three years.) He was overweight, smoked, had high blood pressure, and was depressed from the death of a child a year or two earlier. To make matters worse, he was highly suspicious of any health-care system. This was a tough customer.

I saw him almost every month, and he began to trust me. I started him on medications for his depression. I urged him to stop smoking. He did. He lost weight. His blood pressure came down, and he needed less medicine. After we got the lower hanging fruit dealt with, I began to send him to specialists for other screening needs that had never been addressed—colonoscopy, eye exams, and so forth. I was his doctor, and I was helping him; this went on for nearly three years.

Then one day he came in to the examining room for a regularly scheduled visit and took off his shirt so I could listen to his lungs. I almost fell over when I looked at him. Down the middle of his chest there was a sternotomy scar—the "zipper" you get when you have cardiac bypass surgery.

"Bo, did you have heart surgery since I last saw you?" I asked him.

"Sure did," he said. "Came to the emergency room with chest pain, and they squirted some dye into my heart through a tube in my leg; told me I'd need a surgery or I'd die. Did a fine job, they did," he said appreciatively.

"Gee, Bo, I wish you would have asked the doctors taking care of you to call me; I might have been helpful," I told him. "But I'm glad you're okay. I need to get a copy of your discharge summary and speak to the cardiologist and surgeon who looked after you so I can understand exactly what they did. This will help me best care for you now with your new plumbing. What hospital was this done at?" I asked him.

"This one," he said.

After I picked myself up off the floor, I called the medical records department and had his chart delivered. (This was before the Internet or any significant electronic medical records existed.) Indeed, a month earlier he had spent nearly two weeks in my hospital in what appeared to be quite a "touch-and-go" situation. Although it was clear that he was a patient in the residents' clinic and had been followed there for some time, no one bothered to call me. Thankfully he was well cared for by other specialists and subspecialists and did well, but I must say, the whole episode got me pretty hot under the collar. I took great responsibility and pride in caring for this man, yet I was left "out of the loop."

At the end of the day, it's what happens to the patient that matters, and this one did fine. I'm not sure if I would have had anything medically substantive to offer at that point. His wife, however, whom I had gotten to know during his many visits, had clearly been frightened by the whole hospitalization and asked me why I hadn't come to see him. There I could have provided something of value: support. That's why I always tell patients to call me if something significant happens to them medically, even if they think it's beyond my purview. This certainly qualified!

I'm telling this story because I've seen errors in miscommunication like this occur over and over again in health-care settings, sometimes with no adverse effects and sometimes with devastating ones. And while the story is somewhat dated by the absence of electronic medical records that might have averted the situation (now I often get a "robot e-mail" every time one of my patients appears in the ER), electronic medical records can compound these problems as well (such as when you're cared for in different health-care systems served by electronic medical records that don't talk to one another).

In this chapter I will take a look at how and why medical errors occur generally, but I'll also focus on their increasing frequency and worsening impact on us as we get older. Then I'll provide highly prescriptive advice on what you can do to avoid them. As you'll soon see, at their core, most medical errors involve communication problems.

To Err Is Human

In 1999, the Institute of Medicine, under the direction of Congress, released a widely quoted report entitled *To Err Is Human*.[1] The report estimated that approximately ninety-eight thousand Americans die each year due to medical error, and many more are significantly injured. What was not mentioned in enough detail is how this phenomenon collides with an aging America. Buried deep in the data is a disquieting truth geriatricians have been screaming about for decades: As we age, we become more at risk for medical error because it becomes a "one-two" punch.

Let me explain. Simply getting older places you in harm's way more frequently—that's punch one. It's a law of nature: On average, older people have more chronic medical problems than younger people and therefore have more interactions with the health-care system. Rates of every major medical procedure increase in an incremental and proportional fashion with each additional year of life you tack on. Half of all cardiovascular procedures performed in the United States last year involved patients over sixty-five. Between the ages of twenty-one and eighty, rates of just about every medical procedure (except childbirth) increase with each successive decade of life—joint replacement, colonoscopy, cardiac catheterization, you name it. The more medical problems you have, the more doctors you see, the more medicines you're prescribed, and the more tests and procedures you undergo. And with each additional year of age, your potential for collisions with the health-care system increases. It doesn't start suddenly at some specific or magical age; if you're reading this, it probably has already started.

This truism starts playing out with the first chronic condition you develop in your twenties or thirties (hypertension, for example) and continues as the list of diagnoses, physicians, treatments, and medications lengthens. Put very simply, "punch one" provides the opportunity for trouble. Think of it as the "miles-driven" analogy your insurer uses in trying to price your automobile insurance. You pay more if you drive one hundred miles to work every day on a dangerous freeway in comparison to someone who drives a mile to the station each morning and takes the train.

What is "punch two"? You've already heard about this one from me: the loss of physiologic reserve. Given the same incorrect dose of a medicine, a longer time under anesthesia, a delay in proper treatment and/or diagnosis—any medical error—an older person is far more likely to suffer a complication that creates significant hardship; there's simply not enough extra gas in the tank to withstand new medical conditions, procedures, and/or complications. A twenty-five-year-old oversedated for a surgical procedure will likely wake up groggy; a sixty-five-year-old may not wake up at all. The rapid heart rate in response to an infected surgical wound after an appendectomy will be tolerated just fine by a college student, less well by a forty-five-year-old man with narrow coronary arteries. Rehabilitation for a dislocated shoulder is more difficult for a sixty-year-old man rendered confused by the required pain medication in comparison to his thirtysomething counterpart.

So to recap, as we age, we are at higher risk for medical errors and their consequences because (a) we have more problems and procedures and have higher odds of experiencing medical error and (b) when we do experience a medical error, we have less physiologic reserve to cope with it.

This chapter is mostly about avoiding "punch one"—staying out of harm's way. When you minimize the risk of medical error or prevent it altogether, you never even have to learn whether you have enough spare gas in the tank to tough it out. Why tempt fate?

If at this point you're wondering what in the world you could possibly do to influence your interactions with the health-care system to avoid medical error, I understand your confusion. That's the doctor's job, right? You're the patient (or the relative of one). You didn't go to medical school. Am I asking you to second-guess your doctor about which scans he's ordered, or stand in the operating room to assist in your dad's surgery to make sure the surgeon doesn't leave a sponge in him? Of course not! But as you're about to learn, patients and family members can play a significant role in ducking punch one. And that brings us to the subject of care transitions.

Why You Should Care About Care Transitions

"Care transitions" have been an incredibly hot area of aging research over the past ten years or so. What exactly is a care transition? It's when a patient gets "handed off" either from one care venue to another or from one physician to another. It could be your orthopedist sending you back to your family physician after he scopes your knee for a torn ACL (anterior cruciate ligament). It could be when the emergency room doc sends you back home (perhaps with an illegible instruction sheet) after a night of nausea and vomiting that was treated with intravenous fluid, basically transitioning your care to you. It could be a move from the hospital to a rehabilitation facility after a knee replacement, or vice versa when you develop bleeding from the blood-thinning medicine you're given to prevent a blood clot from your new knee. A care transition could also take place within the same hospital building, such as when you are admitted through the emergency room and a bed finally becomes available on the medical floor, or even when the resident taking care of you goes off duty and "signs you out" (that's what they call it; I'm not making it up) to the new guy "covering you" (along with a few dozen other people he has responsibility for).

We've established that as we age we need more care and have more interactions with the health-care system. In today's medical world, that means we're not simply interacting with some general practitioner over and over again (which might be preferable, actually). We're interacting with many physicians, health paraprofessionals, pharmacists, hospitals, nursing homes, HMOs, and other entities, allegedly all acting on our behalf. So we have lots of care transitions, and study after study has shown that these are high-risk moments for medical error.

The king of care-transition research is my colleague and good friend Eric Coleman at the University of Colorado. In the 1990s we both had the honor of being selected Paul B. Beeson Physician Faculty Scholars in Aging Research—sort of the "Fulbright" of geriatrics. My particular area of study has been elder abuse. Eric's is care transitions and how older people may get "dropped on their heads" when they move through health-care environments. Recently I've come to wonder whether or not we've been studying the same thing all these years.

What I love about Eric's work is its practicality. He has studied the minutiae of medical error, dissecting how and why older people get into trouble when they move from facility to facility or provider to provider. Much of his work has been supported by the John A. Hartford Foundation (one of the fairy godmother foundations that have funded aging research when no one else would). The return on their investment? The discovery that the risks of care transitions are incredible but also that they can often be prevented.

Here are some findings from Eric and others that will get your dander up:

Upon discharge, nearly half of hospitalized patients—of all ages—experience at least one medical error, involving a medication, a follow-up appointment, or a test;[2] In a related study, patients who experienced a medication discrepancy were three times as likely to be readmitted to the hospital within a month than those who did not.[3] In a study of the receiving end of hospital discharges, primary care physicians were unaware of 62 percent of tests that were pending on their patients at the time of discharge.[4] This is a huge and growing issue, because the tests are ordered by "hospitalists" (the physicians who care for you only in the hospital) and may never reach your primary care doctor. And we're not just talking hospital discharge as a moment ripe for mishaps: Admission is another opportunity for problems. In one study, 54 percent of patients had medication discrepancies—many of them potentially life-threatening—between what they were given in the hospital upon admission and what they believed they were taking at home.[5]

And before I forget, let me add one more thing to this "perfect storm" of potential medical error: "physiological" communication impairment in aging patients. As if having more to keep track of—medicines, doctors, instructions—weren't enough, as we get older there's a tendency to develop a bunch of problems that make getting and understanding directions a bit harder: hearing loss, visual impairment, cognitive processing speed. I'm in my late forties, and I find myself squinting at my own prescription bottles more and more each year—as I've been saying, these problems don't begin magically at sixty-five.

Here's the good news: There's a ton you can do to make sure that you don't become a victim of care transition shenanigans. And you don't need an advanced medical or engineering degree to do it.

You can greatly help your health-care professionals ensure your safety or that of a loved one by minimizing the problems caused by care transitions, because at the end of the day, all the information about you must reside with you.

Avoiding these difficulties is about managing data and communication, and as you'll see shortly, this cannot be done exclusively via computers, personal digital assistants, or fancy cell phones; there are necessarily both technical and human aspects of storing and conveying health data. As we age, the details of care become too nuanced to rely exclusively on e-mailed numbers or digitalized images. There are just too many personal preferences and personalities involved (doctors, patients, and families); and the ways in which information is subtly conveyed (and who is in the "loop") can change the entire tenor of a major health-care decision. Technology helps, but no matter how small, fast, or fancy computers get, I believe that this will always be the case. Frankly, I take comfort in the old-fashioned idea that health care will always rely to some degree on human interaction.

My colleague Dr. Coleman has also taken the bull by the horns and created training programs for both patients and providers to minimize care-transition errors. He's even created a Web site, www.caretransitions.org, that outlines some very useful strategies providers and patients can use during these periods to minimize risk. But to start you off, I'll outline a series of "core competencies" you or an older loved one should master if you want to stay out of care-transition quicksand.

How Not to Be a Victim of Care Transitions

First things first: I urge patients, whatever their age, to keep a one-page "greatest medical hits" list on their person at all times. It should be available for any interaction with the health-care system: seeing a new consultant for a specific problem, getting an insurance physical, visiting the ER, or getting treated for a jellyfish bite or ski injury while you're on vacation. The page should include the following.

- **A complete list of your medications:** List them by both brand and generic (chemical) names, including the dosage and dosing schedule. I can't emphasize how important this is. One of the more common errors I see in care transitions is a patient discharged from the hospital with a medication prescribed by its chemical name (e.g., furosemide) that he had been taking before admission under its trade or brand name (e.g., Lasix). You can guess the rest: The patient takes "both" medications, effectively doubling the dose. Depending on the drug, the results range from annoying (as with laxatives) to life-threatening (as with diabetes medicine). If you travel internationally, that's another good reason to record chemical names. Many of the meds sold in America have brand names that are unfamiliar to doctors and pharmacists overseas, but we're all taught the chemical names of these compounds in medical school. Thus if you need a refill of your diabetes medicine in Romania, the pharmacist or doc will more likely know what you're talking about if you give the chemical name. When you transition from one care environment to another, make sure you pull out the list so the discharging docs fully understand what you were taking before you got admitted, and make him or her go over each and every medication on the list.

- **A list of your allergies:** Include any sensitivities to medicines, foods, or contrast dyes (used in medical testing). This is pretty self-explanatory.
- **A list of major medical problems and surgeries you've had:** This is especially important for problems that are in any way active. I'm not talking about your tonsillectomy at age five. You should have a bulleted list of the major medical problems you've faced over the last several years—angina, arthritis, diabetes, and so on. Surgical procedures (with dates) are important to list if they could impact treatment decisions that come up in certain situations. For example, patients with artificial heart valves are at risk for certain kinds of infections during medical procedures and need preventative antibiotics that would not be given to patients without such a history. Patients who have had stents placed in their heart arteries recently may need to be on blood-thinning medications that an unaware physician might try to stop before the anticipated surgery.
- **A photocopy of your most recent cardiogram:** If you have heart problems or have had abnormal cardiogram results, attach a photocopy of your most recent EKG. Should you be traveling and develop chest pains or other cardiac symptoms, you're sure to get an EKG at whatever hospital or emergency room you visit. If it's abnormal, it may well buy you admission

to that hospital. But here's the problem: Most patients with heart problems (and many without) have EKGs that are in some way not perfectly normal. The critical issue is whether your EKG has changed since a new symptom developed, and the only way to know that—you guessed it—is to have an old one to compare it with. Not a problem if you decide to get sick at a hospital where they have all your records. But if you're far from home and there's nobody at your doc's office to fax your latest EKG over to Tunisia in the middle of the night, it's really handy to be able to just pull a copy out. (Helpful hint: These can be reduced in a copy machine to the size of a large index card, and for this purpose, they're still readable.)

- **A description of any abnormal lab findings you've had for some time:** This is similar to the EKG logic. Many of us have minor lab abnormalities that have been evaluated by our docs long ago and found to be trivial—a minor degree of anemia, mildly elevated liver function tests, a shadow on a chest X-ray that has been judged benign. But if a doc who has never seen you before runs into one of these curveballs in the course of evaluating something else (for example, finding an anemia during an ER visit for belly pain), you might get sent down an unnecessary path that could be at best inconvenient and at worst life-threatening (for example, when the doctor, unaware of your anemia history, assumes you're bleeding). The solution: Simply have a copy of the abnormal result with you or a description of it on your "greatest-hits" card.

Some of my "high-tech" patients have been putting their hits list on a USB necklace that can be read on any computer. A former geeky patient (his words) has a Web site where this stuff resides, so he doesn't have to carry anything on his person. A woman I know keeps the list in her AOL file cabinet so it's accessible wherever she can log on to her account. If you like these ideas but aren't techno savvy, there are companies that will do the work for you.

But you don't need to spend much money to have a greatest-hits list—a neatly transcribed index card that fits in your pocket will do just fine!

You can also consider subscribing to a Web-based system of medical recordkeeping. Companies like Google and Microsoft have developed products you can use to enter your health data from any browser and then access it when needed. Google's is free (go to www.health.google.com). I say "consider," because you're going to have to balance your concerns about electronic privacy with the cost and the convenient and ubiquitous access this will afford. And make no mistake about it: There is nothing more private than your health information. I'm okay with Amazon recommending books and movies based on my previous purchases, but it would indeed be disconcerting to someday be surfing the Web and see a banner add for hemorrhoid cream based on health information you're provided. If you're imaginative, I'm sure you can think of other, more chilling scenarios.

Now, here's the most important part: Keep the list updated. However you maintain it and no matter where it resides, this little health summary is going to change. Medications will be added and removed. Dosages will change. New medical conditions will surface. Others will resolve. It's critical that you keep the information—especially regarding medications—as up-to-date as possible and that, as you move from venue to venue, you share it with every health-care provider you come in contact with in a way that is proactive but not pushy. There is simply no substitute for this low-tech approach to reviewing your medical record. Relegating the job to a computer (in the form of electronic medical records, which are becoming popular) in my experience creates as much error as it corrects. As I always say, the most important primary care provider is you.

And if a parent or spouse has any form of communicative or cognitive impairment—vision loss, hearing loss, memory loss (and let's add computer illiteracy)—they are going to need your help. That may mean not only organizing the information into some readily available and usable fashion but also collecting the data from doctors, hospitals, laboratories, and other providers. That can be a trying experience, but it is well worth the effort.

Not for Your Eyes Only: Squinting at Your Medical Record for the First Time

Throughout this book and this chapter, I've suggested that you take a more active role in interacting with health-care professionals, particularly with regard to shepherding your medical information from place to place. That's probably going to mean that you're going to get to see your actual medical record or big pieces of it—discharge summaries, correspondence between physicians, a radiologist's interpretation of your CAT scan, and so on—which you're probably not accustomed to. This experience can potentially be frightening, so allow me to provide a little prophylaxis.

In general, physicians use technical terms when they correspond with one another or dictate notes, not expecting that the subject of their prose (you) will ever see the document. Furthermore, part of learning to think medically involves opening one's mind to all the diagnostic possibilities when a patient presents with a series of symptoms or we're asked to interpret an abnormal test result. In conveying that information to patients, we try to censor ourselves a bit, because the list of scary possibilities would be overwhelming and send most patients into a tizzy. Anyone who has gone online to look up the potential side effects of a newly prescribed medicine knows exactly what I'm talking about.

When you look at your medical record, you get to see doctors at our uncensored best, so brace yourself. The effects of this access on patients range from offended (one patient still hasn't forgiven me for the discharge summary in which I described her as "obese"— even though she qualified for that label by very explicit body mass index criteria that are universally accepted in medicine) to terrified (as when you read the radiologist's interpretation of your brain MRI). As we age, there is almost no such thing as a completely "normal" CAT scan or MRI of any body part. Most people's brains, for example, undergo a loss of volume; get a CAT scan or MRI of yours after age sixty-five and there's a good chance the report will say it has atrophied (shrunk). This might not be a pleasant revelation without the benefit of a consultation with your doctor (today he's seen ten atrophied brains and wouldn't even yawn at yours). A chest scan may reveal small old nodules or scars. A belly scan may find cysts in your liver and kidneys. All these findings need to be interpreted in a clinical context. Most often they are incidental, but when you read your records, you are seeing them unfiltered by a medical interpreter. Google some of the terms used and you could scare yourself to death.

Physicians are famous for laying out any number of medical possibilities in their dictations, letters, and reports to describe findings that are quite often trivial. Famous musings in radiological reports include "cannot exclude . . ." (fill in the blank—multiple sclerosis, Crohn's disease), "not inconsistent with . . ." (how's that for a double negative?), and my personal favorite, used by radiologists, "clinical correlation is advised." This last means "I haven't actually laid eyes on your patient (just his films), but here's something he or she might have based on this X-ray I just took." (Medical joke: What is a radiologist's favorite plant? Answer: A hedge.)

Clinical correlation is advised? Well, of course! When doctors treat numbers and images instead of patients, everybody suffers. X-rays reveal images, not pain. Laboratory values convey numbers, not suffering. Some of the most profound mistakes are made when doctors let "data" like these trump the living and breathing person sitting across the examining table from them. And when patients who don't have a medical degree have direct access to these numbers, a good deal of anxiety can result. When these concerns are communicated to a physician, he or she can follow up with the proper (if time-consuming) therapy: reassurance and education.

My suggestions: Develop some thick skin when it comes to viewing your medical record. Don't try to interpret it without a translator (your doctor, not *Stedman's Medical Dictionary*). And make sure you understand why any test is being ordered in the first place.

A quick recap: I don't expect you to obtain a medical degree in order to protect yourself from medical error and the consequences thereof; that's your doctor's job. But you can play a very important role by making sure that with every changing of the health-care guard, the proper information is conveyed to the next regime.

Remember that most care-transition errors are, at their core, errors in communication. Don't assume that anybody has communicated with anybody else in conveying your medical situation, and you'll always be one step ahead of the game.

In the words of George Bernard Shaw, "The single biggest problem with communication is the illusion that it has actually taken place."

Chapter 10

No Place for Sick People

Hospitals as We Get Older

An elderly lady telephones the hospital. "Can I speak to someone who can tell me how a patient is doing?" she inquires.

"What's the patient's name?" asks the operator.

"Her name is Mildred Stein," the lady replies.

"She's on the fifth floor. Hold on while I connect you with her nurse."

"Can you tell me how Mildred Stein is doing?" the lady asks the nurse.

"She's doing very well. Her blood tests are normal, her X-rays are better, and her doctor plans to discharge her tomorrow."

"Wonderful news!" the old lady says. "Thank you so much, I'm so relieved."

"You're welcome," says the nurse. "Are you a relative?"

"No," says the lady. "I'm Mildred Stein, and nobody here tells me shit."

About once a month, a concerned adult child of one or another of my patients will call with a very specific medical request. Worried about Mom or Dad and perhaps bearing witness to unfolding frailty or some worsening medical problem, they will entreat me to do something I consider truly radical. "Can't you just admit Dad to the hospital, Dr. Lachs?" they implore. "I'm so worried, and he'd be so much safer there under your care."

Man, do I have an earful for them.

Before I launch into one of my favorite rants, some disclosures. First, as I've mentioned, I direct the geriatric medicine program at one of the finest hospitals and health-care systems in the world. We have some of the most innovative programs for older people anywhere, including a dedicated floor we call the ACE (acute care of the elderly) unit. Second, though I make the case in this chapter that the hospital is "No Place for Sick People," I am, of course, being a bit facetious. The truth is, I admit older adults to the hospital all the time. Even when you give older adults great outpatient care, they still use hospital services far more frequently than their twentysomething counterparts—it's just a law of nature.

But as we get older, the risk of *getting sick from hospitalization itself*—regardless of the symptoms that put you in the hospital in the first place—increases. Sometimes I joke with the medical residents that simply driving by a hospital can be hazardous to older adults.

Why is this? Think about some of the things we do to folks at our grand institutions.

• **We put you to bed.** The *Marcus Welby* image of the hospitalized person (young or old) is someone who is sent in for some R & R. Bedrest is good, right? Well, no, it's not. Things in motion tend to stay in motion; things at rest tend to stay at rest. Imposing forced immobility on a person who may have been flirting with immobility is a bad idea, yet bedrest is one of the first hospital admission orders doctors write. Bedrest wastes your muscles, causes blood and other fluids in the body to redistribute in ways that can cause dizziness and balance problems, and can lead to the development of pressure sores, just to name a few of the negatives.

• **We keep waking you up.** You don't think we put you to bed so you can sleep, do you? We wake you at ungodly hours for anything from taking your temperature to drawing your blood. This sleep disruption is thought to play a significant role in the development of what geriatricians call "acute confusional state," or delirium, an alteration in consciousness that occurs in as many as half of all hospitalized older people but occurs frequently in younger folks, too. (I'll talk more about that later in this chapter, because it turns out that the interventions geriatricians use to prevent delirium also prevent a number of other hospital-related problems.)

• **Since we keep waking you up, would you like a sleeping pill?** We've got plenty of sleep medications for when our nocturnal workings keep you from falling asleep. Here's the problem with that: Now additional psychoactive medicines are being introduced at a time when you're probably sick and other medications have been started (such as antibiotics for pneumonia or narcotics for pain from a fracture). This creates a huge potential for adverse drug effects, drug-drug interactions, and related misadventures.

• **Sometimes we pee for you.** One common medical intervention for older and younger hospital patients is the insertion of a bladder catheter to collect urine. There are good medical reasons to do this in certain instances—for example, when we need to measure the amount of urine you're producing if your kidneys are failing, or if we're trying to get fluid out of your lungs using diuretics. But well-meaning nurses and nursing assistants struggling with an increased load of sicker patients (and often encouraged by well-meaning family members) may inadvertently become enamored of catheters because they obviate the need to walk a patient to the bathroom, an especially useful fix if a floor is short-staffed. And let's face it: For many of us, urinating into a shot glass is no small feat—even if you're not sick as a dog with heart or kidney problems. If a patient is intermittently incontinent, an indwelling bladder catheter prevents accidents in bed (and the need to change sheets). So what's bad about this? A lot.

I'm sure you already know about the risks of infection when patients have indwelling catheters. But they also can make some patients incontinent indefinitely. How? Think about my "biology of aging" graphs in chapter 3: Before hospitalization, a person may struggle with occasional incontinence as the muscles that control both the bladder muscle itself and the valve that holds back urine approach the dreaded dashed line at the margins of physiologic reserve. What do you think happens to the individual who is barely holding it together with regard to continence at home—forcing himself to control his bladder muscles while he slowly ambulates to the bathroom—who suddenly finds himself with a device that takes care of everything? No need to get up (he's been prescribed bedrest anyway). No need to have any awareness about how full his bladder is. No need to regulate how much he drinks and when, or worry about where the nearest bathroom is. With these pressures removed, bladder muscles simply become deconditioned. Pile on other hospital-related issues— muscular disuse from bedrest that makes walking to the bathroom difficult, medicines that cause more frequent urination, the introduction of intravenous fluids (sometimes for no good reason), and maybe a sleeping pill that contributes to confusion—and you can understand how the wheels completely fly off the continence cart as a result of this seemingly trivial intervention when the catheter is removed.

Oh, and you fortysomethings: Don't think incontinence as a result of hospitalization is something you need to worry about? Those two drops of urine that occasionally slip out when you sneeze or belly laugh from a good joke—no big deal, right? Just wait.

• **It's not just urination . . .** There's yet another seemingly innocuous but potentially worrisome "temporary" medical intervention related to elimination you need to be aware of. One great way to make someone who has an occasional accident involving loss of bowel control is to use an "adult brief" (preferred term) on them. No need to walk (or be walked) to the bathroom. No accidents. The nurse is happy. Housekeeping is happy. The patient is happy. But guess who is not happy—the patient's family when on the day of discharge they realize that Dad can no longer deal with getting himself to the toilet on time. How ironic to be "cured" of whatever disease you were hospitalized for, only to need a nursing home at the end of your stay because of this issue. And I've seen this happen to younger patients, too.

• **All the comforts of home, vanquished.** And just to make the experience a little more impersonal, when you come to the hospital, we'll tell you to leave your cherished possessions at home: knickknacks, pictures of children and grandchildren, that familiar alarm clock that greets you each morning. The absence of these small things can contribute in a big way to the confusion (and boredom) experienced by many hospital patients. Did I mention those fashionable johnnies we make you wear, which never seem to completely cover your derrière?

• **We inflict hospital food on you.** While it has improved dramatically over the past two decades, it's not the food you're used to eating, whatever its nutritional value might be. At times like these, when calorie stores are being called upon to combat the stress of acute illness, I often tell patients that while nutrients and vitamins are critical for recovery, protein and calories requirements trump them. I'm not suggesting that you maintain a hospital diet of deep-fried Twinkies and wash it down with a cold Budweiser— that may be what landed you there in the first place! I'm saying that if you're fighting an acute illness like pneumonia or another debilitating infection, given the choice between starvation and a hamburger, you'd be much better off with protein than becoming more and more malnourished. Dire warnings about America's obesity epidemic do not apply here.

To summarize, the hospital is a place where your normal routine—mobility, nutrition, sleep, elimination, access to creature comforts—gets interrupted. These interruptions can cause or exacerbate illness in and of themselves.

Some Good News about Hospitalization That May Shock You

Amazing things can happen in our great hospitals, and that's a good thing—it's nearly impossible to live a long and modern American life without winding up in one at least once in the course of getting older. This chapter is about staying safe while getting well in the hospital for patients of any age, and the impact you and/or your family can have on achieving that goal.

The following assertion surprises many nonmedical people when I share it with them: As perilous as hospitalization can be for us as we get older, I firmly believe that there is no health-care venue where laypeople—patients, families, concerned friends and neighbors—can have a greater impact on improving outcomes of care. Sounds crazy, you say. Family members don't do the surgery, they don't take or read the X-rays, nor do they select and prescribe the antibiotics to treat the pneumonia. How could they have such an influence on the outcome of medical care?

It's simple: Most of the perils of the hospital don't emanate from the technical details of the tests and procedures. The physicians who perform all those tasks are for the most part superb. Quite often the dangers of the hospital have more to do with the details that occur before, after, or in between the episodes of "technical" care.

As an example, I'd cite a condition with which all geriatricians have great familiarity, and one that all patients and families understandably dread: hip fracture. Family members are anxious when their loved one breaks a hip and must be operated on. Sometimes they try to transfer the patient directly from the emergency room to the hospital where their favorite orthopedist practices. I meet many families of hip-fracture patients in the waiting room outside the OR in a kind of *Ben Casey* moment, as they bite their nails waiting for the surgeon to emerge with good news, whereupon they can exhale, relieved that the storm has passed.

But here's something you may not know: Most surgical problems as we age just don't play out in the way television has (mis)educated us. I have probably cared for thousands of patients with a hip fracture in my career, yet I cannot recall a single one being "lost" on the operating table. After all, we're not separating Siamese twins here. Most hip fracture repairs are the orthopedic equivalent of pulling a tooth for a dentist. Orthopedist buddies have even confided that they could teach me how to pin one in about a week, maybe a month for a talented layperson blessed with some manual dexterity. The problems complicating hip fracture, as for many surgical procedures as we age, occur after the repair and often have little to do with the fracture itself. They include but are not limited to postoperative confusion, depression, malnutrition, mobility—all things that patients and families can have a role in mitigating during the patient's stay in the hospital.

No, the problem is rarely the big surgery or the high-tech MRI or the carefully concocted potion of chemotherapy. Far more often than not, the technical execution of these modern medical extravaganzas is flawless. Rather, the devil (as every wise grandma will tell you) is in the details—the coordination of multiple health professionals tending to you, the aftercare, the communication between providers, the consistency of information during hand-offs, even things like the food, how soon you get up, your familiarity with your care team (who are all those people?), as well as the general itinerary of how you spend each hospitalized day (for example, what tests am I being given and why?). The nuances of this kind of care often don't require enormous technical expertise, just attention to detail. In short, devoted lay assistance can play a role in recovery if you know what questions to ask. After all, your medical or surgical team wants the same thing you do—a complete, speedy, and uneventful recovery.

Fortunately for all of us, a brilliant geriatrician has come up with a highly specific plan to help you make that happen, one that includes substantive roles for patients themselves and for the people who care about them.

The Hero of the Hospitalized and the Enemy of Hospitalitis

Maybe you worship a particular home-run hitter. Perhaps you're smitten with an operatic soprano or a diva of the silver screen. Or it could be you're a devotee of a particular jazz saxophonist, Impressionist painter, or poet. We geeky geriatricians have heroes, too, and one of mine is the brilliant but modest Dr. Sharon Inouye, the director of Harvard's Aging Brain Center. Much of what we know about hospital perils as we age comes from Sharon's work. But more compellingly, she has demonstrated that something can be done about them.

While we were junior faculty together at Yale, she conducted a series of ingenious studies to determine how frequently older hospitalized patients develop confusion (answer: an amazing one third of the time, with doctors usually unaware of the problem despite family consternation; I'll get to that in a moment). If that weren't mind-blowing enough—pardon the pun—two additional findings of hers opened big doors in aging research.

First, though Sharon set out to study confusion (aka delirium) in the hospitalized patient, she discovered that confusion, while important, was only the tip of a series of interconnected icebergs when it came to hospital-related complications. She encountered many other difficulties in confused and unconfused patients that were also amenable to intervention, including worsening mobility, nutrition, mood, and sleep patterns, just to name a few. Furthermore, these problems had the tendency to affect one another in a rather fascinating way. While each was concerning by itself (developing major depression in the hospital is extremely bad timing), many of these conditions were also risk factors for *each other*. There are countless examples: If you're dehydrated upon admission, your risk of developing confusion during that hospitalization increases enormously, but dehydration and confusion are also risk factors for skin breakdown, or bedsores. Bedsores, it turns out, are a risk factor for malnutrition, and conversely malnutrition is a risk factor for bedsores. The more of these conditions that accrue while a patient is in the hospital, the longer he ends up staying. The longer he stays, the more vulnerable he becomes to even more complications and the deeper the hole he finds himself in. What Sharon uncovered was essentially a snowball effect; she postulated that the most rational solution would be to identify patients with these problems as early as possible (or even before they developed them) so that she could intervene aggressively and (ideally) preemptively. She also came to realize that while she set out to study confusion in the hospitalized patient, she was actually studying hospital-related functional decline, of which confusion was simply one component. That's a mouthful, so frequently I'll refer to it simply as "hospitalitis" when explaining the situation to patients and families.

Sharon's second finding (pay attention, boomers) was that, while certainly older age is a major risk factor and youth provides some protection, you can develop various manifestations of hospitalitis at any age. Think of those strapping young astronauts of the 1970s who, on returning to earth after a long stint on the space station, could barely pull themselves out of the space capsule under their own power. In space, there was no gravity to keep their muscles conditioned. Some scientists believe that the changes bodies undergo in space mimic those produced by aging. Indeed, John Glenn's later-life trip on the space shuttle was not simply a political joyride; many of the experiments he took part in were intended to explore the relationship between space and an aging body.[1] (That's right, the astronaut ridiculed as needing a geriatric walker was making contributions to the biology of aging almost forty years after he had made similar ones in aeronautical engineering.)

Dr. Inouye elegantly explains the relationship between vulnerability to hospital-related functional decline and aging this way:

> Any patient, even a healthy young adult, can develop problems through the right series of misadventures. It's simply a function of the "dose and duration" of those assaults. There's a dose of any known sedative that can confuse anybody, even a Nobel laureate. Sleep deprivation? String together several consecutive nights, say three for an eighty-year-old and ten for a forty-year-old, and anybody would get confused. Older muscles waste away faster than younger ones with disuse, but there's a duration of bedrest for every patient after which walking is no longer possible. When these kinds of assaults occur in combination (as they tend to do as the length of hospitalization increases), the risks multiply quickly.

Sharon devised an ingenious series of interventions that can minimize these risks. They are amazingly straightforward and low-tech, and in a moment I'm going to walk you through them.

But first consider this question: Do you know how hospitals work as you get older? You may think you do, but unless you work in one or have a chronic illness that has you visiting one frequently, you're probably thinking it's pretty much like whatever experience with hospitalization you had as a younger person (giving birth, having your appendix out). If that's your perspective, I'm sorry to break it to you, but you're out of touch. Not only have hospitals changed a bit since they gave you all the ice cream you wanted after your tonsillectomy fifty years ago; you've changed, too.

Aging and the Hospital 101

When you're admitted to a hospital, where you physically end up depends largely on who your *attending physician* is and what *hospital service* he or she "admits to." Attending physicians are granted *admitting privileges* that allow them to admit patients to a specific hospital (I can't just waltz into any hospital, show them my license and degree, and tell the lady at the front desk to admit my fishing buddy) and also to specific services (surgery, pediatrics, ob-gyn, orthopedics), usually based on their area of practice. I am board certified in internal medicine, so I have privileges to admit patients to the medicine service at my hospital. Should one of my primary care patients suddenly become psychotic, I have neither the ability nor the authority to admit her to the psychiatric service; I'd have to find an attending psychiatrist willing to do that. Some physicians are given *consulting privileges* so that they can see patients on other services (a dermatologist can be called to see a rash in a patient on a surgical service), but they do not assume ultimate responsibility for the care of the patients; that stays with the attending physician.

That physician is called "attending" because he or she is literally attending to you and your care. His or her name appears above yours on every page of the medical record. Only your attending physician (or someone he delegates, like a consultant, a resident, or a doctor covering for him over the weekend) can write an order regarding your care, be it something as complex as cancer chemo-therapy or as simple as whether or not you're allowed to get out of bed. He admits you by writing *admitting orders,* and only he (or a designee) can discharge you by writing a *discharge order.* The other doctors you'll see (consultants) are determined by the attending. An ophthalmologist can't simply show up in your room, examine you, and write a note in your medical chart because he wants to (or even because you want him to). The attending physician runs the show, and the buck stops there. He is called by the nurses if you get into difficulty; he is summoned by the administrators if the hospital needs the bed and think you've been there too long; and it's likely he'll get named in a lawsuit if something goes wrong during your hospitalization, even if he had little to do with it.

What makes this configuration so curious is the fact that, more often than not, your attending physician, unlike everybody else in the place, is *not an employee of the hospital.* Yet in her relatively brief visit *she directs everyone as to how to conduct every aspect of your care.* Furthermore, she may have responsibilities in many other places, besides caring for patients in the hospital you're staying at. This can vary substantially by specialty, hospital, and geographic region and is also changing with the evolution of the *hospitalist movement* (for more on hospitalists, see below), but it has dramatic implications for older patients. Here's the most significant one: The doctor who is attending to you will not be at the hospital for most of the time that you're hospitalized. He may spend much of his day at his office, at a hospital across town where he has privileges, or somewhere else in an administrative or teaching capacity.

Think about this structure for a moment. Imagine the captain of a cruise ship who appears on the bridge for thirty minutes or less every day and proceeds to bark orders to the entire crew: He tells the engine room how fast to go, the galleys what to cook, and the com-munications room which bulletins to transmit. After dispatching his orders, he jumps onto his speedboat moored to the side of the mother ship and heads home, with instructions to the crew to call him if there are any problems before he returns the next day. Questions from any of the passengers are answered secondhand by one of his stand-ins; if the passengers wish to speak with him directly, they should try to be visiting the bridge at the time he (usually) makes his daily appearance. And one more thing: He also gives the crew his number at home so they can reach him if the ship happens to be sinking so, one hopes, he can get back quickly enough to provide some assistance.

That is precisely the structure of medical care in most hospitals. It's a model that was concocted in an older era of physician shortage (with not much for doctors to do except tell nurses to monitor patients), before the dawn of specialty medicine, and at a time when America was much younger.

And it worked. Why? Because, by and large, the reasons younger people got hospitalized back then were straightforward (like childbirth), usually required a well-defined intervention (delivery), and rarely involved a bevy of consultants (whose fields didn't even exist yet). You came to have your baby; your family obstetrician left his busy office and delivered it, he went back, you went home. No consultants; the two of you. Or you broke your leg playing pickup basketball; the orthopedic surgeon rolled himself out of bed, came to the ER, looked at the X-rays, either casted you or took you to the OR to repair it; and you went home in a day or so with crutches and physical therapy. Ah, the benefits of youth: no coexisting heart disease to worry about, no medications you take that could interfere with the pain pills he prescribed, and an able twentyish spouse at home to help you in and out of the shower.

But with advancing age comes more medicines, more medical problems, less physiologic reserve, and perhaps a more precarious support system at home. There will also be a growing number of people involved in your care—more consultants, more staff with confusing roles (nurses, nurses' aides, technicians, physical therapists, residents, covering physicians). Add to that the different (and often less straightforward) reasons you've been hospitalized—vague abdominal pain instead of pregnancy, fever and headache instead of a broken bone, a complex surgical procedure (like a heart-valve replacement) complicated by other preexisting medical conditions—and the hospital has become a more perilous place.

You've just completed the first semester of Aging and the Hospital 101, devoted mostly to the dangers. The second-semester course coming up covers what you can do about it.

What Patients and Families Can Do

I've seen my share of hospital mishaps, but there's no way I could list for you every way in which things could go wrong (nor would I terrify you with such a list).* In fact, for many years I struggled with how to respond when hospital patients (and their families) asked me about how to "stay well" during their tenure there. The list of potential problems or complications is so long and varied that I wasn't sure how to begin or even provide a theoretical framework on what to do or be on the lookout for.

I've found that the most useful framework comes from Dr. Inouye's work on interventions aimed at preventing confusion in the hospitalized patient, because these same interventions appear to be effective in mitigating many other manifestations of hospitalitis. Not content to simply observe these complications, Dr. Inouye created a series of maneuvers to prevent them, which she called the Hospital Elder Life Program, or HELP. Adopted by several hospitals throughout the United States, HELP makes use of volunteers to assist in preventing confusion and other manifestations of hospitalitis. Other institutions have informally adopted elements of the program (such as aggressive early mobilization of patients).

---

* For interested and intrepid readers, the classic article "Hazards of Hospitalization of the Elderly," by Morton C. Creditor, MD, from the *Annals of Internal Medicine* 118, no. 3 (February 1, 1993): 219–23, can be found at http://www.annals.org/cgi/content/full/118/3/219.

Even if your hospital has no formal or informal elements of HELP at all, you as a patient or the family of one can adopt many aspects of the program on your own.

The various components are so obvious, so simple, and so rooted in common sense (for example, making sure patients have their hearing aids and glasses, ensuring a good night's sleep, quickly recognizing and intervening in cases of malnutrition and dehydration) that you might wonder what's the big deal and assume that hospitals are paying attention to these things all the time—it ain't rocket science. Here's the problem: Hospitals and their staff have become so fixated on real rocket science (lasers, robots, cameras the size of your fingernail) that the "little things" often get overlooked, and what could have been a small problem instead becomes the ember that starts a conflagration.

Every geriatrician has seen this phenomenon, called the *geriatric cascade*: One seemingly small event or medical misstep leads to others, which in turn lead to others, until an irreversible spiral seems to have been set in motion. Eyeglasses left at home become a hip fracture. An ankle sprain turns into a nursing home placement. A new prescription combined with a misread over-the-counter medication bottle becomes an intensive care admission. In the hospital setting, Dr. Inouye found confusion or another form of hospitalitis invited a variety of treatments and/or tests, which in turn created more difficulties, which—you guessed it—invited more treatments and tests. Here are some examples I've seen or heard about during my career:

- An inexperienced but well-meaning resident mistakes his patient's confusion for a stroke and orders a CAT scan; radiology is so busy that she's not called down for the test until later that night. The patient's agitation from being transported (on top of her existing confusion) is so severe that the radiology technician calls the covering resident for sedation (so the patient will lie still in the scanner). Busy with a dozen medical emergencies of her own upstairs, the covering doc quickly complies. The scan is completed (negative), but the patient does not wake up for two days from the sedation and then is even more confused.

- A man with pneumonia becomes confused, stops eating; his anorexia does not improve, even though the pneumonia is getter better. Trays of food go uneaten because there is no one to feed him when they arrive. Dehydration—a risk factor for confusion—results, and so confusion worsens, causing the man to pull out his intravenous line (which is needed for both antibiotics and for the fluids to rehydrate him). The nurse's solution: a wrist restraint—yet another risk factor for confusion. (Thankfully, restraints are becoming less and less common in American hospitals as their risks become appreciated.) Once restrained, not only could the patient not eat; he couldn't walk and had soiled sheets, which led to a bedsore, which led to pain, which led to—more confusion.

- A woman fractures her hip and has it repaired. Because she was admitted as an emergency case, she didn't bring her hearing aid from home, which leads to confusion. Her inability to hear makes it difficult for her to understand the instructions of her physical therapist, who is unaware that she uses a hearing aid. Her rehabilitation is slow, and because of this she cannot get to the bathroom in time. This results in the placement of a bladder catheter by one of the nurses, since the patient cannot be walked to the bathroom safely. Instead of being able to return home as planned, she is instead discharged to a nursing home when her confusion worsens to the extent that she cannot live independently.

Once this train gets put in motion and starts to gain momentum, changing tracks or derailing it gets harder and harder. But you can lower your risk of experiencing this kind of spiral by following three basic steps.

Step One:
Answer the Question: Who the Hell Are All These People?

Job number one for you, your family, and/or your friends is to figure out who exactly is involved in your care, what their role is, and how they got there. Sound nuts? There are no stupid questions with your health on the line, so shed your temerity ASAP and get down to it.

Start by finding out who is the captain of this ship. By that I mean, who is your attending physician and to what service are you admitted? It may be obvious if you get admitted for a bypass operation (your surgeon would be in charge), but the situation is often not so clear. A patient with a hip fracture and lots of medical problems may be admitted to an internal medicine service with the orthopedist as a consultant or to the orthopedic service with an internist consulting. A patient with a gallbladder flare-up could be admitted to a surgical service with the GI (internal medicine) docs consulting or to internal medicine with a surgeon consulting, whether surgery's planned or not. Find out immediately by asking your nurse in the ER or once you reach the floor you'll be staying on. As discussed, that physician or someone he or she designates 1. admits you, 2. sees you every day, 3. writes all your orders (from medications to consultants), and 4. discharges you unless you are transferred to another service. When another physician appears on the scene, expectedly or unexpectedly, find out who he is, who sent him, and why he's there. There are really only three possibilities as to how and why a physician appears in your hospital room:

1. He or she is your attending physician or someone covering for your attending physician. (You should ask, "So you are covering for Dr. Smith while he is away for the weekend?")

2. He is a consultant "ordered" to see you by your attending physician (or his coverage) for a specific problem. (Ask, "So you are a dermatologist Dr. Smith asked to see me for this rash I developed, which may be due to a drug he prescribed for me?")

3. If you are in a hospital with a training program (residency), the doctor is a resident (trainee) under the supervision of either the attending or the consultant he called. (Ask, "So you are a surgical [or dermatology] resident on Dr. Smith's service?") In teaching hospitals, much of the role confusion arises from the presence of residents, who themselves have covering residents due to work-hour restrictions (a very desirable thing, trust me). At a major teaching hospital most of the physicians you meet will be residents, and there may be many different ones, from many different services.*

This is a good moment to revisit the concept of *hospitalists,* discussed earlier in chapter 7. Hospitalists are attending physicians (usually internal medicine physicians) who do nothing but care for patients in the hospital; they have no other responsibilities (like having to run off to an office full of patients while you're gasping for air). In general, I view this as a good thing; it's the antidote to the cruise ship captain who jumps off the boat after making a brief daily appearance. When you are on a hospitalist service, your family doc relegates your care to this physician while you're in the hospital. The downside is obvious: the loss of continuity. You're handed back off to your primary care doc once you're discharged; it is imperative that information flows back to him about what transpired while you were hospitalized. (You have a role here, too, as you learned in the last chapter, on care transitions.)

We've now dealt with the physicians you might encounter during a hospitalization, but we're not done yet. We still have to talk about the people who do most of the real work: the nurses. They are the day-to-day and minute-to-minute angels who follow physician orders, take vital signs, assess new symptoms, and deal with suffering in the trenches: your nausea, your pain, your shortness

---

* Physician extenders (physician assistants and nurse practitioners, discussed in chapter 7) are also used in hospitals, where they primarily function as residents would and report to the attending physicians of record.

of breath, your anxiety—the list is endless. Nurses educate you about your condition, interact with your worried family and friends (typically more so than the docs), and use every resource at their disposal to innovatively troubleshoot a range of medical and non-medical problems. In most hospitals you'll be assigned a *primary nurse*, who has primary responsibility for your care. She's the one who's supposed to know you best, does most of your assessments, and describes your condition to the next nurse coming on duty (or any nurse covering for her). In short, she is the nursing equivalent of an attending physician.

You're also likely to meet a bevy of people who could easily be confused for nurses (by both their uniforms and what they appear to be doing) but are actually there to provide assistance to the nursing staff. They go by a variety of names, such as *certified nursing assistants, patient care technicians*, and *patient care assistants*. These dedicated staffers are often the heaviest lifters, providing direct service to you (such as bathing you, walking you to the bathroom, even taking your blood pressure) so that your nurse can tend to some of the more technical aspects of patient care (like mixing medications or starting an IV).

Finally, there are a bunch of other people who may show up. Depending on why you're hospitalized, you may meet *nutritionists, physical therapists, occupational therapists, speech therapists, social workers*—the list goes on. Many of them also have subordinates who assist them in your care (like physical therapy technicians). With all of them, your strategy is the same: Ask who they are (their names, their titles), who asked them to see you, and why they are there—and for goodness sake, don't be bashful. One more suggestion: Write it all down. It doesn't matter how good your memory is; even if it's perfect, this would be a confusing ensemble cast of characters, so after you've figured out who someone is, make a note in case you need to remind yourself who's playing what role.

Many hospital floors that care for older people (mine included) have a list of providers posted in the common area, with pictures of every person who might participate in your care (this is an explicit component of the HELP, by the way). In our patients' rooms, we write every team member's name on a whiteboard in direct view of the patient. What a great way of preventing problems before they occur or knowing exactly who to call when problems arise.

Step Two:
Figure Out If You Are at High Risk for Hospitalitis

Who's at risk for hospitalitis? As we get older, everyone. But some people are at particularly high risk. Dr. Inouye has developed two simple bedside evaluations, requiring no fancy apparatus, to determine how likely you are to develop confusion and other hospital-related problems. The first takes place when you pass through the hospital door; the second, as your hospitalization progresses and more risk factors get piled on.

Upon admission, your risk for delirium and hospitalitis increases with each of the following: a previous history of cognitive problems or dementia,* dehydration (determined by simple lab and/ or urine tests that virtually every hospitalized patient gets), corrected vision of less than 20/70 (tested while you're wearing your best glasses), and your general level of illness, based on a severity-of-illnesses scoring system.[2] *After you're treated for a day or two*, you may accumulate a bunch of problems and treatments that—if you are still clearheaded—increase your risk of confusion even more.[3] They are the use of restraints, new or ongoing malnutrition, adding more than three new medications, use of a bladder catheter (sound familiar?), and any "iatrogenic event" (a problem related to hospitalization itself, such as a fall or a medication error). I won't bore you with the details,** but there is a striking

---

* Many patients may not have been formally diagnosed with dementia or cognitive problems before their hospital admission, but these problems cannot be formally excluded unless they have been screened for. A patient is probably at risk if he has experienced memory loss, disorientation, or other symptoms in the past year that could signal early dementia.

** Give yourself a point for each of the delirium risk factors and add them up. For the test that takes place after admission, with 0 points you have a 4 percent risk of delirium;

dose-response curve that predicts the likelihood of hospitalitis based on the number of factors you bring with you or develop once you're there.

Figuring out whether you're at high risk is important for two reasons. First, it tells staff to sit up and take notice with a little extra vigilance. Second, when we start to understand what risk factors you have, we can begin to tailor interventions to mitigate them.

Step Three:
If You Are at Risk, Try These Simple Interventions

Okay, you're snug in your hospital bed, recovering from whatever illness brought you there, but you've discovered you're also at risk for hospitalitis. These suggestions from the HELP Program can help you lower that risk. (For more details, see http://elderlife.med.yale.edu.)

Encourage regular visits. What HELP calls "substantive and regular visiting and visitors" can keep patients engaged and socially interactive. When hospitalizations are long, there are often throngs of visitors on the first day or two (often all at once), but these tend to peter out as the stay drags on. Someone should be there every day. (Many older people have no visitors at all.) Assign a family member to coordinate visits, almost in shifts. Rather than sit and watch television, engage in substantive, engaging mental activities with the patient, like playing cards or a board game or discussing current events.

Keep the patient oriented. Anyone who has spent time in the hospital knows that days can melt into one another without home

---

with 1–2 points, a 20 percent risk; with 3 or more points, a 35 percent risk. It's a bit like the points you get on your driver's license each time you get a ticket; accumulate enough and you lose your license (or, in this case, your mind).

or work structure. The times for sleeping and being awake can become blurred. It may sound silly, but simply reminding patients what day of the week it is, what time it is, who is taking care of them, and what's in store for the day with regard to tests and physician visits can be helpful.

Mobilize as soon as possible. As I said earlier, the R & R many people expect in the hospital isn't always a great thing. Be aggressive about asking your doctor when it is safe to get out of bed and into a chair and/or when you can walk. As soon as you get the green light, start moving! HELP volunteers are trained to help patients walk safely as soon as possible after the okay from the medical team, but you can have a role here, too.

Use nondrug approaches to restoring sleep. If you're having trouble sleeping, don't rush to ask for medication; it's a risk factor for developing confusion. Ask for warm milk or herbal tea. Bring your relative an iPod with soothing music. Think about a massage rather than a sleeping pill to promote normal sleep patterns.

Remember glasses and hearing aids. If you wear them, bring them, or send someone to get them if you've left them at home. Some programs offer "loaner" adaptive hearing devices in hospitals to make sure patients can hear to the best of their ability. (I describe these temporary devices, which have headphones like an iPod, in chapter 13.)

Plan visits around meals. Assistance and companionship during meals is critical, but never feed your relative or friend without the okay of the staff. (Some patients have swallowing difficulties that could make this dangerous.) HELP volunteers are trained to safely assist patients at mealtime, making sure that the food tray doesn't get returned unused.

In a large clinical trial, patients were randomly assigned to receive either the HELP program or "customary" hospital care. The results were clear (and published in the *New England Journal of Medicine*): The rate of confusion among patients was a third less in those receiving these simple interventions, and they experienced many fewer episodes of it on many fewer days.[4]

Unintended Consequences

HELP interventions mitigate other forms of hospitalitis as well. Patients who received them were half as likely as those who got customary care to experience functional decline (for example, losing some of the ability to walk or care for themselves they had before admission).[5] They were less likely to develop bedsores. And there were other benefits beyond the clinical. The costs of hospitalization dropped, probably because patients wound up being less confused and impaired and needed less testing to figure out what was going on. Also, HELP patients had a decreased risk of needing a long-term nursing home stay after their hospitalization, in comparison to their customary-care counterparts. And staff members were delighted to have a cadre of volunteers to assist them—an extra pair of cheery, well-trained hands is always welcome in these environments. Talk about a program a hospital administrator or insurer could love! These savings more than offset the cost of administering the HELP program.

But to me, one of the most remarkable things about the program was not the impact it had on patients but, rather, *the impact it had on volunteers who participated in HELP.* Sharon intentionally created a highly professional training environment for these people; because she explained the rationale and importance of the interventions, they understood the contribution they were making. At our medical center, a volunteer coordinator provides exceptional training and feedback; we even have a volunteer newsletter!

HELP Lite?

If you're in a position of influence at your local hospital, I suggest using that influence to encourage starting a HELP program there; Sharon's Web site describes how to get started. (Each year, programs from across the United States convene to share ideas and strategies.) Besides being a good health-care idea and the right thing to do, HELP also saves money, not only by reducing the cost per patient but also by avoiding complications that the government is now making hospitals pay for.

On the other hand, I'm a realist. I recognize that many hospitals may not yet have the vision, motivation, or resources to implement the program. So are there elements of HELP that you can safely implement on your own for a parent or a loved one? Sure there are. Of course, you're not your parent or spouse's admitting physician (or your own), so you can't control things like which medications are prescribed. But you can certainly provide helpful input and participate in a serious set of interventions that no reasonable doctor or nurse could argue with. The key is coordinating your efforts with the doctors so you're seen as a helpful part of the team, rather than an irritant. Here are some suggestions from the HELP experts who have modified aspects of the program so that they can be applied in just about any hospital setting whether there's a formal HELP program or not.[6]

Easy Ways to Help Yourself or a Loved One in the Hospital

By taking these eight steps, you may be able to reduce the risk of confusion and other hospital-related problems for you or someone you care about.

1. Bring your complete medication list to the hospital, with your regular doctors' names and contact information.
2. Bring glasses, hearing aids (with fresh batteries), and dentures to the hospital. People do better if they can see, hear, and eat.

3. Bring in a few familiar objects from home. Things such as family photos, a favorite comforter or blanket for the bed, rosary beads, a beloved book, and relaxation tapes can be quite comforting.
4. Help orient the patient throughout the day. Speak in a calm, reassuring tone of voice, and tell the patient where he is and why he is there.
5. When giving instructions to patients, state one fact or simple task at a time so as not to overwhelm or overstimulate them.
6. Massage can be soothing for some patients.
7. Stay with the patient as much as possible. During an acute episode of delirium, relatives should try to arrange shifts so someone can be present around the clock.
8. If you detect new signs that could indicate delirium—confusion, memory problems, personality changes—it is important to discuss these with the nurses or physicians as soon as you can. Family members are often the first to notice subtle changes.[7]

I hope I've convinced you that the hospital is indeed no place for sick people, and that this "truism" becomes even truer as we get older. But I'm a geriatrician—an optimist by constitution—so I also hope I've convinced you there are highly effective steps you can take to mitigate the problem.

How ironic that the American medical palaces we call hospitals—constructed to improve the health of our citizens—can become pernicious places as we age. Even more ironic is the fact that it is often the alluring technology itself—scans, tests, blood work—that distracts us from the actual work of healing, when we reflexively employ them rather than think straightforwardly about what's happening to the patient in front of us.

But as a geriatrician I must admit there's also something deliciously fitting and fulfilling about the scientifically proven antidote to this modern medical quicksand. It's rooted in common sense and compassion, and potentially deliverable by family members, friends, or any volunteer who cares about older people.

No, it ain't rocket science, but it works.

Chapter 11

You Could Become Geriatric Just Waiting

How to Emerge from the Emergency Room Unscathed

No valet parking in the ER? That's got to be the biggest oversight in our solar system! Okay, you go in! Tell 'em you're shot. Ask 'em if they validate!

—Brian Regan

A number of years ago I was a visiting professor of geriatrics at a university in Canada, something I do every couple of years, though usually at a U.S. university (and, if I'm lucky, somewhere warm). It's a fun gig that typically involves a formal lecture or two, making rounds in the hospital with residents to see interesting patients, and, one hopes, imparting some geriatric know-how in the process. But on this visit my Canadian hosts were the ones providing the education. During my tour of their emergency room, I got an international crash course in both comparative public policy and population demographics. There were two things I will never forget about that visit.

The first was the scene when I entered the ER. A group of residents excitedly hovered over the bed of a young patient in a trauma bay.

"What's going on over there?" I asked one of the supervising physicians in my miserable French.

"Great case!" he replied.

Now, in New York City a "great case" in the emergency room conjures up some pretty exotic scenarios: Fugu poisoning at a trendy new sushi restaurant. A case of malaria that just walked off an airplane at JFK. Third-rail subway electrocution.

What was the great case here? A gunshot wound. This would have elicited nary a yawn in most U.S. inner-city hospitals. That got me thinking about the public health arguments relating to gun control in the United States and the endless public policy debates about whether European-style restrictions would have any effect on rates of injury.

The other unforgettable thing about my visit to the ER hit me after I had absorbed that initial scene and taken in everything else going on around me. In this emergency room, when it came to age, the young gunshot victim was the exception; most of the other patients I saw were not only old but *very* old. And they filled the halls and corridors. There were so many of them that it seemed as if they were choking off the flow of other patients through the system. In fact, if you were younger and needed care, you'd better have a gunshot wound or you'd be sitting in the waiting room a long time.

In the midst of this odd intergenerational chaos—think *Grey's Anatomy* meets *The Golden Girls*—was a clear-eyed woman with a white coat who was kindly but efficiently ministering to all manner of medical and social emergencies and barely breaking a sweat. I assumed she was the chief of emergency medicine until she put out her hand to shake mine. "I loved your lecture this morning, Professor Lachs," she said. At that moment I spied the "GNP" credential embroidered above her left coat pocket. She was a geriatric nurse practitioner who was assigned exclusively to the emergency room. I had worked with many such nurse practitioners in many different roles, but I had never heard of this before.

She went on to explain why she was there. Her hospital administration had seen a steady increase in ER traffic in the past decade, and much of it was driven by an increase in the oldest patients. Furthermore, these patients were creating a kind of gridlock in the health system because of the overlapping medical and social issues they brought with them; it was a situation that required her particular skill set. Sure, there was the usual smattering of bona fide medical problems—asthma, chest pain, lacerations—but a substantial proportion of older patients found themselves either arriving at the

ER (or unable to safely leave) because of compounding psychosocial or "health systems" problems that would have posed no difficulty for a thirty-year-old. Cases in point: A seventy-three-year-old with a mild gastrointestinal bug who would have gone home if not for the fact that she was recently bereaved and therefore had no one who could make sure she could safely "force fluids"; instead, she endured two days of intravenous therapy in the ER. An eighty-two-year-old man who'd had a fall, and hip fracture was suspected; fortunately there was no break, but his resulting gait was too unsteady to permit his return to his apartment, which was on the second floor of a nonelevator building. A sixty-six-year-old who had no medical problems at all; he had been evicted from his home and sent to a shelter, where he became so fearful he called for an ambulance to bring him to the hospital.

The GNP was there to unclog the system using everything in her masterful toolbox. As I described in chapter 7, geriatric nurse practitioners are not only superb clinicians; they also help patients navigate broken health-care systems, because they see the fractures up close and often have the luxury of at least a little more time than their harried physician counterparts. Curious, I politely ditched my hosts for an hour, deciding instead to shadow her. She moved effortlessly between highly technical medical interventions, like putting in an IV and dosing intravenous antibiotics, and "system" maneuvers, such as begging a local home-care provider to see a patient that night so she could safely send him home (and finally get to sleep herself). In short, she was practicing geriatric medicine as we all do: with sticks and gum.

That night at dinner with my hosts, this scene was all that I could think or talk about. How did this Canadian ER find itself overrun—literally—with mostly older patients? I thought to myself, the ER must be a final safety net for a failing health-care system.

My hosts, proud of their government-run health insurance program, which covers all Canadian citizens, bristled at my hypothesis. Then they gave me the real skinny. What was driving this geriatric tsunami was simply demographics. Montreal was "grayer" than most U.S. cities: The average age of its population was six or seven years older than that of an analogous U.S. metropolis. As a result, there was a much higher percentage of people over the age of eighty-five living in the community served by this hospital. (This would also seem to invalidate the critique that a system of national health insurance would be of poor quality; the people in that ER had grown up under such a system and survived into their eighties and beyond.)

As I left for the airport, my host, who was familiar with the American health-care system, warned me that the scene I'd described from the Canadian ER was like a peek into my future. "Coming soon to a theater near you," he said. That was more than a decade ago.

He was right: Visit most American hospitals' emergency rooms and you'll find that the tidal wave of elderly patients has made landfall.

What Do You Get When You Cross an ER with a Nursing Home? The Perfect Storm

---

The previous chapter discussed hospitalitis and how it occurs. Here's what you need to know about the emergency room vis-à-vis aging: The various forms of hospitalitis that get patients into trouble are exponentially magnified in the ER, because the factors that lead to them are concentrated there to an unusually high degree.

If hospitals have been constructed for younger people—clinically, architecturally, and operationally—then the emergency department, with its focus on trauma, acute illness, and rapid intervention, takes this ageist bias to the extreme. Attention to detail? Patient histories and physical examinations can take just ninety seconds. Continuity? Access to previous medical information may be unavailable or inaccurate, especially if you're typically cared for in another city or health-care system. Customer service? Dozens of other patients may be simultaneously vying for the attention of the ER physician caring for you, and the most pressing needs are often dealt with first—heart attacks or life-threatening injuries trump the mundane questions and complaints of boomers and their parents. Communication? Even if you are conscious enough to tell the ER doc who your primary care physician is, there's no guarantee they'll reach your doc or even try to. Lights are bright, equipment is beeping, people are shouting drug names or Latin phrases or both. If you have to stay overnight, I promise you it's not going to be a Ritz-Carlton sleeping experience. The potential for medical error is also higher in this cauldron of chaos, simply because many serious things are being done to an enormous number of very sick people in an awfully short space of time. Cars get into accidents more often on busy freeways than on empty back-country roads. If the hospital is no place for sick people, then the ER is *really* no place for sick people. The catch is that if you get really sick in our increasingly fragmented system of health care, going to the ER may be the best (and only) potentially life-saving choice.

In this chapter I'll offer some very specific advice on how to negotiate this potential hornet's nest. But first a few words about the process of getting admitted to a modern hospital and how the ER figures into that process.

We'll Keep a Light on for Ya

Over my twenty-five-year medical career, the route by which people are admitted to the hospital for an overnight stay has subtly evolved in ways that most patients (and even many doctors) may not realize. Specifically, the proportion of patients who walk (or wheel) themselves through the hospital's front door at their doctor's recommendation and are whisked directly to a bed upstairs has declined precipitously. Conversely, the percentage of patients who are admitted to the hospital via the emergency room has increased just as dramatically.

There are several reasons for these trends. First, when you're sick, you want and often need to address the problem as quickly as possible. If you can't find your regular doc to figure out how sick you are or what to do, the ER is the only reasonable alternative. There are very few incentives (in fact, there are a ton of disincentives) for your primary care doc to say, "Sure, bypass the ER and come on over right now." There's operational risk to his practice (he has patients scheduled every fifteen minutes for the next eight hours; treating you could result in the cancellation of many appointments), economic risk (tending to patients with complicated situations doesn't get him much more income than the five common colds you've just displaced), and legal risk (he's the guy who diverted you from the ER—what if you have a heart attack on the way to his office?). Why would any primary care doc want to ruin his day with potential ulcers like this?

Another force driving this trend: Insurers simply won't pay for many of the elective tests and evaluations that "semisick" people used to get as part of a hospitalization; they believe that these can be done on an outpatient basis. Gone, for example, are the days when you could be admitted to the hospital for a leisurely evaluation of weight loss, wherein your doc brought you in for a few days of scans, X-rays, and blood tests. In my opinion, this is a mixed blessing; you already know about the many ways older people run into difficulty in the hospital and why most geriatricians will tell you to avoid going if you can. On the other hand, sometimes the complicated series of tests and consultant opinions I need to evaluate a spot on a chest X-ray, intermittent belly pain, or some other new symptom can be logistically overwhelming even to young patients with good mobility and access to transportation. I often find myself wishing I could bring my older patients into the hospital for less than twenty-four hours just so the four or five tests they need could be done efficiently and without taxing their bodies, memories, and travel budgets. On a positive note, a trip to the hospital is unnecessary for many of the things we used to do there (such as a simple hernia repair), which can now be handled in outpatient surgery centers or even some physicians' offices. That's a good thing.

So now more than ever, if you need to be admitted to the hospital, there is a high likelihood that it will be through the emergency room. Unless you're having a major scheduled surgery, it is increasingly difficult for your physician to call ahead to reserve a bed for you, as if it were a table for two in a restaurant. And anyway, if you've been to the ER recently, you know it's more like the department of motor vehicles or the supermarket deli counter than a fancy restaurant—you'll probably be "taking a number" and waiting. (And what's worse, you can't tip the maître d' to cut the line; it's going to take a sucking chest wound to get immediate service.)

But as a geriatrician I can help you here. I've spent thousands of hours in emergency departments—as an ER physician myself, as a geriatrician ministering to my patients there, as a family member hovering nervously over a loved one, and even as a patient from time to time.

Here, then, are my rules on how to emerge from the emergency room unscathed.

Rule #1:
Try to Avoid the Emergency Department

You think I'm kidding? The best way to avoid bee stings is to navigate past the hive entirely. For all the reasons I've described, the ER is the last place you want to get care, particularly if you sense that going there might be "overkill" (i.e., that you or a parent come to the ER for what you thought was a life-threatening problem only to find after an eight-hour wait that it was absolutely trivial). But of course, the problem with trying to gauge this is that if you're not a doctor, you're really in no position to tell if a tummy ache is indigestion from a bad piece of fish or a ruptured appendix that requires immediate surgery.

The bottom line: Only your doctor, after you've conveyed the symptoms to him or her in the office or more likely on the telephone, can reasonably recommend or dissuade you from going to the emergency department. By the way, I'm a pretty good doc and I've been wrong on this in both directions: I've kept patients home over the weekend after they described what seemed to be trivial issues on the telephone, only to find on Monday that they had roaring pneumonia requiring hospitalization. But I've also sent patients to the ER with what I was sure was a heart attack, only to find that they had pulled a chest-wall muscle doing yoga. So suffice it to say, making these decisions is rarely an exact science. However, I still can offer some good guidance.

If your symptoms occur during "business hours" (a rare convenience, I've found), do call your doctor and ask if she can see you. But be mindful of all the disincentives I described earlier that might make her less inclined to do so. The best way to bring down the firewall is to tactfully make your case to your doc or the nurse or the receptionist that you want to be seen.

A corollary piece of advice: Sometimes a resourceful primary care physician can route you to a subspecialist over the phone if the issue is very straightforward. For example, this week a patient called me to say that she had cut her hand, needed stitches, and was on her way to the ER. I had just passed through our ER and knew it was a madhouse that day. After getting more details from her and deciding that she was not spurting blood, I called one of my surgical buddies at his office, who told me to send her right over. She was spared a lengthy emergency room wait for a ten-minute suture job. (Medicare was also saved a considerable sum of money.)

Another patient earlier this month fell and was concerned about an ankle fracture. Since she called me in the late morning, I was able to send her directly for an outpatient X-ray and then to my office, where I could see the films via the Internet. She had not broken anything, and I was able to prescribe appropriate treatment in my office (a compression bandage, anti-inflammatory medicines, and crutches) without the need for the ER.

As I've described, in most systems of care, there are usually nominal incentives for physicians to orchestrate service like this, so it rarely gets done properly. There are, however, two situations, often facilitated by financial incentives, that can create this kind of care coordination to avoid the ER. One is concierge medicine, covered in chapter 7. The other? Certain kinds of managed care. I understand that that may sound counterintuitive, but in many HMOs or similar organizations, physicians bear the costs of their patients' visits to the emergency room (where it can cost a thousand dollars to sneeze). In those situations, systems have often been put in place to avert ER use.

Whatever kind of system of care you're in, a physician who goes the extra mile for you in these situations to avoid unnecessary ER use, no matter how he or she is paid, is an absolute keeper.

Rule #2:
Don't Dawdle in Calling Your Doctor If You're on the Fence

One of the things that leaves patients (and their doctors) with little or no choice about using the ER is a delay in communication. If you are experiencing some symptom as the day starts that you think you can "tough out" but soon discover that things aren't improving, your doc needs to hear about it ASAP. Every primary care doc will tell you that he or she dreads the 4 p.m. phone call about a problem that has been brewing all day long. (These also somehow always seems to occur on Fridays.) When you delay things in this way, you've tied your doctor's hands. The earlier your physician hears about what's going on, the more likely he can cobble together a plan of care that could potentially avert the ER.

And by the way, say specifically that that is your goal—push your physician about this gently, as in: "Couldn't you send me directly to a radiologist to get my foot X-rayed, and then he could call you with the results?" Or "I've gotten something in my eye. Is there an ophthalmologist you know who could see me quickly? I don't wear glasses, so I don't have one."

Rule #3:
Sometimes You Just Have to Take It
Like a Man (or Woman)

The prior "avoid the ER at all costs" soliloquy notwithstanding, there are several situations in which you simply have no choice. The first, of course, is when you call your doc and describe your symptoms, and he tells you they merit immediate ER evaluation. Respect his or her judgment, and don't dawdle. Another situation is one in which he has been monitoring you either in his office or over the phone; you've given it the college try, and your doctor finally says it's "ER Time." You need to suck it up and go. Last, there's the transfer scenario, common in my business, where you're sent to the ER from another health facility, such as a nursing home or a rehabilitation center where you've been convalescing. Perhaps a physician there has been managing a worsening medical problem, like asthma or a urine infection, that is exceeding that facility's ability to provide care. In those situations, your admission to the hospital is not elective, nor is it really an emergency (you are not at death's door, but a doc following you who has been trying to avoid that has just cried "uncle"). Almost invariably you are sent to the ER rather than to a bed upstairs.

In these situations there is an understandable impulse to try to avoid the ER and be directly admitted to a floor of the hospital. Sounds reasonable, right? Why weather the indignities of the emergency room if it's clear from the get-go that you'll be staying overnight anyway?

I've tried to schedule a number of these "direct admissions" over my career at several great institutions, and somehow it almost never seems to work as planned. In my ideal scenario, the patient goes from the ambulance bay to a nice, quiet hospital room, and the evaluation that would have been done in the ER gets started on the floor by an intern or resident. The problem: Access to both technology and physicians differs between the floor and the ER, and often when patients get to the hospital, we find that their medical conditions and needs are "not as advertised." This means that, at that moment, we may not have the resources on the hospital floor to provide the patient with adequate care. In fact, in smaller community hospitals there may be no physicians present in the hospital after hours other than the doc in the ER; so if you're directly admitted, your care may be overseen by physicians who are at home. One might not appear and lay eyes and hands on you until the next day. (I know this from experience, having been an ER doc in a community hospital where I was the only physician in the house. I'd be stitching up a kid's chin laceration in the ER, only to be interrupted by a patient crashing upstairs in the ICU who had been admitted that day but not yet seen by his physician.) Bypassing the ER in some situations can actually undermine your care.

Case in point: Last month I was in my office seeing a patient in her eighties with severe bronchitis who was not responding to oral antibiotics. I was worried that she was developing pneumonia. She wasn't deathly ill, but she wasn't in great shape, either. When I suggested to her two adult daughters that she be admitted to the hospital directly from my practice for stronger intravenous antibiotics, they were furious at the notion of having to do this through the emergency room—their previous experiences there with her hadn't been so great. I called to see if a bed was available for her upstairs, but the hospital was crowded, and there was none to be found.

Now, these were well-connected ladies who immediately whipped out their cell phones and began calling bigwigs at several local hospitals, hoping to use their influence to make a bed magically materialize. (By the way, I wasn't angry about this. I just love this kind of advocacy when it's properly channeled.) It turns out that even good connections can't manufacture a hospital bed where none exists, and the patient went from my office to the hospital in an ambulance. I called ahead to say she was coming, but let's just say nobody was too happy with me. The family had no interest in the ER and wanted her up in a cozy bed; I simply could not produce one.

When the patient got to the ER, she received a chest X-ray that showed pneumonia, as I suspected, but there were other subtle abnormalities that a heads-up emergency medicine resident thought might suggest another problem: pulmonary embolism, a life-threatening blood clot in the lung, which would require an entirely different treatment in addition to the antibiotics. Diagnosing this problem definitively required a fairly sophisticated test called a spiral CAT scan, which she received less than thirty minutes after the possibility was raised. She did indeed have a blood clot and was started immediately on blood-thinning medicines in addition to the antibiotics.

My point here is that had the daughters' advocacy worked and the ER been bypassed, the diagnosis of pulmonary embolism (and its treatment) could have been seriously delayed by many hours, perhaps even a day. She would first have had to be seen by the admitting physician upstairs, who may or may not have considered pulmonary embolism a possibility. She would have gotten a plain old preliminary chest X-ray and would have had to go downstairs for it, intravenous lines and all. Then she would have returned upstairs to her bed while the radiologist read the film; he may or may not have had the benefit of consulting adjacent ER physicians who were caring for the patient (and looking over his shoulder as he read the film). If he had, and decided that the patient needed a definitive CT scan, he would have had to bring her back down in the middle of the night, and the scan could have taken many more hours to conduct and interpret. (ER patients seem to get higher priority in these circumstances because they are "emergent" by virtue of where they're coming from.) All this would have caused a long and potentially life-threatening delay.

The moral of the story: Health-care manpower and technology are physically located near emergency rooms for a reason. By design, ERs enable patients to rapidly access these resources when they need them. In a situation where your diagnosis or course of treatment is not precisely defined, the ER is a place where you can often get answers more quickly than you might elsewhere. So if your doctor decides that it's best for you to go to the ER, it's best to let these guys do their job!

Rule #4:
If You're Coming to Dinner,
Ask Your Physician to Reserve a Table

Emergency rooms take the sickest patients first; after this "triage" (French for "sorting") those whose illnesses are roughly equivalent in terms of severity generally get taken in order of arrival. But if you're able to speak with your physician before going to the hospital, his call to the emergency room can make a world of difference, particularly if he speaks directly to the ER doctor. I'm not saying this will move you to the front of the line; a patient with major injury from a car accident will get seen before you and your hangnail. But in making such an overture, your physician is not only providing information about your clinical and personal history that could expedite decision making about the kinds of tests you need; he's also implicitly conveying that your journey through the ER is being monitored by another health-care provider to whom there is accountability, and that after your emergency care there is a feasible "discharge plan" involving an engaged and interested doctor. All this goes a long way in keeping the ball rolling. As an ER physician I always found that patients whose primary care docs called ahead to provide history and context, and who followed up during the ER visit, got better care; I appreciated the doctor's help, and I reciprocated ardently as a result.

To be clear, this strategy should not delay you in getting to the ER if you are experiencing serious acute symptoms. As I tell my patients, first call 911, then call me.

And while we're on the subject of physician intervention that expedites your emergency room care, let's not forget the "above and beyond the call of duty" award. This is given to the primary care doc who actually shows up in the ER while you're there—sadly, a rarer and rarer occurrence these days, as many physicians have abandoned their rounds to "hospitalists" and almost never come to the hospital. (You should be aware of whether this is the policy when you join a new primary care practice.) If your doc appears at some point during your ER stay—especially if it's unannounced and unprovoked by you—she gets super bonus points, and you've probably found a keeper. Furthermore, there's absolutely nothing wrong with calling her office to let the staff know that you've been languishing in the ER and to inquire whether your doctor might be popping by, perhaps during other hospital obligations, to see if she can jump-start your care.

Rule #5:
Squeaky Wheels Get Grease, So Speak Up
(Respectfully)

A personal observation: The meek do not inherit the earth when it comes to health care. In every environment I have ever practiced in—hospitals, offices, clinics, and nursing homes—patients and families who advocated for themselves got better care, so long as that advocacy was not obnoxious. The key is finding the sweet spot between wallflower and irritant.

I marvel, therefore, at how some of the most successful and assertive people clam up when they enter the hospital. I'm not sure if it's unfamiliarity with the environment or the concern that asking a question of a health-care professional is somehow pestering him or distracting him from his duties. I've had older patients who were about to undergo surgery sign a consent form after a discussion with the surgeon, only to call me afterward with a litany of questions they were too timid to ask the doctor—important questions, like "How many of these have you done before?" or "Will you actually do the surgery, or will it be a resident?" You've got to be kidding! I've seen people get more engaged in a discussion with their dry cleaner over why a stain didn't come out than with their doctor about a life-altering procedure they were about to have.

But no other hospital environment seems to produce temerity

in patients and their families like the ER. This is understandable in one respect: If a physician or nurse is in the process of caring for patients with life-threatening trauma, it's natural to feel a bit hesitant about disturbing her. On the other hand, because of the general climate of chaos in most American emergency rooms these days, if you can't or won't speak up for yourself, it is very easy to get lost in the shuffle. Let me say it even more bluntly: While the ER is a very confusing place for someone of any age, it can be downright perilous for boomers and their families. It is essentially a four-alarm fire. And if you're not in flames, you will take a back-seat to someone who is.

As a result of this, older people in the ER can languish needlessly as more pressing cases displace them. Compounding this problem is the tendency of many people as they age to develop communicative difficulties or mild confusion when they get sick. They may not be able to articulate a problem as precisely as a much younger adult. Providing details about history and medications can be harder. Physicians may subtly withdraw and move on to the next customer when this happens, perhaps ordering some nonspecific tests or X-rays while they try to figure out what to do.

The solution: I always urge patients to bring a friend or family member with them to the ER. I'm well aware that many emergency departments do not permit this (except for children), but that is also changing. A patient who is confused or agitated is at high risk for falling or other injury, and there is simply not enough staff to babysit patients; what ER wants you to end up with a broken hip on top of whatever else you've got? If you're accompanying an older person and you get heat from the nursing staff in the ER, calmly explain the rationale for your involvement: You fear that your friend or relative might injure himself or become agitated, and you're trying to avoid troubling the very busy staff who are dealing with more urgent cases. (By the way, if your child were injured and brought to the ER and no parent was found sitting next to him, what do you suppose would happen? You'd probably be referred to the division of youth and family services for the investigation of child neglect.

How ironic that we toss adult children out on their ear if they're trying to provide the same service for a parent!)

So it's important to be (politely) vocal. But even this has its limits. There are squeaky wheels and there are out-of-control Mack trucks. While I've had patients and families who became docile upon entering the hospital, I've also had the opposite experience: patients and family members who breathe down the necks of staff and question each and every decision to the point of health-care paralysis. This is not going to endear you to anyone, I assure you, nor will it improve the care Mom, Dad, you, or your significant other gets. You need to find a balance between being a facilitator of care and being a pain in the ass—just imagine trying to do your job while someone was in your face every minute questioning your judgment and intentions. The best way to communicate effectively with ER staff is to approach them as a partner in care, not an independent auditor or the inspector general. Explain that you want to help expedite care and offload the work of the busy staff to the extent that it's permitted.

Rule #6:
Understand the Game Plan
(and Make Sure There Is One)

One of the frustrating things about emergency care for older people is the lack of a plan when symptoms aren't discrete or tidy. If you're twenty-two and come to the ER with a facial laceration, it will get stitched and you'll go home. A sixteen-year-old with appendicitis is getting admitted to go to the operating room, period. An intoxicated college student is spending the night to sleep it off. The goals of ER care in these situations are very straightforward.

Not so when the older person comes to the ER for something more difficult to wrap one's head around—a fall, confusion, a vague decline in function. Many older adults compound this problem by remaining silent for fear of bothering the doctor.

Sure, the doctor treating you or your loved one is busy. But in your brief, episodic interactions with her, you're allowed to play a game medical students sometimes call "What Am I Thinking?" At every juncture during your ER stay—when you arrive, when tests come back, when consultants visit—ask the physician to update you (quickly) as to how the latest result changes the list of diagnostic possibilities and what the next step is. Ask goal-oriented questions like "If that X-ray shows I have a fracture, does that mean I must be admitted?" or "How long does it usually take to get the neurologist to come to the ER to evaluate patients, and what specifically is he looking for?" Also use the strategy I described in the last chapter, on hospitals, of identifying each and every professional you come in contact with (you will have an ER attending physician, too, and he's responsible for your care until you're admitted, at which point it is transferred to the admitting attending physician).

Both *hospital* and *hospitality* derive from the Latin *hospitalis*, referring to a guest, as at a hotel or inn. How ironic—what place could be more inhospitable as we age than some of our modern-day hospitals? And within their walls, what department could be more inhospitable than the emergency room? But beyond the medical perils and the lack of amenities, I think what most terrifies patients and families about the ER is the loss of control. Not only are you sick, which is tough enough, but you're sick unexpectedly. In this chapter I've given you a game plan to help you cope. Use it and you'll improve the chances of emerging from the emergency room unscathed.

Chapter 12

In Search of an Honorable Discharge

Flying is not dangerous.
Landing is another story altogether.

As it relates to health care, many laypeople think *discharge* describes one thing: leaving the hospital for home. The truth is, you can be discharged from any number of health-care settings or treatment programs: hospitals, home-care agencies, nursing homes, emergency rooms, and physical therapy and radiation treatments. In addition to being points of departure, these can be postdischarge destinations as well. For example, you can be discharged from the hospital to a home-care agency where a visiting nurse will take the baton from his or her hospital counterpart.

As we already know from our discussion of care transitions, these takeoffs and landings are uniquely vulnerable moments in your health care. In this chapter I will offer advice on how to weather the four most common discharge scenarios you're likely to encounter (which, as it turns out, are also the ripest for disaster): from hospital to home, from hospital to subacute rehabilitation in a nursing home, from subacute rehabilitation back to the hospital, and from the emergency room to home.

There's No Place Like Home

If you've completed your hospitalization and they've decided you're going home, congratulations! As I've said, the hospital is no place for sick people, and most certainly no place for (almost completely) well people. There's no place like home for recuperating, provided you and the health-care professionals springing you from the joint have a reasonable expectation as to what kind of environment you're being discharged to.

Here's the problem: Unless your care providers are geriatricians, they rarely do. I'm amazed that physicians aren't required, as part of their medical school training, to visit the homes of a few of the people they've treated in the hospital and decided are ready for discharge. I don't understand how you can divine whether a patient you're releasing is going to sink or swim based solely on a series of medical tests or X-rays without having even a nominal understanding of what their home is like. Is it heated? Crowded? Smoky? Are there stairs? Is it well lit? Safe from crime? Free of domestic abuse? Every day older people in hospitals get wonderful care from the most attentive doctors and nurses, who coddle them for weeks, only to one day suddenly be told to "fly" as they are shooed from the hospital doorsill. How can anyone possibly make a thorough determination about a patient's "suitability for discharge" without an appreciation of where they're being sent?

Nor do many docs have a full understanding of the kinds of services provided by various home-care players—visiting nurses, home physical therapists, hospice nurses—who can make a discharge safer.

With the rush to get people out of the hospital, many mistakes get made in the discharge process. When these problems are minor, they may be fixed or adjudicated with a call to your doc (if you can reach him). When they're major—you took too much blood-thinning medication, the pharmacy was out of the antibiotic you were prescribed upon discharge, the home-care company forgot to deliver the oxygen your doc ordered—the results can land you back in the hospital or worse. This is certainly not good for you, and believe it or not, it's not good for hospitals, which are increasingly being asked to bear the costs of readmissions and other misadventures under health-care reforms.

Here are some specific steps you should take when you're being discharged from the hospital to make sure you don't wind up back there prematurely. They apply to most or all of the discharge scenarios I will discuss in this chapter, but they are most relevant to hospital discharge. (If you want to make sure you don't miss anything, you might check out my friend Dr. Eric Coleman's "Discharge Preparation Checklist" at www.caretransitions.org/documents/checklist.pdf.)

Know which doctors you're following up with and when. This should include both the subspecialist (if there is one) and your primary care doctor, and you should have a specific date for follow-up, if possible. Now more than ever, with the advent of hospitalists, it is critical to have a very clear understanding of who's running the show when you get discharged and when you will see her. In most cases, a vague instruction to "call my office when you get home to schedule an appointment" does not cut the mustard, unless this was a very straightforward medical problem or a highly elective admission (for example, a hernia repair). And if the hospitalization involved any significant complexity, you should be seeing your primary care physician sooner rather than later, ideally within a few days or a week of discharge. The problem with that: Unless your doc was caring for you in the hospital on a day-to-day basis, she may have little or no up-to-date knowledge on what transpired in the last days of your hospitalization. The solution:

Get the name and phone number of the person to contact if problems arise. "Call your family doctor" is another unacceptable instruction, unless your family doc discharged you or got an extensive debriefing from the hospitalist who cared for you. If you've been under the care of several physicians during a hospitalization, this is a very important question; when you ask, you might find that the answer is not only unclear to you but also to the docs taking care of you (the "six characters in search of an author" phenomenon).

Make sure your follow-up doctors get copies of your discharge instructions and discharge summary. Both are crucial documents. The nurse gives you a paper with your *discharge instructions* when you leave the hospital; it lists your medications and other follow-up information and is essentially a "lay" document. Your *discharge summary* is usually a dictated note that describes why you came to the hospital, what the hospital docs (including your attending) thought the diagnosis was, what happened during your stay (including the results of major blood tests and X-rays), who cared for you, and what the discharge plan is (including medications and treatments). If the physician you're going to see in follow-up did not care for you in the hospital, this is an especially critical document, because that doc is going to be clueless when you show up on his doorstep without a clear sense of what happened during your stay. You should also be aware that there are often delays in dictation that prevent your postdischarge doctor from having a copy of your discharge summary in time for your visit. Ask if that's likely; if it is, then ask your discharging doc to pick up the phone and spend five minutes with your primary care physician explaining what happened to you in the hospital. This is a vital step, and it also gives your primary care doc an idea of whom to call if questions subsequently arise. Most hospitalists now do this routinely, but it's worth your effort to make sure.

Consider getting a copy of your discharge summary for yourself. Ask that it be sent to you as well as your follow-up doctors. Rarely do patients request one, but it can be extremely useful to have on file. As we age, hospitalizations are often "pivot points," when new medical problems are identified, goals of care are more clearly articulated, and new medications or treatments are introduced. Bring a copy to your follow-up appointment in the event that your doc has not gotten one yet. As a physician, I can't tell you how frustrating it is to see a patient in follow-up from a hospitalization without any information about his stay. In those situations I frequently wind up spending the entire office visit on the phone with doctors, doctors' secretaries, and medical-record clerks trying to hunt down information when I could be talking with or examining the patient. It's not a good use of anyone's time. (A warning, though: Seeing a copy of your medical record or correspondence related to your health care for the first time can be a jarring experience. See "Not for Your Eyes Only" in chapter 9 for how to cope.)

Make sure those discharging you understand your home environment. A hospital social worker or discharge planner will probably ask you about your home environment before discharge, but if someone doesn't, find them and talk to them about it. You'd be surprised how many times people get exemplary medical care in the hospital, only to be sent home to environmental issues that completely undermine all that good work. I've seen it all: a patient treated for a pelvic fracture discharged to a fourth-floor walk-up apartment, a patient with confusion sent home on a complicated drug regimen with no one to assist, even a patient with visual impairment sent home after eye surgery with no one to help with cooking or their medicines (which included eyedrops!).

Reconcile your medications carefully. The process of checking each and every medication a physician puts you on versus what you believe you're supposed to be taking is called *medication reconciliation*, and it may be the most important thing you can do with a doctor or nurse upon and after discharge. Some of the biggest discharge blunders get made when people have their medications changed during a hospitalization and then are sent home to encounter a cabinet full of medicines they've been taking for years. This leaves them unsure as to how to reconcile the old drug regimen with the new one. In chapter 9, on care transitions, I told you about some of the major mistakes: accidentally taking a double dose of a drug because your hospital doctor has prescribed it using the brand name and your version at home has the chemical name (so you go home and take both); your hospital doc is unaware of medication or vitamins you take at home, so he prescribes meds that interact poorly with what you're on; or medication strengths that were changed in the hospital but not properly conveyed to your primary care doc or other prescribers- or dispensers-to-be.

And while we're on this topic, let me reiterate another helpful hint from the care-transition chapter: Hold on to your medication list as you do your wallet. Occasionally, hurried health-care professionals will walk off with it as a "time-saver," leaving you with just a memory. Always make a photocopy of your list in case of inadvertent (but well-intentioned) poaching by the doctor. (We're also famous for walking off with borrowed pens and other writing implements—I plead guilty here.)

Before you leave, understand where everything you need upon discharge is coming from. I don't have enough fingers on my hands to count the times I've discharged a patient on a critical medication (an antibiotic to treat their pneumonia, for example), only to discover when they came to see me in the office that it was not taken because the pharmacy didn't have it and the patient "didn't want to trouble" me. Make sure that you'll have the medicines you need as soon as you get home! This may mean asking your doctor to write prescriptions the night before your discharge and having a relative fill them, or having him or a nurse call the prescriptions directly into the pharmacy from the hospital floor. This way you'll know ahead of time what they're out of! And when it comes to being unprepared for discharge, I don't mean just medications. Equally disastrous are the accoutrements that fail to show up—hospital beds for home use, bedside commodes, and even oxygen.

Don't forget the other home-care "players." Your discharge plan should include not just your doctor but any other professionals who may be seeing you at home—visiting-nurse services, physical therapists, medical-equipment providers. Who's coming, when are they coming, and for how long? Although the plan may change depending on the speed of your recovery, you should have a sense of it before you leave the hospital. And all these folks need to be communicating with the "traffic cop"—your primary care doc. As I've said, it's essential to have someone conducting the many players in this medical symphony.

Get advice on postdischarge symptoms that should give you real concern. Again, "Call me if you have questions" gets a C-minus in the spectrum of modern hospital-discharge instructions. There should be specific instructions on what to look out for, based on the condition for which you've been hospitalized. If you're admitted for pneumonia that's been improving, then your triggers to call the doctor might be more breathlessness or new fever. If it's a hip replacement, they might be sudden pain or new redness or swelling around the incision site. If you've had new stents placed, it might be chest pain or breathlessness upon exertion. Getting advice on your key symptoms is not only good medicine, it's also good psychiatry. Patients and families can avoid much anxiety by learning before discharge that certain potentially terrifying symptoms are absolutely normal after some procedures, like coughing up a small amount of blood after a bronchoscopy (lung procedure) or experiencing headaches after a lumbar puncture (spinal tap).

Find out what tests are pending and who will follow up. As hospitalizations have gotten shorter and shorter, nearly every patient is discharged with some test result not yet in. This could be a biopsy result or a urine culture that has not yet incubated, or an X-ray that was read quickly by a resident but has not yet been formally reviewed by the senior radiologist. Find out what's still cooking test-wise, and make sure all that information will be conveyed to your primary care physician (who should be cc'd on everything).

Taking "the Long Way Home": Discharges to Subacute Rehabilitation

---

In the next chapter I'll talk about nursing homes (as well as assisted-living and life-care communities) as a place of residency. But nursing homes can also be a place to temporarily recuperate—and I don't mean only for Grandma. Here are some statistics to chew on: If you make it to age sixty-five, odds are at least fifty-fifty that you'll spend at least some subsequent part of your life in a nursing home. And if you take solace in believing that this eventuality is a long way off because you're only fiftysomething, better think again.

Here's why: If you're hospitalized at any age for any reason and cannot return home after a few days, there's a good chance that a social worker, a discharge planner, or some other cheery individual in a white coat will soon be appearing in your room, trying to get you to consider spending the last several days or weeks of your recovery at a rehabilitation facility or a nursing home in one of their postacute- or subacute-care units. If it's a nursing home, when you get there, you may well find the patients to be a curious mix of relatively younger, high-functioning people like yourself and what you've probably come to think of as "traditional" nursing-home residents—elderly patients with cognitive and/or physical impairments, for whom the facility may well be a last address. One of these folks may even be your new roommate. Unusual bedfellows indeed!

What's driving this bus? Money, of course. In the 1980s, hospitals began to get paid by the disease, rather than by the day—a lump sum for a specific diagnosis, no matter how long you stayed or how many tests you got. This led to patients' getting discharged "sicker and quicker"; many went home only to be quickly readmitted. Concerned about this, Medicare began paying for services that might prevent readmission. This is one of the factors that led to the expansion of home care (such as visiting-nurse services) under Medicare. But soon hospitals and insurers realized that there was a potentially safer destination for their patients who were "too well to stay but too sick to go home." That destination was—you guessed it—nursing homes. For their part, the nursing homes were delighted. Their major funder for long-stay permanent residents, Medicaid (I'll get to that in chapter 17), pays them meagerly. The advent of a new group of patients with more acute medical needs—for which insurers were willing to pay more generously—was welcome news for an industry under incredible cost pressures. In many nursing homes this has created two distinct populations of patients: those for whom the nursing home is an extension of the hospital (thus the terms *postacute* or *subacute*) and those for whom it is literally a home.

The problem is that this situation can create more than just poorly matched bedfellows. Sure, while agitated roommates and vacuous dinner companions may be unpleasant and a big quality-of-life issue during your short (one hopes) stay, the relatively recent clash of nursing-home and hospital cultures can play out in ways that could be hazardous to your health.

The use of nursing homes for the last stage of convalescence is not, in theory, a bad idea at all. In many ways, they are far more focused on the things that are critical for recovery, things that hurried hospitals do less well: staying attentive to nutrition, mobility, mood, and ability to function in the community as independently as possible. These days, many of these issues understandably get shortchanged in the hospital, where patients are so incredibly sick that the emphasis has to be on the broad strokes of rescuing them from the medical abyss of a stroke, heart attack, or major trauma. Once that's accomplished, it's off to the next demanding case. The mundane daily chores of simply getting stronger—physically, psychologically, and nutritionally—may not receive the same in-depth attention. (These are among the many contributors to hospitalitis I described in chapter 10.) Transferring to a nursing home for these kinds of basic interventions—once your most pressing medical needs have been dealt with—could be just what the doctor ordered.

What to Do When They Try to "Subacute You"

So how do you evaluate the potential of a subacute-care situation, especially if you're being asked to leave the hospital posthaste? Many patients and families find this an incredibly stressful experience, mostly because of the pace of it. When you get admitted to the hospital for a scheduled admission like an elective surgery, you have an established relationship with the physician caring for you there as well as with the facility; unless you suffer a complication, you have a good idea as to when you will be discharged and where you'll be going (home). But when you're admitted with an unexpected illness that has a vaguer time frame for recovery and prognosis—like pneumonia, a stroke, or a hip fracture—things rarely run on a schedule. Your life and the lives of the people who care about you were probably turned upside down by the admission itself. And now, just as you're getting acclimated and feeling better, you're being asked to shove off to a new facility, sight unseen, that you may never have heard of. What's the place like? Can my friends and family visit? Do I still keep my doctor? What if I need readmission?

Take a deep breath. I'm going to walk you through this unfamiliar world. The cornerstone of my counsel here will make me sound like a travel agent, but here it is: "Know before you go." And to further extend the metaphor, know what to pack. (You'll also discover that these steps help keep you safe if you need to come back to the hospital.) Here's what to do:

Raise the issue yourself. Don't wait for the hospital or the doctor to broach the subject of subacute care. As soon as you hit the hospital—and I mean day one—start a discussion with both your physician and the social worker or case manager assigned to you about whether some kind of rehabilitation might be needed before you return home. What I'm talking about is called discharge planning, and it's never too early to begin. Even if your inquiry is perceived as overkill (which it likely won't be), you've now opened a dialogue about what is needed once you get home—a visiting nurse, a bedside commode, a visiting physical therapist. This is good stuff.

Send a scout ship. It's perfectly reasonable to send a spouse, child, or friend to "scope out" the places your doctors are proposing to send you to. Early in my nursing-home experience, the facility "tours" given that would wind by me were mostly attended by people contemplating a permanent move for a frail parent. These days, there is always a decent smattering of people with relatives facing imminent hospital discharge.

Lower your expectations. I'll just say it: There are exceptions, but most families find the transition from the hospital to subacute care to be jarring. You're leaving an environment with a large professional staff and daily physician interactions for one that moves at a much different pace and may be physically and aesthetically less appealing. You'll also encounter chronically ill patients with cognitive and physical problems that may not exactly be mood-elevating. You need to dig a bit deeper and understand that your needs can probably be better met in an environment like this, especially if you can't care for all of them at home at this stage of illness.

Don't judge a book by its cover. Be wary of crystal chandeliers and marble floors—that's not the basis for determining the quality of a facility. These are often accoutrements that do more to assuage family guilt than help patients get better. Some of the best subacute facilities I've been to were nothing to look at, and some of the worst have been palatial. Drill down and get the facts. If your mom is coming for rehab after a hip fracture, meet the physical therapists and ask them what their experience is. If your husband had a stroke, find out what the speech and language therapist is like. Ask to see a room. Ask to see a private room if there are any.

Ask questions. Be prepared to ask the facility about continuity of care, especially as it relates to the nature and frequency of physician visits. Start with how many subacute patients from your hospital they care for monthly. Often facilities have very structured relationships with the hospitals they work with most frequently; this is generally a good thing. One of the worst nightmares occurs when your family member needs to be readmitted to the hospital and is sent in the middle of the night to *a different hospital*. I have seen it happen dozens of times, and the result is sometimes a disaster. Every nursing home must have a transfer agreement with an acute care hospital. Make it clear to staff where your family member should go if he or she needs to be readmitted, and make sure they know how to reach you in the middle of the night if the need for transfer arises.

Other critical questions: Who will be my wife's physician? How often will he visit? Are there physicians on call in the facility? What if she needs to be readmitted in an emergency? One of the most frustrating things patients and families describe about the transition from hospital to subacute care is the dramatically deemphasized role of the physician. Find out who will be the doc in charge of subacute care; it is unlikely to be your hospital physician. It's also important to understand how the subacute physician will communicate with the physician who provided hospital care. If there is to be subspecialty follow-up, such as with an orthopedist, find out whether the patient will be taken out of the facility for an appointment or if the doctor actually visits (preferable unless there is some technical apparatus that is not available at the facility but is available at the physician's office).

Ask about the nursing home discharge. You may have been so focused on getting *into* the subacute facility that you haven't thought about getting out. How are patients discharged to their homes? My facility often makes a home visit with the patient to see if he or she can negotiate the environment (bathroom, tub, kitchen). Find out what services are available from the subacute facility after you finally do make it home.

Consider proximity to friends and family. I know I've harped on facility quality in much of my earlier advice, but it's also important to be close to the people who'll want to visit. As hospitalization wears on, visitors become less frequent; the crowd gets even thinner once you enter subacute rehabilitation. Often distance is a barrier.

Maintaining your spirit is key during this phase of recovery, and nothing helps more than visitors. If it's a coin toss between two facilities, this is certainly the tiebreaker for me.

Understand your rights regarding subacute rehab. The law varies from state to state, but when your hospitalization ends and you're being sent off to subacute rehab, you do have rights. Most states give you some choice in the process, often asking you to select a few facilities that would be acceptable. If you feel that you're not being listened to, find the social worker responsible for your case and explain your concerns. It may be that a bed is not available in the place of your choice. While you should not have to enter a facility that you dislike or one that is hours from home, you do need to have some flexibility. In many communities subacute beds are hard to come by and you might need to grab a good one when it is made available. Also be aware that the hospital is not simply tossing you out to save money; an acute-care hospital bed that is occupied by a patient who doesn't need acute services could be used for someone who really does.

Failure to Launch: The Hospital Bounce-Back from Subacute Care

---

Because many nursing homes on the receiving end of hospital discharges have not yet adopted the necessary medical infrastructures to adequately care for really sick patients (they are still in "custodial mode"), you may be put at risk for hospital readmission, often on an emergency basis, should your condition worsen. As I said, these places are great at things like rehabilitation, nutrition, and recreational therapy, but when you get sick, you need a doctor, not an art therapist. Whoever said "laughter is the best medicine" was full of shale; when you're truly ill, medicine is the best medicine.

This is the mirror opposite of the problem with hospitals, where the emphasis is on the acute and high-tech while the "softer" aspects of convalescence are often overlooked. On the receiving end, everybody wants their mom's nursing home to have a home-like, noninstitutional feel, and I have no problem with that. The trouble occurs when homes become so deinstitutionalized that they no longer can provide adequate health care to their residents and to the even sicker ones who are being sent from the hospital.

The best example: physician presence and accessibility. In most states, the mandated frequency of physician nursing-home visits is once monthly. Imagine transitioning from a three-week hospitalization, during which you were seen at least daily by your physician and multiple consultants, to a situation in which you'll be seen only once a month. Meanwhile, as you desperately wait for a doctor to examine you and explain what's going on, you may very likely get the full nine yards of paramedical and psychosocial assessments meant for patients who are coming to live at the facility indefinitely: an eye exam, a life review, a dental consultation—important stuff for sure, but not the highest priority if you just had your hip replaced and are trying to learn to climb stairs again so you can return home.

And if the doctor doesn't come, or doesn't come in time, you can become sick to the extent that you require rehospitalization, maybe even repeatedly. To give you a sense of the impact that this all-too-common form of institutional Ping-Pong can have on patients and families, I'll tell you another story.

Mr. J was a very high-functioning lawyer in his midseventies who slipped on the ice one January morning on the way to work. He was not your typical hip-fracture patient insofar as he was male and young (males who develop osteoporotic hip fractures do so a decade later than women, on average). I felt that the fracture was a result more of the trauma than of the state of his bones.

With little else in the way of medical problems, he sailed through the hip repair effortlessly and within a few days was being encouraged to leave the hospital. Since he was a widower and his kids lived in Europe, he was encouraged to get a few weeks of rehabilitation in the subacute unit of a local nursing home.

A very gracious and proper man, he was not one to complain, but later he confided in me that he was unprepared for how impaired other residents of the nursing home were. Over the ensuing weeks I got reports from his family on his progress. He went to therapy and tried his best to integrate himself into the social fabric of the facility. When a social worker invited him to a group arts-and-crafts session, he accepted, even though most of the participants suffered from fairly advanced Alzheimer's disease. He ate in the main dining room, but none of his dining partners could participate in a meaningful conversation because of their memory loss. This was a man who only weeks earlier had argued complex legal matters before a judge.

Still, things seemed to go pretty well, at least at first. But then the dreaded geriatric cascade was set in motion. His mood began to deteriorate after the first week (the surroundings didn't help), and his appetite declined. He became dehydrated and started to develop low-grade delirium. This made him eat less, and he grew even more dehydrated. He was seen only twice by a doctor during a three-week period. When he spiked a fever in the middle of the night, the physician was called and instructed the nurse to send him to the emergency room; this was done by telephone with almost no on-site evaluation (after all, this was a nursing home, not a hospital, right?).

I didn't get to see him during this unraveling, because he was not in a facility where I had privileges. (You remember privileges, right? Doctors need them to admit and/or consult in nursing homes just as in hospitals.) His family had wanted him to have "the best" subacute nursing-home care and had chosen a fancy facility that had no relationship with my hospital, my medical school, or me. I hasten to point out that this was a care-transition problem facilitated by a well-meaning but misguided (and, I suspect, slightly guilt-ridden) family.

Both the medicine and the sociology of what happened in the subsequent emergency-room stay were fascinating. The triage nurse relegated him to low priority because he was not as sick as many of the trauma victims who were there at 3 a.m. When the ER physician called me, he had no awareness of the history of this man; he saw a "confused nursing-home resident" who he thought had dementia rather than delirium. I can't really fault this doc—he had many other priorities to deal with and probably just assumed that the patient had lived at the nursing home for years and confusion was his usual "baseline." To the doc's credit, he noted that I was the man's former doctor when glancing at his electronic medical record; otherwise I would not have been called at all. The patient was certainly in no condition to volunteer this information; he barely knew he was in a hospital.

When I went in to see Mr. J that morning, he was in a corner of the ER, motioning for help. He was thirsty. He didn't know where he was. He needed to use the bathroom but couldn't get off the gurney by himself.

When he got upstairs, I was able to provide a larger life context to the staff caring for him. As his delirium lifted he became more engaged. One of the medical students he interacted with had been a lawyer before switching careers, and my patient took an avuncular interest in him. It was quite sweet and probably lifted his mood as much as a newly prescribed antidepressant. Soon he was well enough to go back to the nursing home for subacute care. This time everyone was more attuned to his "station" in life, and his new med-student buddy made periodic friendly visits to him. Eventually Mr. J got well enough to go home.

How could this patient's second hospitalization have been avoided? His well-meaning family could have done the due-diligence I advised earlier about selecting a rehabilitation facility, especially with regard to physician coverage and transfer policies. Don't pick a facility based on accoutrements and furnishings first; find out about the medical presence there, the facility's relationship to the hospital you're being discharged from, and how things work when the you-know-what hits the fan. In a nutshell, consider this: If you were to get sick in the facility you're considering, who would care for you and where would they ship you if your problem can't be managed on-site? As I said, every nursing home is required to have a primary transfer agreement or relationship with at least one hospital. Find out which one it is!

And Finally, the "Nail-Biter": Discharge Home from the Emergency Room

---

Okay, I've covered going home from the hospital, going to subacute rehabilitation from the hospital, and even coming back to the hospital from subacute care. But there is one more movement to this concerto that I've so far avoided. Maybe that's because it's the one that gives physicians caring for aging adults the biggest bellyache. I'm talking about the discharge home from the emergency room. *Discharge*, of course, is a relative term here, because you haven't actually been admitted to the hospital, just the "cattle chute" (as one of my patients likes to call his ER experience).

Why do geriatricians loathe the ER discharge to home? I guess that falls under the heading of "damned if you do and damned if you don't." I've spent an entire chapter regaling you with ageist misadventures that can occur in the hospital and yet others that spring from the same landmines in the emergency room. As a geriatrician, you'd think I would be delighted when a patient is declared fit (by me or someone else) to be sprung from the hospital, especially from the ER.

Well, yes and no. Sure, it's always a good sign when someone of any age seems well enough to go home from the hospital. But with nearly every older emergency-room patient I've discharged (and I'm excluding patients with straightforward minor problems like poison ivy, bee stings, or minor cuts and abrasions), I always get a gnawing feeling that I'm missing something and that he or she would be better served by a little more observation. Or I worry that if something goes wrong at home, no one will be around to notice and bring the patient back to see me. One of my "gero-friendly" emergency-medicine doctors nicely summarizes his experience with many older people this way: They're too well to be sent upstairs to a hospital bed but a little too sick to go home. Or, as I like to say, "You can go home now, Mr. Smith, but I'm going to be biting my nails!"

Earlier I made the case that many of the worst problems older people face in the hospital are compounded in hurried ER environments. It should be no surprise, then, that the problems patients face during hospital discharge are compounded in ER discharge, and for the same reasons: ER physicians know patients for a matter of hours instead of years. They have no inkling of what kind of home or family you're being sent back to (and no time to find out). Their ability to coordinate the kinds of home-care services and follow-up I alluded to earlier is more limited. It's harder for them to get you oxygen at home from the ER. And they can't promise that the visiting nurse will come tomorrow, as they might be able to if this were a hospital discharge. There's no real "discharge summary" from the ER in most facilities I've worked at, and even if there were, it's unlikely that it could be expeditiously dictated, typed, and conveyed to your primary care doctor before you saw him the next day.

How does one address these additional layers of potential calamity? All of the previously described strategies apply—most notably, taking matters into your own hands. Make sure that there is direct communication between the ER doc and yours. Understand exactly what tests are pending, including X-rays that have not been officially read by the radiologist when you go home in the middle of the night. If you are to see a physician for follow-up, make sure that those X-ray films are available to him when you leave the ER—ask to take copies with you, as they belong to you. And understand exactly what symptoms should be cause for concern and might result in a return ER visit.

No doubt about it, getting safely and honorably discharged from any health-care environment reminds me of the famous air-travel joke I used to open the chapter: Flying isn't dangerous; it's the landing that's the problem. The irony, of course, is that every significant health-care interaction has to end with a landing somewhere, and that's where a good deal of your due diligence needs to happen.

So I prefer to think of another good news/bad news air-travel metaphor when I consider the hospital-discharge process, one that emphasizes the control you can have. It also has relevance to any aspect of aging.

The bad news: Time flies. The good news: You're the pilot.

Chapter 13

Maybe You're Not the Problem

Disability Caused by Places and Not People
(or Their Diseases)

A man is distressed over the expense of a prostate operation his doctor has recommended, so he seeks the advice of a friend who had the procedure.

"You should do what I did," says the friend. "Go to Home Depot."

The man looks at him, incredulous.

"They do that there?" he asks.

"Yup," his friend replies proudly. "Any operation for $199.99!"

The man decides to go through with it, and months later they see each other again.

"How did it go?" the friend asks.

"It was okay," the man replies curtly.

Now concerned about his referral, the friend inquires, "Any side effects?"

The man responds sheepishly, "Well, every time I pee, the garage door opens."

I don't care if you're fifty or a hundred: The time to think about where you'll be living for a thirty- or forty-year period after retirement—and how you're going to pay for it—is now. Yes, I said now. It may seem like a long way off, but trust me, it sneaks up on you, and a big boomer mistake is not thinking about this question soon enough. It's a bit like the problem of saving for retirement, except for this exercise you need to devote emotional and intellectual capital in addition to the green stuff.

Believe me, I recognize that your preference (unless you're the most unusual patient I have ever encountered) is to remain in your own home for the rest of your natural life. This chapter is about working to achieve that goal. You have the best chance of remaining in *the least restrictive environment* (big geriatric catch-phrase) if you think about this sooner rather than later. Making your current home (or the one you're building or about to purchase or rent) "aging friendly" should begin when you're relatively young and should take into account the kinds of medical problems you may have already developed or are statistically likely to develop. This way, as they occur, you'll be prepared to meet them head-on, not only with nonageist medical care but with a home environment that minimizes excess disability.

As a geriatrician I often have the task of recommending that people move from their lifelong residences to a new environment. And I hate it. (The only thing I hate about as much is telling people they cannot drive.) But long before this, there is a whole range of things I do to try to keep them right where they are, often for long periods of time. Here's the kicker: These interventions are under-publicized, underappreciated, and underutilized. What's more, while some of them are expensive, many are dirt cheap. And most are so simple and straightforward that even a kid could figure them out and implement them. But we adults often miss them, I believe, because the topic of potentially leaving one's home or losing some degree of control or independence is so emotionally charged that we go immediately to an irrational place when the subject is so much as broached.

This chapter is about interventions aimed at keeping you as independent as possible for as long as possible. Much of this can be accomplished with some clever tweaking of your environment than can be incredibly unobtrusive if done correctly. A large part of what I do in my practice as it relates to long-term care is trying to get patients to understand my mind-set and rationale. In asking them to consider accepting more help at home, modifications to their home, or even a new living environment altogether, I'm not trying to take away their independence, which is what they understandably fear most. Rather, I'm trying to protect it. Dangerous living environments, in addition to producing anxiety disorders among spouses, adult children, and geriatricians, almost invariably result in more disability than you started with, either from direct injury or from a complete blowup of existing medical problems that are neglected in unsanitary, unsafe, or unmonitored home environments. Often when this happens, a nursing home—admittedly the most restrictive of all living arrangements—becomes the only option, and that's a real shame if it resulted from avoidable problems. As I said in an earlier chapter, geriatricians hate excess disability because it is avoidable.

Both the physical structure and the location of the dwelling you call home—and in which you hope to spend your later working or "preretirement" years—should be chosen and modified with forethought if you want to stay put as long as possible. Think about who you really are, functionally; not who you would like to be. If you're in your fifties and have been diagnosed with a chronic illness, it will likely progress, even if you take really good care of yourself. Don't build a chalet in the Himalayas if you have emphysema. If your spouse is newly diagnosed with and in the earliest stages of rheumatoid arthritis, that multilevel brownstone you're renovating should be zoned for an elevator; otherwise stairs may eventually force you to move. A colleague of mine—in her thirties, mind you—refused to take a job at a prestigious teaching hospital in a relatively inaccessible suburban area because she suffers from a congenital eye disease that will someday, probably twenty years from now, render her unable to see well enough to drive. She wanted a big city with taxis everywhere so she could raise her kids in the same place over the next two decades. These are tough things to think about—a bit like buying life insurance. But it's the responsible thing to do, and in this case, *you* are the beneficiary, not your heirs. (In fact, as I'll explain in chapter 17, if there's anything left over for them when you kick the bucket, I contend that you may have done some serious miscalculating.)

The first place to make a down payment on your future independence? The floor under your feet and the roof over your head.

The Role of Home Modifications as We Age

Every year at our annual geriatrics picnic for the faculty and their families, my wife makes a beeline for her favorite faculty member. No, it's not one of my superbly trained internists with years of experience and clinical wisdom, nor one of our unusually empathetic social workers, nor even a nurse with exemplary patient-advocacy skills. No, my wife heads directly for Rosemary Bakker, the most unusual faculty member in my program. You see, Rosemary has dual degrees: one in gerontology and another in interior design. She has dedicated her life to making sure that homes don't produce excess disability by making sure they're age-appropriate. My wife invariably manages to get a little complimentary consultation from Rosemary and usually emerges with swatches of fabric in tow.

Rosemary began her career the way most interior designers do: using her exquisite taste to help people furnish their new digs. But when her mother developed Alzheimer's disease and subsequently broke her hip, Rosemary became obsessed with trying to find ways of bridging the seemingly disparate worlds of aging and interior design. I'm convinced that she has not only bridged them but is now starting a commercial revolution. And I believe that someday every Home Depot and Target in the United States will have an aging section with products we've tested together. We'll have freestanding stores with all manner of aging-friendly products for boomers. And I'll know that Rosemary's ship has really come in when fancy streets like Madison Avenue and Rodeo Drive have high-end purveyors of these products next to Armani and Bottega Veneta. The rest of us can shop at the local "Gray-Mart," where they roll back the prices to the 1970s or '80s.

To watch Rosemary walk into someone's home and scan the landscape for accidents waiting to happen reminds me of those brainteasers on a restaurant kiddie menu, where you're asked to identify the small differences in two virtually identical pictures. In less than three minutes she'll find the throw rug that slides across the floor, the room with inadequate illumination, the floor glare that's dangerous for a patient with cataracts, as well as five other time bombs I never would have considered or even heard of before.

Rosemary will tell you that the design of most dwellings in existence today was intended for twenty-one-year-olds, even though that's not who's living in them. The result: excess disability and problems in daily functioning that result as much from the environment as from the effects of disease or other physical conditions. Just a few of dozens of examples she loves to point out:

- Windows or doors that require too much force for an older person to open safely. I've seen several osteoporosis (thinning bone) fractures in the spines of older New Yorkers who were simply trying to open windows that had been "painted shut" over the winter.
- Lighting levels that are fine for thirtysomethings but pose a fall risk in patients with macular degeneration or other eye problems. In one study we conducted among our homebound house-call patients, we took a light meter into their homes to measure illumination at critical spots like the bathroom sink, where many people take their morning medicines. The result: The average level was less than 10 percent of what lighting experts recommend—*for younger people without visual problems.* Pretty scary, given that we asked people to turn on all their lights before we measured!'
- Treacherous walking surfaces—rugs or floors or sills between rooms that cannot accommodate our changing gait as we age.
- Doorbells and telephones that cannot be heard by patients with even a mild degree of hearing impairment, leading to greater social isolation.

- Tubs you can't get into or out of when you have arthritic hips or knees. You either fall and break your hip or stop bathing altogether. I assure you that either outcome will shrink your circle of friends.
- Stair widths or heights that can't be negotiated safely by people with neurological problems like Parkinson's disease.
- Appliances and utensils that people with manual-dexterity issues can't operate. If you can't use your old can opener, you may not eat. I've seen more than one patient get a million-dollar evaluation for weight loss (e.g., CAT scans, colonoscopies, and multiple subspecialty consultations) when the culprit was not medical and the solution was disarmingly low-tech (in this case an electric can opener)!
- Dwelling layouts that are impractical as gait or mobility slows. One of my patients was in the midst of invasive bladder testing for new urinary incontinence when I realized that he had just moved and his bathroom was too far down the hall for him to make it there in time. His urologist was unaware of this and ordered the studies. How's that for excess disability created by the environment?

Rosemary's Web site www.environmentalgeriatrics.com walks patients, families, doctors, and other health-care professionals through the process of making a home more gero-friendly. Another of her Web sites, http://thiscaringhome.org, is geared to families trying to modify homes for patients with Alzheimer's disease and those with "normal" memory loss as well.

Home Modifications That Can Save Your Life (and Don't Involve Moving Walls or a Home Equity Loan)

Youth, as I've said before, is indeed wasted on the young. It's difficult for twentysomethings to imagine their own mortality or even minor disability. Sounds like *their* problem, right? Unfortunately, that's not quite the case. Guess who's dreaming up designs for the "places" and "things" for an aging America. Yup, it's those fear-nothing youngsters. Most dwellings in existence today were designed by young people for young people. And that's a recipe for excess disability.

Far too many people (or their medical conditions) are being "blamed" for their inability to function safely and independently at home, in the workplace, and in society, when the problem may be mostly (or entirely) due to the environment. We've been building things for generations expecting few people to live past fifty, but when they do, we're surprised when the environment becomes unmanageable. And again, you don't have to be that old! If you're fifty-five, try opening the freezer of a high-end refrigerator. If you're sixty, try timing your hotel entry through one of those hotel revolving doors with a small piece of luggage. If you're over sixty, have you ever tried to cross a wide city street before the light changed and found that it's a close call? I'm a relatively younger man, and sometimes I find myself suddenly unable to easily maneuver in the kitchen: There are more jars I don't have the strength to open, more manual can openers I can't operate, more recipes I can't read without glasses, and I find myself standing on chairs to reach shelves—the same shelves I swear I could reach just a few years ago.

Sure, it would be easy to blame my worsening balance, eyesight, and manual dexterity for any of these situations, but if my external world had been crafted with someone my age in mind (and why not—fifty is as good an arbitrary age for product design as twenty), the thought would never cross my mind (or anyone else's) that I had a problem. I could argue credibly that my "disability" was created by my home and its accoutrements and had little to do with me. It would be like blaming an Olympic swimmer for losing a race when there wasn't enough water in the pool, or booing a supermodel's runway performance when the designer made her wear a dress that was two sizes too small or too big.

Yet when I make these arguments to families and patients, many refuse to adopt simple changes in their home that could minimize disability. The reasons range from expense (no excuse, see below) to ageism. Yes, ageism. Several of my image-conscious patients have decided against making home modifications (such as installing higher toilets or grab bars), but not because they don't believe these will help. They do. Amazingly, they're concerned that people coming into their homes will think them less youthful and "hip." Well, I'd rather suffer from not being "hip" than from getting a broken one!

Most dwellings in existence today can be modified to meet the needs of just about everyone at every age. What's more, you don't need to spend a ton of money to do it. Here are some quick fixes that can extend not only the useful life of your home but maybe your own life, too.

The bathroom: This is the most dangerous place in the home, what with hard surfaces, water that makes floors slippery, nothing but your birthday suit between you and the tile and tub, and, to top it all off, poor access to a telephone should something go wrong. Even if money is tight, this is the one place where spending more may be worth it (for example, changing to shallower tubs or replacing them with walk-in showers so you don't have to be an Olympic hurdler to bathe). A simple fix, installing grab bars, will make it easier to enter and exit the tub or shower and use the toilet, and reduces your chances of a preventable fall. (Hate the industrial-chrome look? Well, they now come in a variety of tasteful colors to match your décor, so you can be safer without feeling like you're in the disabled-access stalls at the public library's restroom. One of my patient's artistic daughters even described her "rails" as "cool.") Many people find it easier to bathe while seated in a bath chair, using a handheld shower hose that attaches to the tub spout or shower arm. Be sure the bottom of the bathtub has antiskid strips or a mat. And one more thing: Don't forget to equip your tub faucet or boiler with antiscald devices, which either prevent your water from getting too hot at the source or sound an alarm to tell you that the bath you're about to sit in is dangerously toasty.

Lighting: As we age, we need more light to compensate for changes to the visual system. When was the last time you updated the lighting in your home? (And I'm not talking about sconces and lampshades; I mean the *actual illumination*.) Simple changes like using higher-wattage bulbs (make sure they're safe for the fixture you're putting them into) or adding additional lights in strategic locations can make a world of difference. And don't overlook "path lighting" in corridors, as many falls occur not in rooms but en route from one to another.

Flooring: The surfaces on which we walk can interact with gait changes to produce potential difficulty. My preference: Use the same or similar surfaces throughout the dwelling, because it is often at "transition points" between rooms (and surfaces) that falling occurs. Area rugs can be a huge danger, especially if they slide or have edges that curl up to produce trip hazards. If you insist on area rugs, use double-sided carpet tape to make sure they lie flat at every point and don't slide. Deep carpeting is a bad idea. (Most geriatricians and physical therapists are not expecting "shag" carpeting to make a comeback anytime soon, and we're just delighted.) A better choice is a nonslip flooring surface that can be easily installed. And while the slipperiness (or "grippiness") quotient of the flooring surface is important, there are other factors you should be thinking about, too. Vinyl has more "give" on impact in a fall than porcelain tile, for example, and lowers the chance of a fracture if you do slip. (Like a glass or an egg that you might drop, you want to "bounce" rather than "crack.") Vinyl also is warmer than tile and easier to stand on for long periods of time. And let's not forget color and glare: Shiny surfaces are tough for people with certain kinds of visual problems, and darker surfaces may make any obstacles on the floor difficult to see.

Bright colors: The use of color in almost any home furnishing, surface, or item can work wonders as we age. It can make it easier to find items (like a red coffee mug on a white coffee table) or avoid missteps (a bright-colored bedspread that contrasts sharply with the floor color so the edges can be safely identified). Never choose the same color for a seating surface and the floor: Your butt could easily miss the target.

Furnishings: Chairs should have arms and not be too deep, so that it's easy to rise from them; the same goes for couches. Rather than replace what you have, get higher cushions that you can't sink into. Again, contrast the colors of seats with the colors of floors to avoid accidents.

Kitchen items: Can openers, potato peelers, jar openers, scissors, and other utensils are available in ergonomically designed models that are easier to use as we get older—less force and manual dexterity is needed to get the jobs done. A great Web site that includes reviews of these products is run by the National Resource Center on Supportive Housing and Home Modification: www.homemods.org.

Simple technology fixes: Some incredibly cool technology is on the horizon to keep us boomers happy, healthy, wise, and safe, but you need not wait to get cracking. Right now there are simple and inexpensive technological improvements you can take advantage of to make your life easier and better. For those with visual impairment, there are telephones with large number buttons. For those with hearing loss, there are doorbells and phones that flash lights rather than "ring" and clocks that vibrate your pillow instead of sounding an alarm. If you don't want to spend money on an expensive hearing aid, Walkman-like devices available at your local electronics store for less than fifty bucks can change your life—a great way to test-drive a hearing aid.*

---

*These devices can be found on the Web, but if you're not an Internet consumer, Radio Shack has a version. It's called amplified stereo listener with 3-band equalizer (model: 33-1097 | catalog #: 33-1097). http://www.radioshack.com/product/index.jsp? productId=2104057&cp=&sr=1&origkw=amplifier+listener&kw=amplifier+listener& parentPage=search.

Many state and local governments and private community agencies that serve older adults can provide financial assistance for modifications like grab bars or for simple apartment repairs. To find out if there are low- or no-cost government services for eligible adults, check with your local department of aging, found either in the phonebook or through the Eldercare locator, which can be accessed by calling 800-677-1116 (weekdays from 9 a.m. to 8 p.m.) or found on the Web at www.eldercare.gov.

Deciding When It's Time to Move

I love the idea of staying at home, and I love environmental modifications with that goal in mind. But I'm also a pragmatist. Even if you're Bob Vila, you may ultimately run up against the simple fact that the effectiveness of modifications wanes over time if your mobility and/or other problems outstrip them. And that, my friends, brings us to one of the most difficult responsibilities of an aging specialist: knowing when to encourage a patient to pick up stakes and move, or helping people get older loved ones to come to the realization that the time has come. And even if you've gotten everybody on the same page, the story's not over. You've got to know what the options are. Which brings us to the next chapter.

Chapter 14

Homes Away from Home as We Age

Where thou art—that—is Home.
—Emily Dickinson

Environmental modifications can go a long way toward keeping you or a parent in your own home, but sometimes health issues or other problems leave us with no other choice but to shove off for new shores. In some cases the decision to leave your house or apartment is cut-and-dried, dictated by medical or environmental circumstances that are unfortunate and completely beyond your control. An acute devastating illness such as a stroke might make independent community living no longer possible. Sudden bereavement can mean the spouse who did all the day-to-day property maintenance is no longer present. Adult children who were pitching in may need to move out of the area, and you simply can't do the things they helped you with. Or financial reversals can make upkeep of a large property impractical or wasteful. Another common instigator of a move is that the safety of a neighborhood has deteriorated over a fifty-year period of home ownership; perhaps a parent was even the victim of a burglary or other crime that set this very important discussion in motion.

Far more common, however, are slowly developing medical or social issues that put the question of "a move" somewhere on the horizon but without a precise time frame. This can be a mixed blessing. On one hand, you have the time to plan and think through the multiple economic, social, and medical issues in the light of day and in the calmness of a noncrisis situation, perhaps as early as in your fifties. The downside is that human beings tend to procrastinate when there is no fire pressing them to action, especially when it comes to issues that are not terribly pleasant to think about.

Having presided over literally thousands of dwelling transitions in both urban and suburban environments for patients of all ages and their adult children, I urge you—no, I plead with you—in the strongest terms to think preemptively about these issues. If the very thought of moving to some new environment where you'll be getting some enhanced services (ranging from lawn care to medical attention) makes you feel as if you're losing control, you have no idea how much control you might have to relinquish when a move has to be made abruptly without any prior planning.

In this chapter I'm also going to talk about something else that is bound to spook you: nursing homes. Don't think a chapter about nursing homes or other long-term care facilities applies to you? Perhaps you think you're immune because you're one of those people whose spouse or kids promised you they'd never put you in a nursing home. I've got news for you. As someone who has spent thousands of hours working in assisted-living facilities and nursing homes, allow me to describe the people who live there: They are people whose family members promised them they would never place them in a nursing home.

But with regard to moving, this chapter is not just about nursing homes, which most people always associate (understandably but erroneously) with a complete loss of independence. It's also about environments that afford some assistance while promoting as much independence as possible, so you or a loved one can live safely and comfortably. The goal is finding what geriatricians like to refer to as "the least-restrictive alternative." This is one of the central ideas in geriatrics, whether we're talking about which walking aid to prescribe or which assisted-living facility to recommend.

So let's look systematically at the places boomers and their parents think about when considering housing options—what they are, how they're paid for, and what kinds of patients are appropriate for each one. It's a useful exercise to go through with me, because if you do this on your own, you'll encounter a bewildering array of terms that will only confuse you, especially if you're getting your information from people trying to sell you something—like a spot in an assisted-living facility or long-term-care insurance. Lucky for you, you've got a geriatrician to take you on this little real estate tour to give you the "big picture."

Some of the most common terms you'll encounter as soon as you begin to research living options are "life care," "assisted living," "skilled nursing facility," "continuing retirement community," and "senior campus," describing different kinds of facilities. In the following sections I'll discuss them all, in reverse order with regard to the amount of independence they offer, starting with those that cater to the most functionally impaired residents.

Skilled Nursing Facilities

A skilled nursing facility, or SNF (sometimes pronounced "sniff" by people in the industry), is probably what you think of when you think of long-term care—a nursing home. Yes, these are for people with Alzheimer's disease, stroke victims, and those with other diseases that have rendered them unable to live independently. Of all long-term-care residents, those in nursing homes are generally the most impaired when it comes to activities of daily living (ADL),* such as dressing, bathing, and eating. And yes, most nursing home residents are there for an indefinite stay. But as I described in the chapters on hospitalization and discharge, nursing homes have also become important places to get rehabilitation or extend recovery after hospitalization.

Among many other names you might hear to describe a nursing home are *long-term-care facility, custodial care,* and *home for the aged.* Also, because subacute rehabilitation after the hospital is a far more lucrative business than the care of long-term residents, many nursing

---

* ADLs (activities of daily living): bathing, dressing, eating, mobility from bed to chair, using the bathroom, grooming. These are generally rated as (1) needs no assistance, (2) needs some assistance, or (3) needs total assistance.

homes these days have names that emphasize the rehabilitation component to the extent that you can't tell they're a nursing home (even
though they continue to quietly house a group of long-term residents).
So expect to see nursing homes with *convalescence center* and *rehabilitation center* in their names, even though they do not technically meet
the criteria for a formal rehab center (I'll describe that shortly).

Nursing home care is expensive and getting more so. No matter
how much money you've saved over a lifetime, you can blow through
it in no time at all if a stay becomes prolonged or indefinite. In fact,
nursing home care at some point impoverishes the vast majority
of people who live there, whereupon they apply for Medicaid (the
same program that pays for medical care for younger indigent people
in general). As a result, the major "payer" for nursing home care
in the United States is not families (at least not directly), nor is it
Medicare (the government program that pays for health care once
you turn sixty-five). Rather, it's state governments in the form of
Medicaid dollars. (Medicaid, unlike Medicare, is a jointly funded
state and federal program, whereas Medicare is federally funded.)
I'll talk a bit more about Medicare and Medicaid in chapter 17.

There's one big exception to this setup: Medicare does come into
play in nursing home care for a limited nursing home stay, but only
on the heels of a hospitalization. The government (the nation's single
largest purchaser of health care) figured out that just about *anything*
is cheaper than being in the hospital. Some of the patients who may
have been flirting with the need for a nursing home prior to their
hospitalization never regain enough function to return home, and
the majority of these folks eventually enter the Medicaid rolls.

Assisted Living

The next most restrictive place on the hit parade is the assisted-
living facility, or ALF. Watching the evolution of assisted living
over the course of my career has been fascinating. When I was a
young buck in geriatrics, the mission and clientele of ALFs were
pretty straightforward: They took on people who weren't quite sick

enough for a nursing home (or still had enough of their "marbles") but not quite well enough to live alone safely. This filled a real need for many guilt-ridden adult children who, on the one hand, felt just terrible about sending dear old Mom to the nursing home before her time (where she would be the undisputed valedictorian of her profoundly impaired class) but, on the other hand, did not have the time, room, resources, or marital fortitude to have her move in with them. These early ALF residents had minor or no impairment in ADLs but significant fraying of their IADLS* (instrumental activities of daily living), such as preparing meals and handling money.

All these folks needed was a little supervision, basic house-keeping services, maybe some assistance in getting to the dining room, and someone to respond almost immediately in the event of a true emergency, such as a fall or an unexpected acute illness. For them to live alone meant hiring twenty-four-hour live-in help to be around for the rare misadventure—wasteful if people don't really need ongoing minute-to-minute assistance.

And it worked (and still does) for the right older adult and his or her family. Peace of mind for both is a large chunk of what you're buying when you enter assisted living. Most of my patients in good assisted-living environments love the housekeeping and laundry services. They don't have to pick up after themselves or worry about clean linens, and they like the fact that they can still cook if they want to, without being obligated to prepare a meal if they can't or prefer not to. (Note to self: Write business plan for high-end assisted-living facility for teenagers, as opposed to the not-for-profit one I currently preside over with Mrs. Lachs.)

For the most part, this arrangement worked pretty well in the 1980s and '90s. Patients stayed in assisted living for as long as possible. Once ADL impairment or general frailty became too severe, there was really no choice but to move to a skilled nursing facility,

---

* IADLs (instrumental activities of daily living): preparing a meal, shopping, handling basic money chores, housekeeping.

and those beds were plentiful. Medicaid or other reimbursement was available when patients needed to move to nursing home care. A new crop of mildly impaired older people moved in to fill the vacated space at the assisted-living facility.

But a funny thing happened as America got older and nursing home care became more and more stigmatized: No one wanted to leave assisted living, even long after they became too sick or frail to stay there. Exacerbating the situation in some communities was a shortage of nursing home beds (whose numbers are highly regulated because they expand the Medicaid rolls and therefore state budget deficits) coupled with profound overbuilding and overexpansion of assisted-living facilities. Many ALFs could not fill their beds and began losing money or went bust. Those that did stay in business had every incentive to keep their beds full rather than have their tenants leave for nursing homes, so they sometimes kept patients whose frailty exceeded their ability to provide care; these folks probably would have been better served by traditional nursing homes. Families, for their part, were delighted, because they were not responsible "for moving Mom or Dad to the nursing home." In the same way that nursing home residents were sicker and becoming more like the hospital patients of a decade earlier, assisted-living facilities had patients who would earlier have been placed in nursing homes in that same era, and they needed more than the occasional helping hand. They needed to be turned to prevent bedsores. They needed help not just with preparing a meal but sometimes with eating it, or getting in and out of bed, or with medication supervision.

These "care mismatches" still persist in many parts of the United States and have left the federal government wondering whether they should be overseeing assisted living with the same vigor and scrutiny they give to regulating nursing homes. In fact, many of us who work in the field of elder abuse believe that the headline-grabbing nursing home scandals of the 1970s (which helped lead to their regulation) are about to happen again with assisted-living facilities.

How is this relevant to you or a loved one who is considering assisted living? It serves as the basis for several of the medical questions you should be asking the staff of any assisted-living facility you're checking out. Later in this chapter I lay out specific advice on how to evaluate a long-term-care facility at any level of service—a skilled nursing home, independent housing—but the tendency by patients or families to over- or underestimate their medical needs is most dangerous in assisted living, because medical services can be so limited and vary from facility to facility (and from state to state). This is also true of staffing and the quality of staff training.

So with apologies to David Letterman, here are . . .

The Top Five Mistakes Patients and Families Make in Evaluating Assisted-Living Facilities

1. **Underestimating care needs:** Often adult children have not lived with a parent for some time, and social gatherings and other nonchallenging settings are not good venues for getting a clear picture of how marginally (or well) someone might be functioning. It's often only when a caregiving spouse dies or needs to be hospitalized that the full extent of impairment becomes unmasked, because that spouse may have been quietly filling in the gaps for some time.

2. **Overestimating care needs:** Here's the other side of the coin: I've seen patients placed in nursing homes when they could easily have been cared for in a good assisted-living facility or even at home with some augmented services. Families often believe that getting Mom or Dad "the most care possible" is the considerate thing to do, but this also may put him or her in an overly restrictive environment. When patients are "overassisted" their skills can decay. The best example: A patient gets a beautiful new wheelchair and then stops walking. It's easier than physical therapy, and many of my patients love it, but it creates excess disability. Tough love is good here.

3. **Overemphasizing amenities and decor:** Suffice it to say that some of the most impressive long-term-care facilities I've seen were nothing to look at. Conversely, some of the most "well appointed" left much to be desired on the medical front.

4. **Failing to consider the impact of geography and social networks:** Can you recall a time in your life when you had to pull up roots and leave your friends for a job, school, or other life circumstance? Having to make new friends is difficult and anxiety-provoking at any age—ask any child who has had to make such a move during the school year. When we move, we leave not only our physical dwelling but also our friends and daily contacts, increasing the risk of social isolation. This risk grows more severe when you go to a new long-term-care facility. I won't be coy about it: Many people don't like visiting these environments. (I've got some ageist theories about this.) Thus, the buddies you've left behind may have two barriers to overcome if they want to visit: distance and prejudice. And as we've discussed, social isolation can cause big problems as we get older, yet I often watch families select distant facilities over ones nearby because of the décor, the view, or some other similarly less-critical parameter.

5. **Overall poor due diligence:** This is a big decision, one of the biggest you'll ever make, and needs to be treated with the utmost seriousness and thoroughness. Later in this chapter I'll give you highly prescriptive advice on how to approach this issue with eyes wide open and armed with the right information.

Independent Senior Housing

Next on the list are the housing alternatives available for the most able-bodied older people. I'll refer to these generally as "independent senior housing," but in this basket I'm lumping a huge number of living arrangements. They include NORCs (naturally occurring retirement communities), in which a population of individuals who have grown older together decide to "stay put" in an apartment building or housing complex so they can remain socially integrated and have access to "aging-friendly" services (such as a transportation van to shopping facilities or a blood-pressure clinic on-site). Other examples include housing sponsored, introduced, or supported by a local not-for-profit agency or a local government that believes its older constituents are part of the community and should be able to remain there if they wish to. This kind of support sends a terrific message to everyone. "It takes a village" doesn't just apply to raising kids. Anytime communities rally around their most vulnerable citizens, everybody benefits. An outstanding example of this commitment is Beacon Hill Village in Boston. The community's Web site, www.beaconhillvillage.org, describes its remarkable efforts to bring services to older adults in their home and even offers advice on how you might export its model to your own community.

Another form of independent senior housing is a development designed as a community for older people because that's the lifestyle they want. Such developments aren't "naturally occurring" but are planned and built by for-profit companies and real estate developers. There is also government-sponsored subsidized housing for middle-income or low-income older people who cannot afford local rents. The best way to identify such resources in your community is through the local agency on aging (AAA), which should be listed in the blue pages of the phone book, or through the national AAA Web site at www.eldercarelocator.com. The U.S. Department of Housing and Urban Development has a Web site (www.hud.gov/ groups/seniors.cfm) that can help you identify subsidized senior housing, but expect a waiting list in most cases. If you're in the market for high-end senior housing, the real estate section of your local paper is a good bet.

The Whole Enchilada: Life-Care or Continuing-Care Retirement Communities

Finally, let's talk about the "everything under one roof" approach to housing for older adults: so-called life-care communities or continuing-care retirement communities (CCRCs). These, too, come in a number of permutations and configurations, with various ways to pay. In general, I'm a big fan of CCRCs when they're planned and managed correctly.

In the classic CCRC, all levels of care are offered. At the highest levels of functioning are older adults who are completely independent; their homes often resemble private apartments or town houses. They may choose to come to a communal area for meals or use other services offered by the CCRC (such as housekeeping) if they wish. On the same campus are patients with more medical or social frailty who receive more extensive care. This might include the assisted-living component, where residents have all meals provided and have assistance in their apartments with some basic care needs; or traditional skilled nursing care, where residents are highly ADL-impaired and require assistance with dressing or grooming. Many CCRCs also provide day care for adults, so their children can work during the day but still keep Mom at home.

In general, there are two ways to pay for CCRC care: a monthly fee (much like rent) that varies based on the intensity of the services you require; or an *equity model*, in which a substantial up-front fee is paid, along with some monthly carrying charges. There are also combinations and permutations of the two. In the most comprehensive model, the entry fee keeps you in the facility for the rest of your life—from independence to hospice—irrespective of the particular resources you require. This usually means you can have the reassurance of knowing exactly what your housing costs will be for the rest of your life and cease worrying about someday having to find another place to live or another level of service somewhere else. I always encourage families to consider an option like this if they have the resources, not only for the economic peace of mind but for a more powerful reason as well: When a life-care facility has made this deal with you, it's in its very best interest to keep you as healthy and as independent as possible. Why? Because the frailer you become and the more you need the labor-intensive parts of the CCRC (such as the skilled nursing facility), the more your care costs. So it serves the facility's interests to conduct wellness programs, exercise classes, and a whole variety of activities intended to keep you fit and independent. It is one of the very rare situations in American medicine where the goals of health care and the goals of finance are completely aligned: Good medicine and good business meet, because the healthiest patients are the least expensive ones.

Another benefit of the CCRC model: You're uprooted only once. One move from a lifelong home is traumatic enough for most people. Imagine having made that transition successfully, only to have to do it again a year or two later when a facility does not have the capability to address your worsening medical problems. Most CCRCs permit you to stay on the same campus for the entirety of your stay, over decades if needed. This is especially important if you enter the facility with a spouse; should one of you develop medical problems requiring a higher level of care than the other, a CCRC obviates the often heartbreaking decision to have to move away from a loved one because the facility doesn't offer the range of services necessary to serve you both.

That flexibility can have other benefits. A facility with a full range of services (including postacute care) can permit your recently hospitalized loved one to return to the same campus, easing the transition from the hospital.

The incredible flexibility of CCRCs was underscored for me a number of years ago when I visited one north of New York City in my role as director of geriatrics for my health-care system. A couple in their eighties, both high functioning, lived in a completely independent portion of the facility (basically a lovely two-bedroom townhouse). They experienced a jolt when the husband was admitted to the local hospital after a bowel perforation from diverticulitis. His surgery and the subsequent two-week hospitalization was predictably debilitating, and when it came time for discharge, there was no way he could return to his apartment with his wife; he needed more supervision and care for his surgical incision, which was slow to heal. What he really needed was postacute rehabilitation in a skilled portion of the CCRC to make sure he was supervised during meals, to see that he got his medications, and to check his vital signs. He also needed to have blood drawn periodically. If everything went perfectly, he was at least a month away from returning to true independence and back to their town house.

But there was a snag. Unfortunately, no beds were available in the "postacute" section of the facility. The hospital, eager to discharge him (probably for reasons I described in chapter 10), was about to send him to rehabilitation in another facility across town. This was a bad idea for a number of reasons: They didn't know him at the new place, he couldn't have his usual physician following him there, and worst of all, his wife didn't drive and wouldn't be able to participate in the emotional component of his recovery.

His facility's solution was ingenious: Since this was a full-fledged CCRC with a variety of services—including a home-care agency and a medical adult day-care program for people in the local community—it was able to cobble together a way to keep his recovery on campus. A creative administrator decided that during the day he would place the man in day care, where he could be monitored and have his medications administered, then use the CCRC's home-care service to put a home health aide in the man's apartment at night so his wife could have peace of mind and an additional set of hands to help her until he was back on his feet. This intervention helped to keep the man where he wanted to be—at home with his wife—and at considerably lower cost than if he had been kept in a nursing home full time for his (probably rockier) recovery. And let's not even discuss the possible medical and emotional costs of what could have happened to his wife if they wound up being separated, especially if she became ill.

A well-run CCRC can be just the ticket for the right kind of resident. These places are evolving quickly, and you'll be hearing more and more about them, including innovative programs being developed there that weren't even on the horizon a decade ago. New trends include a "time-share model," in which some national operations with "blue chip" CCRCs throughout the country will enable residents to stay in their facilities in other cities (sort of a Ritz-Carlton vacation club for the graying). Other innovations include the virtual linking of CCRCs on the Internet so that residents can communicate their likes and dislikes and see which programs are working in other communities and which aren't. (If you can find such a message board or blog about a CCRC you're considering, that may be one of the most useful ways to get a true picture of how the place works.) I'm sure some version of "Aging Facebook" is on its way. In fact, social-networking sites for older people are already springing up.

How to "Kick the Tires" of a Long-Term-Care Community

So now that you know all the different types of long-term-care communities, let's get down to brass tacks: What's the best way to size them up?

I'll start by making some overarching (and slightly cynical) comments about the whole industry. At its best, it has some wonderful players who are deeply committed to improving quality of life for older adults. But there are also operators who view the business as little more than a series of real estate transactions, even though they may regale you with stories about their undying commitment to the elderly. As someone who has had to extricate many patients from living environments that were wrong or inappropriate, I have a bird's-eye view of how bad decisions get made, but I've also seen how good ones happen. Here's some advice on how to look at long-term-care facilities in ways you may not have thought about. These strategies apply to just about any of these facilities, any level of care, and any type of patient.

If all things look equal, choose a not-for-profit facility. True, at the end of the day this is a business, and the people in it want and deserve to make a profit for their work. The issue is how much profit is reasonable. When it comes to squeezing profit from the world of long-term care, here's the rub: Show me any housing situation involving older people—assisted living, life care, nursing home— and I will show you a facility that can always be made better (no matter how good it is) by the addition of more staff.

Until every resident has his or her own personal aide, nurse, physical therapist, recreational staff, and private room, spending more money on those things will nearly always improve the quality of care. That creates some pretty interesting dynamics when a CEO has to decide how much to pay his senior management (and himself) when some of those resources could go to hiring more staff. If the company is publicly traded, there's another very hungry mouth to feed: shareholders. And shareholders love it when the cost of running their business drops; the business becomes instantly more profitable, and stock prices rise. So what's the major cost of providing services to older people in these settings? By a mile, the answer is staff. Lay some off and your business just became more profitable.

Let me be very clear: I have seen wonderful for-profit facilities, to which I would gladly send any family member, and I have also seen not-for-profit facilities where I wouldn't board my dog. But extensive literature on this subject says that, on average, by any number of measures—staffing levels, rates of bedsores, state citations, successful and unsuccessful lawsuits, rates of functional decline—not-for-profit facilities are superior.[1] Quite simply, in these places any excess revenues have a better chance of being invested in more staff and better programs.

Understand your care needs and how they're likely to increase. This may sound obvious, but it's essential to be clear about the reason you're considering a change of venue. Is it simply to avoid social isolation, or are there real needs for supervision or assistance with daily tasks, such as meal preparation? Or is the issue proximity to medical services in the case of an emergency?

Next, figure out how the needs you've identified are likely to increase over the short and long term. "I don't have a crystal ball" is an unacceptable answer. Talk with your doctors and other health-care professionals about your *functional prognosis* (not only how long you will live but how long you will live without needing assistance—see chapter 17). When you begin to break it down into digestible bits, you may discover that you can make some highly reasonable assumptions about these issues in some cases but are totally clueless in others. And that's okay! Without at least attempting the exercise you're lost.

Some examples: Loss of mobility that results from a single medical event like an injury or stroke may create disability (such as a slow stride) that remains stable for decades. In that situation, I'm fine with an assisted-living facility or CCRC campus that has longer distances for you to traverse by foot or less skilled care available, because it is going to be a long, long time before you have difficulty navigating those distances or need those extensive services. On the other hand, a patient whose slow stride results from Parkinson's disease is likely to experience a gradual worsening of his gait in a few years. If your facility cannot accommodate you in that situation, you could well be moving again soon. Similarly, a patient with memory loss from head trauma has a far different prognosis than a patient in a similar condition who has Alzheimer's disease. Of course no one has a crystal ball, but looking at the decision through this lens can and should completely change the way you evaluate a facility.

And don't think you have to do this alone. Geriatric assessment programs (usually found at academic medical centers) are ideally suited to helping you make this decision. One of the reasons I frequently see patients in office consultation is to ascertain whether they can live independently, and, if they can't, where they should go. By doing your homework and taking advantage of all available resources, you can often avoid undershooting or overshooting the target.

And please, don't rely exclusively on the marketing department of the facility when it comes to gathering information for your assessment; they may have an agenda, depending on what "inventory" is available and most remunerative. Instead, take the opportunity to get a "medical estimate" as to what services you need now and what you'll need down the road. Would you replace your roof because a guy cleaning your chimney knocked on your door and said he noticed it needed replacing immediately? No, you'd get several estimates, not only about the cost but as to how much useful life your roof had left.

Interact with front-line staff. Facilities may tout their five-star chefs, the award-winning architects, the master yoga instructor, or any number of impressive impresarios, but these are not the people who are doing the heavy lifting. Even before you reach the point of needing day-to-day care, it's the front-line staff who have the most impact on your life, and you should meet some of these people before you commit to a facility. Who are they? In home-care settings, these are the home health attendants; in long-term-care facilities, they are frequently the certified nursing assistants, or CNAs. Virtually every medical service field has a category of paramedical assistant, including physical therapy aides (PTAs) and occupational therapy aides (OTAs). Assess the quality and demeanor of these people. A good question to ask them: "How long have you worked here?" High turnover in the front-line staff is a good sign that something might be amiss.

Visit at night and on weekends. When you go for the guided tour, you tend to get the spit-and-polish version of the facility. What you want to know is what the place is like at its most vulnerable— after hours, when staff are less plentiful and emergencies require a quick mobilization of resources.

Look at state survey results and complaint logs. Nursing homes (and assisted-living facilities in some states) are required to undergo a survey process annually or when a patient or family logs a complaint. Typically the survey results have to be posted for public inspection. Summaries or prior surveys are often available to the public online at www.medicare.gov (click on "compare nursing homes in your area"). While the survey process can be arbitrary and unfair at times (I've participated in or reviewed several), a history of chronic problems in one or many areas should raise questions. These problems do not necessarily disqualify a facility, but they should have you asking hard questions of its management.

Don't be deceived by furnishings and trappings. Just as the chefs and yoga instructors shouldn't be the key factors in choosing a facility, neither should big fireplaces and spacious reading rooms.

Sure, I like amenities when I travel: A nice big marble bathroom. A fancy, well-appointed hotel restaurant. But you're making a huge mistake if you prioritize these kinds of niceties when choosing a living environment for your later years. Unfortunately, it happens all too often. Why? Because these amenities are frequently the focus when facilities market themselves to prospective buyers and their kids. Large advertisements in the Sunday real estate sections for "senior communities" will focus on the marble staircases, the crystal chandeliers, and other architectural wonders. While environment is certainly important, you should be more interested in the level of staffing, the specific expertise of individuals in charge of certain programs, and a variety of other intangibles.

Know who you're doing business with. It is critical that you understand the expertise and history of the owner and operator of any facility you choose to enter. How old is the facility? How many of these facilities does the management own or run? How long have they been in business? In the case of the CCRC arrangement, where you are paying a fixed fee for care for the remainder of your life, you are actually buying two things: a place to live and a form of insurance, insulating yourself against downstream health-care costs that you may or may not be able to anticipate. If this were any other form of insurance—life, disability, whatever—what would be the first question you'd have for the salesperson? You'd want to know about the financial solvency of the company issuing the policy. Yet most people enter a CCRC with little understanding of the underlying financial health of the outfit they are (quite literally) getting into bed with.

Get references. You get them for people who renovate your kitchen, babysit for your kids, or paint your house. So why in the world wouldn't you want to get feedback from people who are actually living in the facility you are considering? Speak to these residents, and speak to their family members. Ask specific and probing questions about what they like about the place and what they don't, and share your concerns with them. Ask about other facilities they may have looked at and how they came to choose this one. In the case of assisted-living or life-care communities, ask if people have signed on for higher-level amenities (more assistance, more housekeeping) and whether they are actually using them.

Take a test-drive. This could be something as simple as going to the facility to share a meal with residents or even spending a few nights there to see how it feels. Many places offer respite services and other temporary short stays that could be used to check out or acclimate to a facility before committing. In the case of nursing-home care, patients and families who have previously used a facility for subacute rehabilitation have a bird's-eye view of how the facility operates and feels. Other services offered by nursing homes, such as adult day care, also provide a possible transition into the facility and offer an insider's perspective.

Ask about access to medical services. This is one area that patients and families often completely overlook when choosing senior housing. Does the facility have a physician on-site, or is the main care provider a nurse? What hours do they keep? If there is a physician, do you still have the option of seeing your own doctor? How do you get to him? Can he come to the facility? What if you need to be hospitalized? Is there an existing relationship with a local hospital, and if so, are you free to use any hospital or must you go to that one?

Get the details on transitioning to another care or service level. How is the decision made? What is your participation in it? What are your rights? One of the thorniest issues in long-term care is deciding when increased frailty has created care needs that exceed the facility's ability to provide a commensurate level of services. Often, that determination is in the eye of the beholder, and when there's disagreement between the facility and the resident (or his or her family), it can have nasty consequences. I've seen these differences of opinion occur in both directions—sometimes families believe more care is needed than the facility asserts, and sometimes less. Let me give you two examples.

Let's say you enter an assisted-living facility, perhaps paying a hefty up-front fee, and at some point the facility believes you can no longer walk safely enough to evacuate the premises in the event of a fire. Their solution is to move you to a nursing home on the other side of town that has more staff but that would also have you living among highly impaired residents, away from the friends you've made over the past three years. Who is right? What solutions are there? If the facility insists, for example, that you must have a twenty-four-hour companion in order to remain, can you appeal? If you cannot, then who pays for that additional assistance?

In the opposite direction, what if you enter a CCRC, pay for "cradle-to-grave" service up front, and then believe you need the next level of service to remain safe and well? Who decides when additional care is actually needed? Or say your mother is in a skilled nursing facility after a stroke and you believe that she has the potential to make additional recovery with more intensive physical and occupational therapy, but the physical therapist says that she has "plateaued" and that additional therapy would provide little or no improvement from her current state. How do you respond? How are these disputes mediated should they occur? You need answers to these questions before you agree to enter a facility.

Consider getting a lawyer for contracts, especially equity deals. As I hope you've gleaned by now, this can be pretty complicated stuff, and the money issues may be the least complicated. What is the definition of *disability*? Who decides? Is there an appeal process? The complexity is exponentially compounded in an equity model, because as we discussed, in that situation you're buying both insurance and housing. So unless you're dealing with a very straightforward and limited episode of care (a brief subacute nursing-home stay, for example, or a simple month-to-month rental situation in assisted living), you probably need a lawyer to make sure all the details get worked out. And there are lawyers who do nothing but this. (A word of caution, though: Not everyone who markets himself as an "elder law" attorney actually is one.)*

Understand exactly what you're buying. It's critical to know exactly what your payments cover, from meals to medical services. Medicare or Medicaid may pick up some of the things your tuition doesn't (such as doctor's visits or ambulance rides), but you need to identify everything the facility is offering for your hard-earned dollars. Are you getting a double room or a single room? Is there transportation to the mall, and if so, who pays? Who is giving you your medications? Only in this way can you identify gaps in services before they get wider and create potentially dangerous consequences.

Have an exit strategy. Sometimes things just don't work out. What happens if the facility is not to your liking, either right away or after you've spent some time giving it a chance? In a pure rental model, you should be able to just walk away without any financial encumbrances. But it's not so easy when you have paid big money up front to secure a lifetime spot. What happens then? Does your "investment" have value that can be bought and sold to the next customer?

---

* A good way to identify someone truly competent in this field is through the National Association of Elder Law Attorneys; visit their Web site at www.naela.org. There is now an actual certifying examination in elder law that is nationally administered that results in the designation Certified Elder Law Attorney (CELA). While finding a CELA-blessed elder law attorney doesn't guarantee you won't get a bad egg—there are people in every professional field (including medicine) with fancy titles, degrees, and certifications who can get you in hot water—this kind of first pass due diligence greatly improves the chances of getting the right kind of help. Another source of referrals is your state bar, most of which have elder law subcommittees. Another place to potentially find an elder law attorney is from your geriatrician if you have one. I know it sounds weird to get referred from a doctor to a lawyer, but every geriatric medicine program, by virtue of its work, has regular interactions with attorneys in their communities over issues like guardianship, powers of attorney, health care proxies, and trusts and estates. If you're lucky enough to have a geriatrician, you might ask him or her about elder law attorneys they have worked with.

Again, arrangements and agreements with more than a modicum of complexity should probably be reviewed by an attorney.

It Ain't Just a Business Deal

The decision to move to alternative housing is usually a highly emotional one. Many investment gurus will instruct you to take emotion out of a business or investment decision, but I'm not sure that completely stripping emotion from this decision—even if it were possible—is the best idea here. Emotion plays an important role in determining where we want to live. Think about falling in love with your first house or getting your first apartment.

Yes, you must perform "due diligence" on what it is you're purchasing. That process certainly involves a careful review of the numbers and details, but the feeling you get about a place and the other people who live there counts, too.

One of my patients likened the process to how his grandson selected his college. Accepted by many upper-tier institutions, he used a simple question as a litmus test: "All things being equal, could I picture myself here?" It worked for him, and it can work for you.

So make decisions about where you want to live with your heart and your head, and give yourself a good amount of time to consider the various issues I've raised here. After all, this decision could affect you for a long, long time. Here's the good news: There are many choices. As boomers we've tended to outfit our pads with creature comforts, and this attention has paid off with a wealth of appealing options when it comes to keeping us healthy and cared for as we age. I, for one, can't wait to see what new living options our creative contemporaries come up with as we get older, just as they've done it in previous eras with everything from feng shui dorm rooms to eco-friendly vacation houses.

Man, it's going to get interesting!

Chapter 15

Medications as We Age

On alternate nights at nine p.m.,
I swallow pinkies, four of them.
The reds, which make my eyebrows strong,
I eat like popcorn all day long.
—Theodore Geisel (Dr. Seuss), *You're Only Old Once*

There are millions of Americans alive today because of medications that did not exist a century ago. Imagine being a newly diagnosed insulin-dependent diabetic before the purification of insulin in 1927, or a child with Hodgkin's disease before the discovery of curative therapies in the 1970s, or a patient diagnosed with HIV infection in the 1980s before the discovery of the drugs that have dramatically slowed the progression of that disease. Your prognosis in those situations would be very poor, nearly as bad as if you ruptured your appendix in medieval Europe before the advent of modern surgical techniques: no gloves, no anesthesia, and no antibiotics. So I'm grateful for the amazing advances we've made when it comes to treating patients with drugs.

On the other hand, few doctors have more issues than I do with the pharmaceutical industry these days. I believe we have become a nation of overprescribing physicians and overmedicated patients. Every day I see patients who feel they're being shortchanged if they leave the doctor's office without a prescription, often because they've recently seen a drug advertised on TV. But piling on the prescriptions can lead to another insidious problem as we age, called *polypharmacy.* Translation: too many drugs. If you're a "child of the sixties," you may remember a time when you thought that could never be a problem. But take my word for it: As you get older too many drugs can mean a world of trouble.

In this chapter I'll give you a gerontological perspective on medications. As you'll soon see, to blame drugs alone for the problems they can cause is a profound oversimplification; it's the collision of those drugs with an aging body that creates issues, and many of these are preventable if you're armed with some basic information.

This Is Drugs; This Is Your Aging Brain (and Body) on Drugs

Before we talk about the stuff you can get without a prescription, let's start with the drugs that require one. A variety of factors lead to an increased risk of adverse drug events as we get on in years, and these range from the highly biologic (like decreased kidney elimination of a drug from the body, allowing its level to rise in the blood) to utterly environmental (like poor lighting, so you take the wrong medicine from the wrong bottle). And as you may have guessed, often these factors exist concurrently, further complicating the picture. Would it surprise you to learn that as many as 25 percent of Medicare hospital admissions may be due in some way to an adverse drug event? You're less likely to become a victim if you understand how and why these occur, so I'm going to give you a crash course in the six ways drugs can get you into trouble and what you can do to avoid them.

1. **Polypharmacy and drug-drug interactions:** These happen because as you get older you see more doctors and they prescribe more drugs, not to mention what you add to the mix with your own over-the-counter selections. One common example: Cardiologist A prescribes the blood thinner Coumadin for a blood clot in your leg, and Gastroenterologist B prescribes Tagamet (cimetidine) for heartburn (or you get it over the counter at your local pharmacy). The Tagamet slows your liver's ability to break

down Coumadin, the blood thinner builds up in your body, and you start to bleed. What's the solution to polypharmacy? Make sure every prescriber knows exactly what you're taking, and keep that list with you at all times; update it when you start a new drug or change your dosage. Use sites like www.drugs .com (a kind of online version of the *Physician's Desk Reference* you might have noticed in your doctor's office while he kept you waiting) to see if new medications interact with your old ones. At every visit, ask your doctor if there are some meds you could do without.

2. **Drug-disease interactions:** Everyone talks about drug-drug interactions, but as we age, drug-disease interactions become equally or more important. Why? Because we develop more chronic medical conditions, and newly prescribed drugs can affect them dramatically. Example: You have glaucoma (a potentially vision-threatening condition in which pressure builds up in the eye), and a urologist prescribes a medicine for incontinence that increases the pressure in your eyes, putting you at risk for more vision loss. Earlier I told you about my patient with well-controlled bipolar disorder who became unhinged when an orthopedist gave him some prednisone for a joint problem. The solution for this should be obvious: Make sure every prescriber knows your chronic conditions, and make sure the doctor who treats those conditions has lectured you on what kinds of meds, if any, to avoid.

3. **Slower elimination of drugs:** Quite simply, many of the organs that are supposed to remove drugs from our bodies do it more slowly as we get older. I've seen the biggest problems of this kind occur with sleeping medications and sedatives, when an older person is given a dose appropriate for a twenty-one-year-old but not a seventy-year-old. The result: You lie down for an hour-long nap and wake up days later. To avoid this, keep a copy of your recent blood work, which typically includes kidney and liver function (these organs are the heavy lifters when it comes to removing most of what we put in our bodies—water, vitamins,

supplements, and, yes, drugs). Keep those test results with you at all times as part of your medical "greatest-hits" document. Anyone prescribing a drug should be able to tell you if the dose is okay or needs to be lowered to meet your level of kidney or liver function; if they don't, ask.

4. **Changes in body composition:** This is one of the reasons manufacturers recommend a lower dose of some drugs as we get older, even if your kidney or liver function is normal. As we age, lean muscle mass is replaced with fat; for certain drugs this can affect the level of the drug in the blood, because some medications preferentially seek out fat. The best example I know of? Alcohol. The same two-ounce drink given to a seventy-year-old and a twenty-one-year-old can produce a higher alcohol level in the older patient, even if they are of the exact same weight and level of liver function. Follow the manufacturer's suggestions for lower doses as you get older, or ask your doc if he's taken this into consideration.

5. **Changes in the "target" organ:** So let's say your doc gets the dose just right, and the level of the drug in your blood is just right, too. The part of your body that the drug is supposed to affect is not the same as it was forty years ago; it may be much more sensitive to the drug than when you were younger. A common occurrence of this is being given too much sleep medication in the hospital the night before a surgery; the resident calculates the right dose, but because you have a more sensitive brain (and less brain reserve), you become delirious, which is not a good way to head to the OR for an elective operation. The solution is to "start low and go slow," as we say in geriatrics. You can always get more medication; it's much harder for me to retrieve a pill that's already in your gullet. Ask your doctor if a lower dose is practical or possible.

6. **Cognitive or sensory changes that preclude you from taking a drug correctly:** And just at the age when getting the dosing and timing of any drug right is more important than ever, your body makes things more interesting by throwing in changes

in memory and vision, or piling on manual-dexterity challenges that can upset the applecart. For instance, you can't read the pill bottle, so you take the wrong drug or the wrong dose. Or you forget you've taken your medications, so you take them again (or not at all). You can't get the pills out of the childproof bottle. Or you do a combination of all the above distributed over six medications. The solution here is organization, with or without technical assistance. I'm a big fan of "prepouring" medications, using one of those containers marked with the days of the week (you can get one in any drugstore for about two bucks) so you'll know if you missed or took a dose and on what days. Coming soon: devices that dispense the meds for you and keep track of whether you've taken them or not (early versions are available but a tad expensive). And there are already wristwatches with programmable medication reminders (see, for example, http:// thiscaringhome.org/products/watch-alarm+reminders.php).

With all these medication perils, it's understandable that patients and families often come to me with a common question: "Why so much medication, doc?" Usually I answer this with two other questions: Are you and your doctor sure you absolutely need all the medication you've been taking? And is the medication you're taking helping or hurting?

How to Find Out if Medicine Is Helping or Hurting

It usually goes something like this: A seventy-three-year-old patient has an orthopedist who prescribed an anti-inflammatory (such as Advil) for his bum knee, a cardiologist who prescribed Lipitor for his cholesterol, a primary care doc who's giving him blood-pressure and gout medications, and a GI doc who has him on meds for his reflux (heartburn). Then some new symptom appears—it could be low energy, insomnia, memory loss, poor appetite—any number of things. The patient has come to see me to determine whether these symptoms could be due to a medication or a combination of medications.

This is when geriatricians are at their best, but figuring out the answer is laborious and detailed work. As I've said, geriatrics is a combination of internal medicine and good old common sense, so the first thing we do is undertake some pharmacological detective work, leaving no nit unpicked. In cases like this, geriatricians have an algorithm we use to get to the bottom of things. You should consider the strategy I'll outline here, *but always in partnership with your doctor.* Think of it as "CSI: Medication."

Let me repeat: Talk to your doctor, and never start, stop, taper, or permanently discontinue a medication without his say-so. If he recommends or approves medication changes, always proceed under his supervision. I know I sound like a broken record, but this is absolutely critical. No one knows you medically like your doc does, and you can't know what he was thinking when he started a medication or changed the dose. The following steps always need to be coordinated and approved by him or her.

Be clear with your doctor about the symptom you think might be due to medication. He's about to do an experiment in collaboration with you, and every experiment needs a clear, measurable endpoint and outcome. This is critical, because many of the symptoms caused by medicines are vague: low energy, loss of concentration, irritability, and insomnia are just a few examples. Get specific with yourself and your doctor. For example, if you believe loss of appetite is being caused by a medication, keep a "before and after" diary of the calories you consume each day, as well as a meal-by-meal estimate of your predining hunger. Nothing fancy is needed, maybe just a simple three-point scale: hungry, not hungry, in between. It's the only way to assess whether subsequent cessation of a medication is having an effect. (This step is less important if you have a discrete measurable symptom like erectile dysfunction—that's a pretty clear endpoint.)

One thing at a time, please! This is another geriatrics pearl and applies not only to medication maneuvers but also to many other interventions typical of geriatricians. The only way you and your doctor can figure out what's going on is to change one thing at a time. If you stop several medications at once and conditions dramatically improve, you have no way of knowing which medication was responsible or whether it was a combination of medications. In a similar vein, trying to ferret out these kinds of issues should not be done when there are other medical, social, or environmental issues going on. What do I mean? Don't try to assess the influence of stopping or starting medications when you're about to go on summer vacation in a new environment (and be miles away from your doctor). If you're recovering from stomach flu or shoulder surgery, that's probably not a good time to be "stirring the pot," as my grandmother used to say. This process is like a scientific experiment, and in science we like to keep all potentially confounding variables constant other than the one being tested. Bottom line: This is complicated enough already. Don't make it more so by changing up other variables during the experiment.

Let your doctor decide which "drug holiday" to take. This part gets a bit complicated. It must absolutely be done under physician supervision and counsel, but I'll give you some insight into how geriatricians think about suspending a part of your drug regimen. Basically, three factors determine which medication gets the heave-ho first: (1) whether the medicine has a known association with the symptoms you're experiencing (although no known association does not rule out the possibility that this drug is responsible; it just lowers the probability), (2) whether any of your symptoms can be linked timewise to when you began taking a particular drug, and (3) how critical the medication is, given your current medical circumstances (that is, would it be dangerous to stop it?). This is complicated, so let me run it by you slowly.

You don't have to be a doctor to know that certain medications are simply not optional, while others are what I'd call discretionary. In the not-optional category, I'd include things like insulin if you're diabetic, thyroid hormone replacement if you've had the gland removed, or medications you take after you've had a stent placed in one of your cardiac arteries to keep it from closing up. You have no choice but to take these drugs—life and/or limb are threatened without them, and if you're experiencing problems, you're probably going to have to put up with them (although another option would be fiddling with the dose or the timing of the dose to minimize side effects).

In the discretionary category I'd include medicines that treat annoying but not life-threatening symptoms like those from allergies, lack of sleep, or anxiety. Whether these symptoms are ruining your life depends on both their severity and your constitution. The drugs' effectiveness is subjective, but if you had to do without them, you'd survive.

And finally, there's the medication you absolutely need to stay healthy but for which there are valid substitutes so chemically different that they have a vastly different side-effect profile. The best example that comes to mind here is blood-pressure medications. If you've got a bona fide case of hypertension, it *must* be treated, given the overwhelming evidence that you lower the risk of stroke, heart attack, and a litany of other medical problems by doing so. But if you're having a side effect from a blood pressure medicine, there are literally dozens and dozens of other choices. Which is not the case if your thyroid gland's been removed and you need thyroid-hormone replacement.

The other bits of logic geriatricians use in formulating the order of a drug holiday—investigating temporal associations and known associations with a specific side effect—seem obvious but frequently get overlooked or given short shrift because they involve a lot of doctor-patient time and communication. It requires both you and your doctor to go back over your history and perhaps your medical records in painstaking detail to determine when a medication was started (it might have been years ago) and each time a dose was escalated or decreased, then to try to correlate changes in your symptom with either the start or the dosage change of the drug.

Prune the medication typically associated with your symptom first. Certain drugs are notorious for producing certain side effects: Antidepressants have been linked to erectile dysfunction, chemotherapy to nausea, steroids to weight gain. But just because you can't find your symptom in the *PDR* for the drug you're sure is the culprit, that doesn't mean you're wrong. Geriatrician's rule: Nearly any drug can cause nearly any side effect. If you dig deep into the medical literature, you can almost always find a case report of a drug causing what you're experiencing.

So pack your things. You're taking a drug holiday.

———

Okay, so now it's time to carry out the experiment—again, *always in collaboration with and under the supervision of your doctor.* Together you've selected a medication that best "fits the bill" using the criteria I described above, but be careful! Certain medications cannot be quit cold turkey. Abrupt cessation of drugs like Valium and Ativan can produce seizures. Stopping beta blockers like atenolol or Toprol can even cause a "rebound" heart attack. My point: You can't simply say, "I'm stopping this medication." Make sure your doctor explains to you exactly how to go about it. This usually involves lowering the dose gradually over some defined period, or "tapering," as we docs like to call it.

Presumably you've been keeping a watchful eye over your symptoms in such a way that you'll be able to objectively assess whether or not the experiment proves your hypothesis. A couple of thoughts here: First, don't rush to judgment. It can take some time for medications to wash out of your system, especially if you've been taking them for a while. Second, you might get an opinion from a spouse or a friend on the effects of the experiment, especially when they're open to interpretation (like changes in libido or irritability).

And while you're doing all this, make sure you keep track not only of the symptom but also of any other problems that wax or wane. Pay attention to your overarching sense of well-being, too.

If the results are equivocal, ask your doctor about the advisability of a rechallenge. Commonly used by physicians when they're not completely certain if a symptom is related to a particular medication, a rechallenge is putting you back on the medication in the hopes of seeing whether the symptoms recur (depending on their severity). Again, you'd do this only under the supervision and advice of your doctor, and you certainly shouldn't be rechallenged if the medication produced a serious or life-threatening side effect. It's more suited to symptoms like fatigue, memory loss, or loss of libido.

If you've definitively solved the riddle of your symptom, congratulations on your fine detective work! But even if stopping a medication has produced no improvement, if at the same time you've experienced no ill effects, you may have learned something almost equally important. Ask yourself this: Did cessation of the medicine produce a dramatic change in the symptom or lab value it was originally prescribed to treat (like high cholesterol)? If it seems negligible, maybe you've discovered another pill you could do without. That would make your life less complicated, safer, and maybe save you some money to boot.

You Don't Need a Prescription to Get into Drug Trouble

I'll talk more about vitamins and supplements in the next chapter, but there's one last point worth making here. In the drug-holiday excursion I outlined, the substances you evaluate should include all your vitamins and supplements along with your prescribed medications. Don't be fooled into thinking that, because something you put into your body is natural, organic, or over-the-counter, it can't wreak havoc. Sometimes it's the supplement or natural compound itself, and sometimes it's materials used to bind the supplement together so it can be taken in pill or capsule form (what pharmacologists call the "vehicle"). In other cases it's the supplement interacting with a prescribed medication.

I've seen this hundreds of times. I've had people bleed from gingko, contract life-threatening diarrhea from certain vitamins, and even suffer strokes from vitamin K in a supplement they were taking. (K's the medical "antidote" to the blood thinner Coumadin, which my patient was taking for atrial fibrillation, a heart rhythm that predisposes one to blood clots, which can be ejected into the brain's circulation to produce stroke.)

In the case of supplements it's a bit more complicated, because their side effects are not as widely studied as those for prescribed medications. Medicines are highly regulated, with a detailed reporting system in place to assist you in determining whether there has been a clear association with your symptom and your medication. This isn't always the case for supplements and vitamins.

Just like all the other interventions modern medicine offers—radiologic imaging, laser surgery, hospitalization—drugs are a profoundly double-edged sword. Judiciously applied, they can save and prolong lives. Haphazardly prescribed and poorly monitored and/or coordinated, they can make patients as sick as any god-given disease. And as physicians get more hurried, drug companies overpromise, and patient expectations rise, I'm not sure the pendulum is swinging in the right direction. One bright spot on the horizon is the electronic medical record, which helps ensure that every health-care provider you interact with knows exactly which medication you are taking. But I believe it will be years before this system is applied across independent hospitals, physician groups, and pharmacies. And when it is, there will still likely be problems; we've talked about the limitations of any nonhuman system and why it will never be a complete substitute for a carefully guarded piece of paper that you keep in your pocket.

In the meantime, the forces that tend to lengthen our medication lists as we age are growing ferociously and unabated, including direct-to-consumer prescription-drug marketing (a horrific development, in my view). And there just aren't enough geriatricians to protect everybody. So in this chapter I've tried to partially immunize you against those forces, whether they come from your own desires, the drug industry, or a well-meaning but busy physician who is all too willing to satisfy your Madison Avenue–induced curiosity for a drug you didn't know existed, to treat a problem you may not even have known you had!

Chapter 16

Complementary and Alternative Medicine, Vitamins, and Supplements

Who Do You Believe?

Never trust a faith healer with a toupee or false teeth.

I'm always amused when a new patient arrives, usually at the insistence of a skeptical family member, for a consultation focused on reviewing his vitamins, supplements, and naturopathic remedies. These patients are invariably (and understandably) not happy to be there, and their demeanor usually reflects that. After all, they've been dragged to an Ivy League internist, an "establishment" doc, to be read the riot act about their irresponsible, tree-hugging health-care behavior. They've usually acquiesced for one reason and one reason only: to maintain domestic tranquility.

Initially, they have barely a passing interest in what I have to say. How could my narrow-minded Western medical education possibly prepare me to hold forth on these nontraditional vitamins, supplements, and other therapies, especially when they've been proffered by an internationally recognized guru who has received major attention and accolades? Yes, these folks have come grudgingly, often ready to defend their regimens with articulate arguments and sometimes even scientifically valid literature to support their assertions. In short, they've come ready to do battle with "the man."

But here's what I find so amusing about these encounters: Where I work, I'm not "the man." Ironically, many of my colleagues see me more as the counterculture figure, the bearded fellow in

Birkenstocks whose mind is open to nontraditional therapies in an environment where they've been generally dismissed, so long as I can marshal some evidence to back up their effectiveness. As you learned in the last chapter, we geriatricians, by constitution, have a general disdain for drugs, because we've seen way too much havoc created by multiple medications in aging patients. We also have more accommodating postures to alternative therapies, including nonpharmacologic interventions like meditation and yoga. I've prescribed peppermint and caraway oil for patients with certain intestinal problems. I use fish oil all the time in the prevention of coronary artery disease and its complications. I've sent patients to yoga classes for a variety of medical problems, including back pain. I believe along with Mrs. Lachs (a spa aficionado and a health-care professional), that massage therapy is one of the best nonpharmacologic treatments for stress ever invented.

When I explain to patients that they need not be defensive about these treatments and that I just have to understand what it is they're taking, it's like a shroud has suddenly been lifted. Most geriatricians I know stop more medicines than they start, and every time I see a new or established patient with a long list of medications, the first thing that comes to mind is "Can I stop any of these?" This is usually the case even if things are going relatively well and there are no problems. It's just the way we're taught to approach medicine. I like to think of geriatricians as culture and counterculture in one package, a posture we adopted long before it became a trend among medical centers to try to integrate complementary medicine into their traditional medical offerings.

This idea permeates geriatrics. I've said that the problems that conspire to cause trouble for older people arise from a combination of complicated medical, psychological, social, and environmental factors. It's insane to think that in all or even most cases a pill is going to fix everything on its own. After all, just about every patient I know (including me) uses a combination of "Western," or traditional, therapies and some form of nutritional supplements or nonmedical approaches to whatever ails them.

In this chapter I'll give you one geriatrician's view of vitamins and supplements, as well as "complementary" or "alternative" medicine (CAM).* Disclaimer: I say "one geriatrician's view" because not all my colleagues will agree with my assertions and ideas about this controversial and charged area of American medicine. That said, I feel pretty confident that I have plenty of support for my views among my peers.

Which CAM Therapies Are Worthwhile?

It's one of the most common questions I'm asked: "Doc," the patient says, "I hate taking medications, and I'm interested in natural therapies, vitamins, and supplements. Do any work? Which ones? Where do you get them? Would you spend your own hard-earned money on 'em?"

The answer to the first question is a resounding "yes." There are, without a doubt, therapies that don't require a prescription, some of which can be found occurring naturally in the environment, that can bring proven benefit to people with certain conditions or prevent disease in patients at risk. This is not a new idea. It extends back almost 2,500 years to 400 BCE, when Hippocrates noted that ground bark from willow trees was capable of reducing fever and pain. The natural substance involved was salicilin, a cousin of modern acetylsalicylic acid, more commonly known as aspirin.

Another note here: "Natural" therapies are not limited to things you can put in your mouth. In fact, some of the strongest evidence for the usefulness of CAM in treating specific diseases involves mind-body interventions like meditation or yoga. Examples include

---

* The nomenclature used to describe these other forms of patient care vary widely, even among practitioners. In this chapter I use the definitions offered by the American College of Physicians, which has published an outstanding and fair-minded treatise on the subject. *Complementary medicine* generally describes therapies that are administered as an adjunct to conventional medicine. *Alternative medicine* usually refers to treatments that are used instead of traditional therapies. Together, the two disciplines are often referred to as *complementary and alternative medicine* (CAM).

mental relaxation techniques to reduce chemotherapy-associated nausea, yoga to treat certain kinds of back pain, and physical activity as part of a comprehensive regimen to treat depression. Some of these natural therapies have been studied as rigorously as drugs or surgery.

So, yes, some non-Western approaches do work. The follow-up question about which ones are worth spending money on is far more complicated. Figuring out the answer will involve some due diligence on your part. Since I don't believe you're going to want to spend money on stuff that doesn't work (notwithstanding a few observations I'll make later on "the placebo effect" as it relates to aging and medications or alternative therapies), it's worth learning a bit more about these issues. For example, there are situations in which both a natural and a pharmaceutical remedy are effective. In those situations you're going to have to get a little more sophisticated than the binary "works/doesn't work" approach to understand what's right for you. If you want to make an intelligent decision, you're going to need a better understanding of just *how much* the nontraditional therapy works so you can compare it to the traditional "stuff" in terms of both effect and cost.*

I suspect you're getting the picture. Wrapping your head around all this requires some sophistication vis-à-vis how therapies of any kind—drugs, supplements, vitamins, surgeries, psychotherapy, acupuncture, exercise regimens—actually work. Figuring this out is complicated at any age, but it gets harder as you get older. If you'd like to jump off here and simply be redirected to a Web site or reference book that does this for you, I perfectly understand—with one caveat: There are various painless ways to outsource this activity, but remember that no one has your interests at heart (or

---

* This entire scientific area of assessing which treatments work and how they compare to existing treatments is called comparative effectiveness research and became a considerable focus in discussions about health-care reform. Why the sudden interest? At least one reason is that the cost savings realized from paying for only the most effective and least expensive treatments could potentially be used to insure more Americans.

understands the nuances of your values and health situation) the way you do. Doing the work yourself is like bypassing a restaurant for a home-cooked meal made with vegetables that you grew in your own backyard. The sense of accomplishment and satisfaction can be enormous. And if you've ever obsessed over more familiar consumer decisions (like which new car to buy next), you may have found that research can be a very enjoyable part of the journey.

Show Me the Data

A major barrier to making intelligent decisions about health-care therapies—traditional or CAM—has to do with the very nature of medical research: It's prone to a virtually infinite number of ways in which it can be screwed up, even when researchers have the best of intentions and are highly conscientious. I'm talking about research that involves actual living and breathing people, with all their foibles, habits, biases, and other characteristics that make them unique. Research of this type goes by a number of names: *clinical research, clinical trials, clinical epidemiology, outcomes research, patient-oriented research*, and *dry-bench research* (to differentiate it from *wet-bench research*, which takes place in a laboratory with test tubes and beakers). I'll use the term *patient-oriented research* in this chapter because it makes it very clear who the potential beneficiary of the science is. When this type of research involves older people, these human variations and eccentricities can become even more pronounced; the potential for errors, even larger. Human beings in medical studies have a nasty habit of not behaving as neatly and predictably as lab rats. First of all, we each bring a different body and medical history to an experiment. While it is possible to breed genetically identical mice and expose them to a drug or supplement (and their "control" counterpart to a placebo), no two sixty-year-olds are precisely alike with respect to prior surgeries, medications, social support, physical activity, and emotional state. There are an infinite number of variables that could cause a condition under study to worsen and might be misattributed to the supplement being administered. Second, human beings may miss doses of medications, fail to adhere to an exercise protocol, or simply not show up to a medical appointment for follow-up. (The mice have little choice in these matters.) Third, many of the "endpoints" human beings are interested in achieving (the reasons we seek out traditional or CAM treatments in the first place) are very hard to measure objectively. If I give a mouse a medication I'm testing to improve mental functioning, I can time how long it takes it to complete a maze, but for humans there are so many other "softer" but important aspects to mental functioning—memory, attention span, ability to use language, mood, irritability—that it becomes far more difficult to assess objectively whether someone is improving.

You could spend a lifetime learning to conduct and interpret studies of therapies in order to minimize error and bias and get the right answer about their effectiveness. There are even physicians who devote a large part of their careers to this area, in the same way a doctor might choose to focus on cardiology or pediatrics. I am one of them; in the late 1980s I spent two years after medical school and internal-medicine training as a Robert Wood Johnson Clinical Scholar at Yale in a program devoted to the design, conduct, and interpretation of patient-oriented research. It is as much a passion for me as the practice of medicine itself.

My qualifications on this issue thusly established, let me break it down for you.

How to Evaluate the Evidence:
"Do-It-Yourself" versus "Takeout"

Understanding the scientific findings about the therapy you're considering can take a lot of work. Even if you have access to medical literature (and you do, see page 242), you first need to have at least some basic knowledge of the relevant medicine and the associated medical jargon and then be willing to navigate many clinical nuances to determine whether the studies have validity and relevance to you. In the case of CAM, evaluating those studies is even harder for many reasons, not the least of which is the fact that CAM treatments aren't standardized the way medications are. An antibiotic is the same whether it is given in Los Angeles or New York. But acupuncture or meditative techniques can be very practitioner-dependent, and an unregulated supplement can have different amounts of the active ingredient (or different purity) in different brands.

At this point you may be saying, "I don't want to get into those kinds of details; just send me to a place where I can get the answer," or "I'm just going to leave this to my doctor; he went to medical school so I wouldn't have to." Here's my take on that line of reasoning. First, as you'll begin to see as we move through this chapter, there is rarely a definitive "answer" to these kinds of questions as we get older. As I said earlier, if you've seen one eighty-year-old, you've seen only one eighty-year-old. Many considerations—other diseases or diagnoses you may harbor, costs, the ability to adhere to a treatment regimen, the quality of the studies—influence the decision about taking a supplement or beginning another CAM therapy. In approaching any medical treatment, I'd urge you to adopt an evidence standard that fits both the severity of what you're trying to treat and the intensity of the treatment. We're willing to suffer nauseating chemotherapy to treat testicular cancer because the evidence is superb that it cures the majority of patients, and because the disease is life-threatening. You'd probably be less enthusiastic about such a toxic therapy for acne.

As for letting your doctor worry about it, be careful. Multiple studies suggest that "evidence-based medicine"—clinical decision making based on rigorous scientific studies as opposed to a less substantiated strategy—has not completely penetrated the rank and file of practicing docs. That inertia is understandable. Between examining patients, doing paperwork, and arguing with insurance companies, many physicians can't find time to eat, never mind read each new issue of the medical journals. That's not to say that there aren't hordes of excellent physicians who pride themselves on staying current, and more modern tools (Internet- or PDA-based systems) that help them do so without going to the library every week. The problem is that, as a patient, there's no way of knowing whether you've been lucky enough to hook one of those doctors.

Regardless, there will always be "do-it-yourselfers" who want to get to the bottom of everything themselves and others who prefer to hire contractors. Therefore, I'll provide some advice for each camp.*

The Takeout Approach

If you're unable, unwilling, or too busy to fetch the scientific article from the medical journal in which it appeared (and that's going to cover the majority of readers), no problem. But in that case you're going to need to rely on some independent adjudicator of the research who can distill it for you in layman's terms. Several outstanding resources exist in this regard:

- The National Center for Complementary and Alternative Medicine, an arm of the National Institutes of Health (the major government funder of biomedical research), has a wealth of consumer information about vitamins and supplements, a list of ongoing clinical trials involving alternative and complementary treatments, and good general advice on how to evaluate such therapies. Visit www.nccam.nih.gov.
- The American Federation for Aging Research (AFAR) is a premier not-for-profit foundation that supports aging science. On its superb Web site, www.infoaging.org, it maintains a huge archive of evidence-based answers to questions about

---

*There is, in fact, an "in between" approach for readers who want to dig a bit deeper into the evidence but not spend all their time in medical research. Several highly regarded summaries of CAM describe the research in more than lay detail. If you can stand the technical jargon, my favorite, *The ACP Evidence-Based Guide to Complementary & Alternative Medicine*, is published by the American College of Physicians (2009).

treatments, both natural and pharmaceutical. Readers can post questions to be answered by some of the most eminent scientists and clinicians in gerontology.[1]

- Medical journals themselves now include lay interpretations of the research, which physicians can give to patients. The best example in my field is a journal called *The Annals of Internal Medicine*.[2] These interpretations are incredibly useful resources that summarize the current thinking on many CAM and traditional therapies. In an appendix, I've included lay interpretations of four CAM trials that were conducted with high-quality methodology: the use of glucosamine for hip arthritis (a negative study), the relationship between green tea consumption and the prevention of certain kinds of diabetes (a positive study), the use of acupuncture for knee arthritis (mixed results in comparison to placebo), and a study of yoga versus commonly employed exercises for back pain (a positive study). These studies appeared in the most prestigious and widely read journal in American internal medicine. Who says traditional docs don't embrace CAM?

- Notwithstanding my earlier comments, don't write your doctor off because he's a traditional MD. He may be familiar with a particular CAM treatment you're considering. Believe me, if you've got a question about it, you're not the only one. I always get phone calls from a number of patients every time an article about a CAM treatment appears in the *New York Times* or another widely read periodical, and so does your doctor. If he *hasn't* heard about it, it's a great opportunity for you to learn about it together.

For Do-It-Yourselfers

If you'd like to be a bit more adventurous (and I highly endorse this), you can nominally school yourself in how research is conducted and actually get ahold of articles on a CAM therapy and try to digest them. Sites like Google Scholar (http://scholar.google

.com) and Pubmed (www.ncbi.nlm.nih.gov/pubmed) are excellent places to search the medical literature for recent articles that may be of interest to you. The former is more forgiving and accessible but also a bit of a thicket: You'll be wandering through a database that contains scholarly articles not only on heart disease but on orchid production, geologic formations, astrophysics, and linguistic anthropology. While the details of how to search the databases is well beyond the purview of what I can cover here, excellent lay tutorials can be found at http://scholar.google.com/intl/en/scholar/about.html for Google Scholar and www.nlm.nih.gov/bsd/disted/pubmedtutorial for Pubmed.

Getting hold of an article on a subject of interest is just the first step. Now comes the difficult part: determining whether it provides any guidance for you. Here are five steps to help you in making that decision.

1. **Make sure that what's being studied is what you're interested in.** It sounds obvious, but often it's not: Studies that attempt to test alternative-medicine treatments may or may not be testing the one you're considering in the same way you'll be administering it. For example, if you're thinking about taking a vitamin or supplement, you need to make sure that the study you've found has the same ingredient, dose, and frequency. Be sure that accompanying interventions aren't complicating the picture (such as a list of other supplements given with the one you care about, or additional treatments like physical therapy). If the study focuses on a physical intervention like yoga, meditation, or an exercise program, make sure it's clearly articulated how the intervention was performed. How long was the session and how many times per week? What exactly were the components? A swimming program intended to improve shortness of breath run by a former Olympian may not generate the same effects when it is "rolled out" at the local YMCA by the guy who works at the front desk. Look for this kind of detail in the description when you evaluate a treatment.

2. **Be sure the patients in the study are as like you as possible.** A rapid-walking program that improves blood pressure and mood in the participants could be great, but what if everyone in the study was a healthy twenty-one-year-old undergraduate? Would the same benefits be realized in seventy-seven-year-old men with arthritis and diabetes? This is what epidemiologists call "generalizability" of studies. While you're never going to find a study with someone *exactly* like you in it, the participants should be at least close to your age, gender, and general health state, or you run the risk of comparing apples and refrigerators.

3. **Assess the quality of the study.** This is done by seeing how many elements of a randomized trial—the Cadillac of clinical research—it has. In these trials, half the patients are randomly assigned the treatment and the other half get a placebo; patients don't know which treatment they received; this is called blinding. Double blind studies refer to those in which both the patient *and* the physician are unaware of who got what; this is highly desirable when feasible. Other desirable aspects of the randomized control trial besides a control group and blinding: formal assessments of the outcome, reporting of side effects, a discussion of study dropouts, and a tally of adherence to the supplement or therapy in the treatment and control group.

4. **Look for self-effacing scientists.** At the end of their papers, the best scientists usually spend very little time discussing their brilliant findings and lots of time discussing potential anticipated and unanticipated problems with their research—and how these might have screwed up the findings. When you find a discussion section with lots of self-back-patting (as opposed to lots of self-reflection), be very, very skeptical. The best scientists are skeptics, especially of their own work. It's the only way science advances.

5. **Involve your physician in this "journal club."** One way to engage your doc (and get a sense of his facility and familiarity with recent medical literature) is to ask him about studies

you've read and consumed and see if he'll opine (by all means, share the paper with him). Some physicians are threatened by this strategy, but I absolutely love it (except when volumes of Internet printouts begin to cramp the limited time I have to spend examining and talking with a patient). This tactic is especially useful in getting your physician to consider alternative treatments he may not be aware of. Providing medical evidence of a type your physician is familiar with can be a great way to engage him on a specific topic and improve your doctor-patient relationship in the process.

One important, final point on evaluating medical evidence before you adopt a CAM treatment or strategy: Some practitioners of alternative therapy contend that, since their interventions are non-Western or nontraditional, the ways in which Western medicine evaluates evidence does not apply to them.

This is utter balderdash and usually intended to obfuscate some other issue—namely, the absence of effectiveness of their potions or ointments. I don't care if we're talking acupuncture versus nicotine patches to quit smoking or guided imagery versus Norvasc for blood-pressure reduction; any therapy given to human beings should be proven safe and effective by the same scientific criteria.

Aging and the Placebo Effect

Any discussion of treatments used in aging or aging-related diseases, especially alternative treatments, would be incomplete without a discussion of the placebo effect. This describes the situation in which patients who have received a "sham" treatment with no pharmacological or medical value—say, a sugar pill for depression or a saline (saltwater) injection for pain—experience perceived improvements in health or relief of symptoms anyway.

If you have any doubt that the placebo effect is real and measurable, let me tell you about the Beta-Blocker Heart Attack Trial (BHAT).[3] This important study, published in 1981, showed that in patients who sustained a heart attack, a type of heart medicine called "beta-blockers" (common examples are Toprol, Lopressor, and atenolol) decreased the risk of death one year later as compared to those given a placebo. The study has been replicated many times, and thus beta-blockers are now given routinely to patients discharged from the hospital after a heart attack.

Let's take a deeper look. In this well-conducted trial, patients who randomly got assigned the beta-blocker and took their medicine every day were less likely to be dead one year after their heart attack than the folks who missed dosages—the investigators counted the pills remaining in the bottles to determine who was adhering and who was slacking. This result isn't surprising; if a medication really works, patients who actually take it are going to do better than patients who forget to (or just don't care).

But for me, a mind-blowing aspect of the BHAT trial was that the people who were assigned placebos also had their pills counted, and guess what? Patients who took their placebos religiously were less likely to die than those who took them less regularly! And the endpoint of this study was not some nebulous factor like mood or energy level. It was cut-and-dried, an outcome that even the most inexperienced doctor or researcher could agree upon: death.

Here's another compelling testimonial to the placebo effect in regard to aging-related diseases: In a study published in 2005,[4] Italian investigators told subjects who had electrical-stimulation devices implanted into their brains to control Parkinson's disease (an effective therapy for severe symptoms of the illness, like horrible tremors) that the stimulators were on when in fact they were turned off. Remarkably, many patients responded with clear improvement of neurological symptoms of the disease, even though they received a type of "placebo."

So what's this placebo thing all about, and why is it so relevant to aging? From a purely biological standpoint, we know that some patients are especially likely to respond favorably to a placebo. In sophisticated imaging studies, certain parts of these patients' brains light up when a placebo is administered; "placebo nonresponders" have less such activity. From a behavioral standpoint, patients who take their placebos regularly (like those in the BHAT study) may demonstrate certain related behavioral patterns (like regular flossing or seat belt use) that lend themselves to better survival when compared to their placebo-slacking counterparts.

My take on it? I think the placebo effect has to do with our expectations about aging as we get older. There is a mountain of data that says outlook and expectation greatly influence longevity and quality of life. I'm sure you've seen it in your own social network. We all know at least one compelling older person whose positive outlook on life is an inspiration to everyone around her, someone who remains upbeat even in the face of overwhelming loss—the death of a spouse, devastating financial reversals, debilitating medical diagnoses that come out of nowhere. People like these somehow put the best face on things and sally forth with amazing courage. On the other hand, we've all met the opposite type: the guy for whom minor perturbations in health or circumstance are perceived as earth-shattering.

When outlook on aging is studied scientifically, you begin to see the power of the mind in healing and the placebo effect. Becca Levy at Yale has studied the subsequent longevity of people in their fifties (that's right, I said fifties) as a function of their perceptions about aging. For example, she asked them if they agreed with statements like "Things keep getting worse as I get older" and "As you get older you are less useful." After controlling for their medical conditions, subjects who were boomer-aged when initially interviewed lived 7.5 years longer on average if they disagreed with those statements in comparison to those who endorsed them.[5] So if you're a boomer and you don't think your current outlook about getting older has any impact on the rest of your life, you might want to give some thought to brightening your attitude a bit!

Many therapies—both traditional and CAM—probably work their magic to some extent through the placebo effect. But because this is often closely linked to patient expectation and belief, it may be most pronounced when it comes to CAM therapies, in which both the purveyor of the treatment and the patient often have strongly held beliefs and expectations about the therapy's effectiveness. Furthermore, patients who seek these treatments out often do so because they believe traditional medicine has failed them—and in many cases they are not wrong. Thus, they may have high expectations for their new self-selected therapy and a vested interest in learning that their decision to go in this direction was the right one.

Is there anything wrong with this? What's the problem with a sugar pill that makes people feel better, even if there is no medical or physiological basis for the improvement? After all, geriatricians are always espousing an optimistic view of aging in which patients are active participants and decision makers in their care; for all the reasons I have described, taking away a patient's hope is one of the worst things doctors can do. A trusted doctor's disapproving look in response to a safe but marginally effective treatment could certainly send that message.

My response: There's nothing wrong with it, as long as you follow some simple guidelines and keep a lookout for the signals that should give you pause about a CAM treatment (or any treatment, for that matter). If you are thinking about seeking CAM therapies for whatever ails you, here are five warning signs that should have you thinking twice:

1. **When you ask for evidence and don't get it.** This entire chapter is about using evidence to make good health decisions about CAM. If you've followed my advice about researching a treatment yourself or going to a credible source of evaluation and you've come up negative, ask the purveyor of the therapy why he thinks the treatment is effective and where you can read more about it. If you're dismissed, talked down to, or discouraged, I'd give him one more chance to give you straight information and then move on. Don't fall for unscientific testimonials, conspiracy-theory arguments about why data has been suppressed, or proclamations that the usual metrics for proof don't apply to this particular treatment.

2. **When the purveyors of such therapies have a treatment for everything.** As a physician in New York City, I try to keep abreast of the goings-on in the CAM world, and I often listen to its purveyors on local and national radio. One host has a remedy for every single caller's problem. Hour after hour patients call in, describing their heartbreaking illnesses. The conditions are all over the map: A man who sustained a stroke a decade ago that left him bedridden, whose wife called to see what therapies could help him. A woman with advanced Alzheimer's disease whose husband wants to know what natural treatments might cure her. A woman with advanced scleroderma who is understandably tired of traditional rheumatologic therapies and wishes for something else. For every caller, without exception, the guru had a definitive recommendation for a natural or nutritional therapy that was "proven to work" but unknown to doctors. I'm the first guy to admit that modern medicine has failed many patients and offers few or inadequate answers for many maladies. But you should ask yourself; shouldn't the same be true of any school of health-care practice, CAM or traditional? How could it be possible that there's a treatment for every last affliction known to man, yet modern medicine missed it? This is no different than the snake oil salesman who asserts his concoction cures everything from athlete's foot to cancer. Be skeptical when you see this pattern of claims around any treatment.

3. **When conspiracy theory is a major selling point.** Samuel Johnson said that "patriotism is the last refuge of a scoundrel." Similarly, the last refuge of people trying to sell you a medical cure is often their noble proclamation that evil forces have kept their breakthrough discovery from wider distribution. As I said earlier, I have huge problems with the pharmaceutical industry and other quarters of the modern medical-industrial machine, but not to the extent that I believe useful therapies are being suppressed, particularly in this information age. Plenty of responsible practitioners of alternative and complementary

medicine quietly make their case with data and balanced arguments and without the need for "me against the world" Don Quixote rants. Many patients who seek these treatments are desperate and vulnerable, and the last thing they need is an Elmer Gantry.

4. **When alternative treatments become an obsession.** If your pursuit of these therapies has shut you down to the possibility of seeking bona fide medical treatments you actually need, or you're spending so much on vitamins or supplements that you have no money left to enjoy yourself, it's probably time to take a step back. One of the first patients I saw as a junior faculty member at Yale was a woman with Alzheimer's disease whose condition had worsened over the past six months, which is why her husband sought consultation; though she had impaired memory initially, he told me that she had gone from highly functional to almost bed-bound. It was the kind of decline I would have expected over a decade, and it just didn't make sense. When I examined her, I noticed she had a thyroid scar on her neck, suggesting that the gland had been removed, but her husband hadn't mentioned this to me; she was not on thyroid hormone replacement, as would normally be the case in such situations. When I approached him about this, he explained that the thyroid surgery had occurred forty years before, around the time they were married. Then he told me this story: After I diagnosed her with Alzheimer's, he became convinced that it was due to some toxic exposure she had sustained from her medications (not a bad thought, actually), so he decided to stop them all and replace them with natural therapies. For her missing thyroid gland, a CAM practitioner suggested kelp (seaweed), since it was rich in iodine and could help a thyroid problem in place of thyroid hormone (iodine is a major component of thyroid hormone). The only problem with that logic is that you need a thyroid gland to convert dietary iodine to thyroid hormone, and she didn't have one. When he reluctantly agreed to let her take a "prescribed" medicine,

the thyroid hormone almost completely reversed her dementia, because it wasn't Alzheimer's disease that caused this worsening mental impairment—it was the withdrawal of hormone that she needed and had been taking for many years.

5. **When they're trying to sell you something besides their medical knowledge.** When any medical provider, alternative or otherwise, starts selling you stuff out of his or her office in which he or she has a financial interest, you should pause and think about this arrangement. I'm all for making a buck, but unless the doc has some excellent rationale for your using this particular cream or other treatment, go buy it from someone without a conflict of interest. The American Medical Association (I'm not a member) has specifically stated that it is improper for physicians to sell nonprescription drugs or merchandise from their offices.[6]

Anti-Aging Medicine

Finally, I would be remiss if I did not talk specifically about one growing movement that largely falls under the CAM umbrella: the "anti-aging medicine" movement. There are many factions to this growing juggernaut, including an academy that certifies practitioners in the field, which is not recognized by the American Board of Medical Specialties (the entity that certifies fields of medicine that you are probably more familiar with, like surgery, medicine, obstetrics, or pediatrics). Definitions of anti-aging medicine are also all over the map, ranging from "the early detection, prevention, and treatment of aging-related illnesses" (sounds pretty responsible to me) to the view that aging is an illness that can be cured and that the potential for the human life span is infinite (sounds less responsible).

Similarly, the scientists and practitioners who have associated themselves with this field range from some highly respected folks who have conducted credible peer-reviewed research to outright snake-oil salesmen who make dubious claims without data. Many of the latter have been subject to license revocation, civil sanctions, and even federal fines. Congress has convened hearings to try to determine how to better protect the public from some practitioners of anti-aging medicine,[7] and the International Longevity Center has published a useful pamphlet on the subject, "Is There an 'Anti-Aging' Medicine?" (see www.ilcusa.org/media/pdfs/bk_antiaging.pdf).

How do practitioners of anti-aging medicine and geriatric medicine see each other? By and large acrimoniously, I think it's fair to say. Many of the former have huge issues with geriatric medicine. They contend that geriatricians have essentially resigned themselves to aging as an inevitable process; they lament the "death culture" of geriatrics; and they actively attempt to forestall or reverse aging through preventative or other techniques that they believe are proven and effective. Having reviewed hundreds of these claims and the data behind them (when I could find such data), I can tell you that, for the most part, they are not proven, and certainly not to the extent that the practitioner typically asserts.

In my camp, there is understandable concern. Every doctor of geriatric medicine with any amount of clinical experience has seen older people harmed physically and economically by a practitioner of anti-aging medicine or products sold under that banner (a claim that I am sure anti-aging practitioners would make of traditional medicine). Research gerontologists, who study the biology of aging, point to any number of groundless claims about miraculous reversals of aging that threaten the legitimacy (and funding) of their own work.

I take a pragmatic view of the whole debate. First of all, I do not believe aging is a reversible disease; virtually every living thing on this planet has a life span that is finite, and I will not insult your intelligence by claiming otherwise. I am also troubled by the high priority many anti-aging proponents place on physical appearance as opposed to actual health. But do I believe that it is possible to lengthen our lives beyond what science has already delivered to us?

Certainly! We may someday be able to manipulate genes and slow the aging process, but I suspect we will never reverse and stop it. For now I think that the science with the best chance of helping patients will result from breakthroughs that treat, slow, or prevent common chronic conditions associated with aging. Many of these interventions are already known to us in the form of diet, exercise, social integration, and access to health care, as well as specific treatments for individual health problems you have developed or are at risk for. I proffer those interventions every day to people of all ages in my practice. If that's anti-aging medicine, then I guess I'm practicing it.

Beware of Misunderstood Gurus Bearing Gifts

The human impulse to seek longer life is certainly an understandable one. But to the extent that it can be at times driven by fear—fear of aging and (dare I say it?) fear of death—I would contend that there is something about anti-aging medicine that is, well, ageist. All forms of prejudice are driven by fear; we mock and deride the things we fear most. So, yes, let's do everything we can with a sound scientific basis to prolong life, but how about a little commonsensical acceptance of aging at the same time?

In a television interview, one anti-aging impresario cited a conspiracy against him and likened his "cutting edge" approaches and radical views of aging to those of previous scientific giants who were visionary but laughed at in their own time. The sympathetic commentator agreed: In every scientific revolution, aren't there geniuses who are mocked by the status quo yet turn out to be right?

Sure there are. But there's also a much, much longer list: the guys who were wrong and we never heard about *because* they were wrong. For every Einstein there were thousands of scientists who proffered ideas and theories that were absolutely bizarre. A twentieth-century Dutch librarian named Bart Huges, who never finished medical school, believed that brain function could be enhanced by drilling holes into the skull to make more room for blood flow.

(He performed the procedure, called trepanation, on himself. There are still strong proponents of the practice, including an international society.) Stubbins Ffirth, an early-nineteenth-century Philadelphia physician, believed that yellow fever was not infectious but was caused by heat because it peaked in summer and disappeared in the winter. (Of course, this was because the mosquitoes that carried it didn't fancy Philadelphia winters.) To prove his point, he ate, drank, and bathed himself in the bodily fluids of yellow fever patients (yes, including vomit) to show that he would not catch it in the winter. (He didn't, because yellow fever patients who survive into winter have late-stage disease and are no longer infectious.) And in the anti-aging realm, there was Russian doctor Alexander Bogdanov, who was apparently a better writer and politician than physician-scientist. He believed that blood transfusions were the key to immortality (or at least life extension) and conducted a series of experiments on himself in the late 1920s, before the advent of blood typing. The first few went pretty well; he thought that both his hair loss and his vision improved. Unfortunately he perished after transfusing himself with the blood of a medical student who had both malaria and tuberculosis.

How will science remember any particular modern anti-aging guru? Time will tell. But let history be that judge, not the guru himself, especially if he is also selling something. Einstein got no commission for his theory of relativity. He did it for the love of science.

Do I believe that scientifically valid techniques will add even more quality years to our lives over the next several decades? Of course! But I also believe that as each of those techniques are proposed and developed, they should be evaluated on the basis of evidence to the greatest extent possible. This chapter provided you with some tools toward that end. You'll need them. As America ages, I have no doubt that the fountain-of-youth claims will come faster and faster.

In the meantime, I'm a geriatrician, and I've got work to do. I have countless patients and families of all ages who need my help in the here and now. They're struggling daily with mobility problems, memory impairment, polypharmacy, and social isolation as they attempt to navigate a health-care system that's often incomprehensible, even if you have "all your marbles" and several advanced degrees from Harvard. That's okay; as I've said, geriatricians are optimists by constitution. And while I can't see myself being put out of business by anti-aging medicine and its proponents anytime soon, make no mistake about it—I'd be delighted to be proven wrong.

Chapter 17

Money and Aging

A shroud hath no pockets.
—Scottish proverb

I'm a doctor, but I'm going to discuss money. And I'm going to do it in a way that certainly no doctor, and probably no financial planner, tax attorney, or CPA, ever has before. In this chapter I'll give you a big-picture look at the relationship between money and health as we age, and how you can use what we know about this relationship to your advantage. With that framework in place, in the next chapter I'll get specific about how this plays out in several critical areas, including health and long-term-care insurance, financial gerontology, and retirement.

I wish I could look you in the eye and tell you that the way we age has everything to do with god-given gifts and what we make of them and nothing to do with money. But the truth is, study after study has confirmed the powerful impact of resources (that's a euphemism doctors sometimes use when they're uncomfortable mentioning "money" in the context of patient care) on longevity, health, quality of life, and many other forms of real and perceived well-being.

My observations from the trenches confirm this. That's not to say I haven't seen or cared for many older adults of limited means who haven't led long and productive lives. Similarly, I've cared for wealthy individuals whose resources did little to combat the effects of bad genetics, unwise lifestyle choices, and bad luck. But on average, given equivalent health and other prognostic factors, economic status confers both longevity and a better ability to weather illnesses when they come along. There are hundreds of studies looking at every stage of life to confirm this, and in our later years the impact of financial health on medical health becomes more profound.

That's an incredibly important point for both boomers and their parents, especially you boomers, who still have the time to plan ahead to avoid some serious mistakes. To help you in that pursuit, you've got two powerful weapons: (1) knowledge that has been gleaned from gerontological research over the past few decades regarding what we know about aging, health, and money; and (2) a set of case studies that's already in your possession—your parents, siblings, and friends and colleagues who have aged "successfully" or "unsuccessfully."

When I talk about "planning," I don't mean simple financial planning. If having money by itself made for a better aging experience, I could have simply directed you to a responsibly written book about handling finances throughout your life. There are some superb books about that,[1] including many that handle some of the emotional issues associated with money that I'm going to discuss shortly. No, the planning I'm getting at is a bit more complicated. It doesn't simply involve looking at a retirement table to determine how X dollars invested monthly at Y rate of return will produce Z nest egg at age seventy. Instead, it requires having some general understanding of not only how long you might live but how well you'll live, what kinds of medical problems you're likely to face, and the kinds of limitations these problems might or might not create. It involves deciding how much money you'd like to devote to basic needs (plus some buffer to assure you of retaining control of your financial and physical health to the greatest extent possible), versus how much you'd like to devote to seeking *meaning* as you get older. If that last idea sounds high-minded or corny right now, you're probably a younger reader; I promise you that it will seem a lot less so as you get older and start having to make some decisions about how much time, energy, and money you'll be sending in that particular direction.

And if there's any money left over after this exercise, it involves deciding how much of it you'd like to leave to entities that are important to you and will survive you; this could be a spouse with a vastly longer life expectancy, several adult children and/or grandchildren, a favorite charity or cause, or any number of outlets that give your life, well, meaning.

And when it comes to that last point—the folks who might get what's left over when you leave, or who didn't bother to wait and may be already at the trough—we get into some pretty complicated emotional territory. The power of money casts a shadow over your health and well-being, but it also affects the folks who will outlive you in decidedly positive and negative ways, both during your lifetime and after it. It can rekindle and fan awful sibling rivalries and old slights, or it can be used to ensure health and well-being for the next generation. It can be used as a manipulative tool during life and from the grave, or it can be used to provide a true safety net for the people and causes that we love while simultaneously teaching children and grandchildren something important about independence. Money is many things over the course of our lives, but I believe that, as we age, it becomes a tool more than anything else. And as with any tool, the more knowledge and experience the wielder possesses, the better the outcome or final product is likely to be.

A Geriatrician's Practical Paradigm for Money and Aging

Traditional financial planning is often viewed in two stages: (1) an "accumulation" or "positive-cash-flow" phase, while you are a working earner; and (2) a "drawdown" or "negative-cash-flow phase," when you live off your nest egg or the interest on it. This model is far too simplistic for our time, when America is older than ever and people are likely to live longer than any actuarial table suggests. In this chapter I'll expand and refine this argument by pointing out the three major flaws of the traditional model:

Flaw one: The "accumulation phase" is far too focused on

accumulating financial wealth. There are other assets that should be stockpiled during this phase of life: larger and better social networks, wisdom about yourself and about aging, and the adoption of evidence-based practices to prolong health and well-being that I have already discussed. In short, I'm asking you to broaden your conception of what a nest egg is actually made of.

Flaw two: The binary notion of these two phases, whatever you'd like to call them—working versus retired, accumulating versus spending, positive versus negative cash flow—are becoming anachronistic for many of us as we age. With a longer average life expectancy and a changing economy come multiple significant career transitions over the life course. (Gone are the days when most Americans worked for the same company or even in the same field over a fifty-year employment history.) Many of the most successful people I know these days seem to have employment schedules and job transitions at every stage of life that defy this model. Many of my colleagues in their forties and fifties have furious work years punctuated by periods of sabbatical that are the result of choice or circumstance (such as layoffs). Conversely, some of the most successful older adults whom I care for have never really "retired," even when money is not a concern. Instead they work well into their later years because doing so brings resources other than money to their "nest egg"—meaning, control, creativity, and ongoing personal interaction with colleagues, to name a few.

The final flaw of the traditional financial planning model? It's the duration of "the phases" that we have come to accept as standard; these, too, no longer describe how we really live. A healthy sixty-five-year-old "retiree" could have a life expectancy of thirty more years, and in the near future the average American may spend as much time in what we used to think of as the "retirement years" as in the so-called working years. This has created huge issues for individuals and for societies, which both must rethink their traditional notions of longevity. Medicare is a great example. When enacted in 1965, it was meant to provide health care to people who had been employed for forty years but were suddenly no longer covered by their company's insurance plan when they retired. Not a problem when life expectancy was sixty-seven or sixty-eight and few pricy medical technologies were available to expend on older people; the idea was that you'd perish (inexpensively) two or three years after retiring. Fast-forward forty years and American medical innovation has extended life but may also bankrupt the Medicare system.

Creating a Personal Business Plan for Aging

There are endlessly nuanced formulas you can use to figure out things like how much money to sock away before retirement, how to take distributions from pensions if you're already in retirement, or how to make financial decisions that affect cash flow at every stage of life. But here's the aging view from thirty thousand feet. There are essentially three "inputs" you need to consider in order to make intelligent decisions about how to save or deploy financial resources as you get older: how long you'll live and in what state of health, what you want to achieve at various stages of life, and whether you want there to be anything left when you're done. Everything else is details—important details, for sure—but details nonetheless.

And as with every financial model, we can run into all kinds of problems with the data used to create it. Sometimes we're forced to make assumptions that may be wrong. Our ideas about what we value can change as we get older. Curveballs can come out of nowhere: unexpected illness or injury, devastating financial reversals (or windfalls), bereavement—the list is endless. In fact, for many people the variables seem so endless, incalculable, or fluctuating that they choose to simply forge ahead without making a plan. This is a bad idea. To let the currents of life simply carry you along the "aging and money" river may send you through a tributary that is unpleasant, avoidable, and perhaps impossible to escape once you're in it.

In my practice I care for many people who have been successful in the investment and finance world. In speaking to them about money and aging, I often liken the process to creating a "business plan" for getting older, because it's a language they understand, and they find it motivating.[2] I suspect that you might find it helpful as well.

All new businesses, or "start-up" companies, have a life span that includes both an early stage, when many resources or investments are needed and no profit is turned; and (ideally) a subsequent period when there is return on investment and the company becomes self-sustaining. In their late stages, the most successful start-ups have enough resources to do any number of interesting things: pursue new lines of business (or buy other companies), perhaps start a not-for-profit arm, or even agree to be acquired by another business, whereupon all those who participated may be handsomely rewarded. They can then choose to do with the resulting windfall as they see fit.

The "business" you're building here is the creation of a medically, emotionally, and financially self-sustaining life as you get older—and only you can articulate what it is you want to be doing at fifty, sixty, seventy, or eighty. In the same way that every successful business fills a unique and unmet "market need," you're going to have to do your own internal "market research" to determine what needs you'll be meeting with your plan and what unique slant your enterprise will bring to the table (in comparison to the business-as-usual approach to getting older you may have been taking). This process of articulating "what the business does" will also enable you to make some reasonable estimates as to what your expenses will be.

Conceptualizing aging as a business plan will also force you to make some educated assumptions about changing market forces that could derail your progress, such as the possibility of a medical illness that temporarily sucks financial and emotional resources from the enterprise—you'll need reserves for that. You'll also need to make an educated guess about whether such curveballs are likely to be temporary ones that mimic a short recession (say, a rotator-cuff injury that puts you on the disabled list for a year) or more protracted ones that portend a sustained and fundamental shift in "the economy" (for instance, being diagnosed with a progressive chronic illness like macular degeneration that might produce progressive and indefinite disability). But as you can see, in an aging business plan, the headwinds come not from "competitors" in the traditional sense but from a variety of random and nonrandom factors in and out of your control.

And finally, all new companies need a management team and a board of directors whose incentives are aligned to help the enterprise succeed. In some cases board members are chosen for unusual expertise that the company needs in its fledgling stages (like a conflict of interest–free gerontologist who is well versed in areas like long-term-care insurance), but in other cases board members are simply long-standing trusted friends and partners upon whose reliable counsel and example we come to depend. These could be older "mentors" who are themselves aging well or adult children who have your best interest at heart. Whoever these people are, they work together with the common goal of creating the new enterprise. At the end of the day, every successful business has a cadre of individuals with different skills, resources, and motivations, all of whom believe in the business plan, the mission, the product, and the founder and therefore rally around his or her vision.

That would be you.

Getting Specific

Enough with the metaphors. Let's walk through the three major elements of a plan for getting older that makes the most of your money, talents, and quality time: functional life expectancy, meaning, and legacy.

Functional Life Expectancy

I won't beat around the bush: You have to estimate how long you're going to be around. Any responsible financial planner will take this into account, as would any insurance broker; it's the reason life insurance becomes more expensive when you've contracted a chronic illness that might cause disability down the road. For these and many other reasons, one of the first questions you'll get asked in a typical retirement-planning exercise is to estimate your life expectancy based on actuarial tables, your health history, and perhaps some element of your family history.

That's a perfectly satisfactory take on financial planning if you're a newlywed in your twenties with a child on the way. But it's an unbelievably simplistic approach when you're at later stages of life, in that it ignores everything we've learned about aging over the past three or four decades. Simply looking up some insurance tables to calculate your remaining life span can be enormously depressing and, more important, inaccurate. Why?

Traditional life-expectancy tables generally ignore *functional life expectancy*—not just how long you're alive *but how long you are alive and able to function independently.* The relevance of this is obvious: The individual who perishes at ninety from a sudden heart attack while jogging will have far different health-care expenditures and resource needs in late life than the ninety-year-old who succumbs to a chronic disease like Alzheimer's, for whom the last five years could be spent bedridden. The implications for both financial and life-course planning are profound, because these circumstances dramatically change the balance sheet of what kinds of resources (financial and instrumental) you'll need. While living a long and independent life is rewarding, it can be expensive; living a long life punctuated or capped with periods of functional dependence consumes even more resources.

Some life-expectancy tables and formulas reflect *median* survival. So while it might be disheartening to know that the remaining life expectancy for a sixty-five-year-old male is, on average, twelve years, half the individuals who reach that age will live longer than twelve years, and many substantially longer.

Finally, life-expectancy tables reflect the remaining survival of "average" people of that age. Let's say you're a seventy-five-year-old woman who is in superb health, with a great family history and access to meticulous medical care: flu shots, stress tests, mammograms, colonoscopy—the works. You want to get an estimate of your remaining years on the planet and decide to use a Web site that calculates it for you. But let's be clear: You're asking the computer to estimate the remaining life expectancy *of an average seventy-five-year-old woman.* But what if you're not? The average seventy-five-year-old has two or three chronic diseases. If you have none from a combination of luck, genes, and taking good care of yourself, the remaining years reflected in the calculations could be an egregious underestimate.

As a result of these and other factors, patients and their families often make huge mistakes in attempting to forecast their futures, in both directions. On the one hand, I see new retirees make the mistake of spending too fast, not realizing that a newly retired sixty-five-year-old in decent health could live thirty more years! They might sell their home and buy a more expensive one in a vacation community; in this case they may have burned through not only financial resources but social ones as well, by uprooting themselves from long-standing friends, neighbors, and colleagues. Similarly, I see patients with serious established chronic diseases who have expectations about longevity that are simply unrealistic; in those cases patients often will unnecessarily hoard resources and deprive themselves of needed care or desired comforts in the erroneous belief that they will need them far into the future. In some cases that belief springs from the patient, but in others it reflects a failure of the medical profession to responsibly communicate and level with people as to the severity of their chronic disease and prognosis.

How does one realistically approach the issue of functional life expectancy? Here's a geriatrician's guide to getting started in a way that hopefully doesn't terrify you.

Longevity Planning 101

- **Start with actuarial life expectancy as a guide, but don't fully rely on it.** Wait a minute, Mark, didn't you just tell me these were of limited utility? Yes, I did, but to understand how these tables work is to understand how the rest of the world (without a gerontology perspective) sees you, and there are distinct benefits to that. Anyone trying to sell you a financial service or insurance product (see the next chapter) is probably using this model, and I'm about to give you a leg up in those interactions. The best example: the Social Security Administration. It knows nothing about you or your health, only your age, and on that basis it's going to start sending you money at a date of your choosing: more monthly if you wait, less monthly if you don't. (This is only one of the reasons that Social Security is going broke, but I digress.) You can make a more intelligent decision in choosing that date by using this exercise. Many such actuarial tables are available online, but why not start with Social Security's (found at www.socialsecurity .gov/OACT/STATS/table4c6.html)? As I said earlier, these tables refer to "average" seventy-five- or eighty-five-year-olds, even though I've never actually seen one. You'll obviously fall in a different place on this spectrum depending on whether or not you have serious medical problems.
- **Refine the estimate by factoring in your health habits and medical history.** This can be done in a couple of ways. Some actuarial tables will include some rudimentary "adjustments" for things like smoking history, hypertension, or other common medical problems. If those are your only medical issues, then this might suffice in terms of capturing the big picture. Another option is to visit Web sites that calculate your physiological age (as opposed to chronological age) based on a variety of variables that are known to be predictive. Good sites include www.realage.com (created by Dr. Michael Roizen and

my New York–Presbyterian Hospital colleague Dr. Mehmet Oz) and www.livingto100.com (created by geriatrician and fellow Beeson scholar Dr. Tom Perls). Using your physiological age, rather than your chronological age, in the actuarial tables will help you make a better estimate of your longevity.

- **Factor in specific medical problems.** If at any age you have a serious established chronic disease (such as rheumatoid arthritis, emphysema, Parkinson's disease), it will tend to have more influence over your functional and general life expectancy than factors like high blood pressure, particularly if it's well controlled. For many common chronic diseases, doctors use specific prediction tools to forecast mortality and disease course; these are well beyond the scope of this discussion but a good jumping-off point for one with your doctor about general prognosis, particularly if you have a trusted subspecialist who has followed a particular problem over time. It is entirely appropriate to ask your doc questions about prognosis over the long haul, in terms of life quality and quantity.

- **Make predictions about your functional abilities as you age.** This is the most important part of the inexact science of determining functional life expectancy. Certainly no one can precisely predict the future, but there are some commonsense approaches to the process that you should embrace. First of all, chronic diseases that are established are likely to progress, even when you take great care of yourself (unless, of course, you're felled by a natural disaster). Progressive arthritis will likely produce mobility problems at some point down the road. Visual problems like macular degeneration will likely produce some visual disability over a long life span, even when aggressively addressed with the best ophthalmological care available. Strong family histories of diseases that increasingly appear to be at least partially inheritable (such as Alzheimer's) should also be considered in this process.

With this exercise completed, you may have a better sense of what's ahead, recognizing the old adage "Man makes plans, and God laughs." You could get hit by a truck going to the post office tomorrow or be struck by a bolt of lightning on the golf course. You could also outlive every scientific prediction made by a slew of talented physicians about your "prognosis." I've been wrong many times when I've been asked by patients and families, "How long do I have, Doc?" But imprecision is not a valid excuse for avoiding the topic entirely; you've got to make some reasonable guesstimate of longevity if you're to plan appropriately.

Man's (and Woman's) Search for Meaning

If the last exercise was a bit sobering, I apologize, but I have a great antidote for you. The next step is where you get to explore the "blue sky" in your aging future, and I urge you to be as expansive and creative as possible in this activity.

My favorite "geriatric" TV commercial is for a financial-services company in which a fortysomething man and woman are talking to someone on the phone and they're frantic. "Now he's in Europe!" she screams to the man, with a worried, sick look on her face. "You shouldn't be doing this at your age!" the man grumbles into the receiver. "You're driving us crazy!" Typical parents going nuts about their wild kid, right? The next camera shot tells the real story: It's not a kid they're worried about; it's Dad. An older man, obviously their father, is shown sitting in a European piazza wearing a beret, earnestly painting the street scene before him on a canvas affixed to an easel.

In this exercise you need to relinquish every ageist idea you've ever harbored about the world and yourself. Yes, I'm talking about making your "bucket list," and you need to do it with nauseating specificity in terms of both content and the time frame for each phase's implementation.

Caution: While it's tempting to undertake this exercise in consultation with a spouse, friend, or other confidante, at the end of the day, no one can do this for you. This is about your "special magic," and the first pass should be done by you and you alone. For some the vision is truly expansive aggressive, and utterly unpredictable; one of my colleagues went from being a surgeon to making exquisite handcrafted furniture and he couldn't be happier. A patient of mine pursued a degree in social work at eighty and had a ball with her twentysomething classmates, becoming the toast of the university. I also have a 107-year-old patient who has become a spokesperson for successful aging.

But the best example of a boomer with this unfettered spirit of inquiry and adventurousness I can think of is my wife, Susan. Her unabashed willingness to identify new things in the world that she wants to experience and then pursue them is simply wondrous to me. Last year, at the ripe young age of fifty, she marched into the local music school and announced to the hipster behind the desk that she wanted to rent a saxophone and buy a series of lessons; he immediately assumed that this was for her child and asked her how big he was and what grade he was in. He almost fell off his chair when she told him this was for herself. "Lady, that's the coolest thing I've seen in a long time," he told her. She got a similar response from a local artist she cold-called to inquire about watercolor lessons for no good reason other than "it's something I've always wanted to do."

You might not think of my fifty-year-old wife as "old" (I certainly don't), but this active stance when it comes to following her interests has been part of her aging business plan since her thirties. She moved early to acquire these skills so in later life she would have a greater sense of meaning, a way of relaxing, an outlet for stress, and a sense of accomplishment. She tells me she has much bigger plans for sixty, seventy, and eighty (she took my advice and doesn't share them all with me), but she has calculated the expense of all of them (time, money, effort, competing priorities) and decided that woodwinds and watercolors were reasonable places to start, given her other life responsibilities at the present moment. Yes, we have three kids to raise, but she's got a plan, and she isn't waiting for an empty nest, more time, or some other real or abstract obstacle that might never materialize.

I've learned a great deal from the woman I married; her "carpe diem" approach to living is identical to that of successful oldsters

I encounter in my practice every single day. They've all got a plan. And while they may not follow it to a "T," it provides a steady and reassuring compass for enduring goals and priorities, especially when life invariably serves up some unanticipated twist of fate.

If there's one kind of book we geriatricians can't stand, it's those "Ten Places/Things/People You Need to See/Visit/Hug before You Die" types. Why? Because those are someone else's lists. Make your own and you'll have a much more meaningful journey. Some things to keep in mind:

- Don't buy into media or pop-culture stereotypes of what older people should look like or be doing. This is about you, not Madison Avenue. Those beautiful gray-haired folks in the Viagra commercials may or may not reflect your abilities, tastes, interests, or proclivities (except maybe for the sex part). If you've been a couch potato your entire life, I'd certainly encourage you to get moving for dozens of reasons I've already discussed, but if your target activity is bungee jumping because you think that's what "cool older people" are supposed to be doing, you're setting yourself up for failure and disappointment.
- Be specific about the things you've always wanted to do, and map out a realistic time frame for undertaking each of them in the context of the "functional-longevity" exercise. Be adventuresome but realistic, and don't necessarily focus on purely physical undertakings. If your mobility is limited, your aspirations might be to learn to be a pastry chef rather than go trekking on a wildlife conservation mission. Time it out: Do the surfing safari in your sixties, not your seventies, and save the more cognitively intensive activities (like visiting the pyramids) for later. And don't overlook the small graces in this planning process. They're goals as worthy as scaling a mountain for many of us.
- It's about the "one thing" (well, maybe two or three things). In one of my favorite boomer movies, *City Slickers*, Billy Crystal is besieged by a midlife crisis and tries to extract the "secret

of happiness" from a sagacious old cowboy, who tells him that it's just "one thing." Unfortunately, the rumpled cattleman keels over before he can provide more details about what that thing is. Crystal then spends the rest of the movie searching for what he believes must be some universal truth. The irony, of course, is that the "one thing" was not a single epiphany applicable to all of humanity but literally *one thing*. That thing is different for each of us—it's an activity, cause, or pursuit that brings meaning and value to life that we can articulate only for ourselves. Research on happiness and life satisfaction consistently points to engagement in a belief, cause, ideal, or mission as a major factor in achieving happiness. I look at the happiest people in my little orbit—at home, at work, in organizations I belong to—and this jibes perfectly with my personal experience. The most fulfilled individuals I know seem to be deeply involved with and committed to one or two things that bring meaning to their lives. The benefits they derive from these pursuits seem to trump so many other forces—money, health, and other life circumstances.

- I believe that role models become more important than ever as we age. Whom do you want to be like at each decade to come, and whose "older" demeanor do you find, well, less appealing? Each of us can identify individuals from both popular culture and our own social network whose life course and outlook seem to resonate with us. Don't make the mistake of focusing exclusively on the physically robust or outwardly beautiful Eileen Fisher–model types. Try to find people who seem to thrive as they age, even in the face of chronic illness, personal losses, or whatever life hurls at them. When you've found these folks, cherish them as a resource, and pick their brains. Ask them about what makes them tick, both in the here and now and as they look into their own futures. How and why have they maintained this outlook and life course when some of their contemporaries have not, especially when faced with similar obstacles and adversity? What advice would they offer you at your age?

Legacy: You Can't Take It with You

The last major decision relating to a business plan for aging is about whether or not you want substantial resources to survive you. If you're superwealthy and unable to "spend down" your nest egg no matter how frenetically you try in your remaining years, many would say that congratulations are in order. I have a somewhat different take.

Certainly the knowledge that those you love and worry about will be adequately cared for after you're gone provides great peace of mind. This is especially relevant when a parent has an adult child with special needs; I have cared for many such heroic patient-parents, and the concern they express for a vulnerable adult child in light of their own mortality is both touching and heartbreaking. They'll get no argument from me over what to do about nest-egg leftovers in that situation. Nor do I have trouble with other acts of kindness, such as a grandparent endowing a child's college education through a 529 plan or similar program.

But money left over in circumstances other than these can often create new problems and/or fuel long-standing ones. I encounter several of these every day when older people speak to me of their concerns about money and family relationships. See if any of them seem familiar to you.

The first is what I would call an adult form of learned dependency. Children who breast-feed into late childhood can develop some truly unusual personality characteristics; the same could be said of adult children who have access to unusual parental resources throughout childhood and adult life. While many heirs to wealth demonstrate extraordinary responsibility with the gift that has been given to them, others never really learn to make their way in the world independently. This becomes a disaster if they ever suddenly find that they have to.

The second problem sometimes generated by an embarrassment of riches as we age is a habit of unnecessary personal deprivation that leads to a failure to use resources wisely. This can affect aging people of any means, modest or otherwise. A pathological need to pass wealth to the next generation can lead one to deny oneself necessary health care, personal services, or other things that would make life easier or enhance its quality or duration. I see this over and over—people who have worked their entire lives, socking away resources for their later years, who are unwilling to access them when a real need arises. Sometimes this occurs through legitimate miscalculation and poor forecasting of future longevity and needs (now that I've taught you how to do that, though, you have no excuse), but in other circumstances it's due to a misplaced sense of duty to leave something to a child or a spouse. In the same way that you must make an earnest attempt to forecast your own needs, you'll need to make a realistic assessment as to whether the windfall you're planning for the kids is truly necessary and even whether it will have the desired effect.

And when it comes to things you need, I'm not just talking about health-care services. If there are life plans and dreams that you've saved for and you have the time and functional abilities to safely undertake them, I say go for it. In this case, the bumper sticker "I'm spending my children's inheritance" would seem to apply.

A third side effect of excess bounty as we age: sibling rivalry revisited. If you have leftover resources as you get older and several heirs, you may wittingly or unwittingly have produced the sequel to Cain and Abel. Several common scenarios can have devastating effects on families, however well-intentioned a parent may be. For example, you might plan (and sometimes tell your children) that you're planning to leave more of an inheritance to one child than another as a way of "evening out" things that have occurred during life—for instance, if one child was favored (financially or otherwise). In other circumstances, an adult child who has provided the bulk of caregiving to a parent may feel that a bigger chunk of inheritance is her due for such devotion; brothers and sisters may not agree.

The last (and furthest from least) problem created by an overgrown nest egg is what I call the "From-the-Grave Smite"—the ultimate act of retribution. I have cared for family members on both the giving and the receiving end of last wills and testaments that are meant to hurt those who survive. Here's my general advice if you're planning to be on the "doling out" end: While I'm sure that you perceive a lifetime of endless hurts—some of which may be very real and horrible—as the justification for such a "Lazarus" move, you're making a huge mistake. Instead of using your egress as a chance to bring about a healing with those who survive you, you're instead pouring gasoline on the family and financial pathology that you probably had some role in creating and that has likely been ongoing for many years. Your last act could either be a petty one that perpetuates the vitriol or an attempt to bridge the gaps. Which way would you like to be remembered?

Every family and every situation is different. My point is that the time to work out these issues and communicate about them is while you're alive, not afterward. If you feel the impulse to be punitive as you consider this difficult matter, I urge you to at least think about these issues and perhaps get some therapy; it could be a way to open a dialogue that is probably long overdue. If you cannot resist the impulse, well, that's another compelling argument for dying broke.

These issues are, in fact, far from limited to the wealthy. Even a meager nest egg can produce similar unintended consequences. I've seen it happen with patients who had neither multinational corporations to divest nor trust funds to distribute.

One final point about legacy, perhaps the most important one: Recognizing and sidestepping these quagmires before you get bogged down in them can have unbelievable benefits for you and the people you love. I have a theory about this. Most psychologists and psychiatrists worth their salt will tell you that money problems in families often aren't about money at all. They're about something else: anger, jealousy, control, insecurity—the list is long. That's why when families address aging-related financial issues in a forthright, head-on way, there's an opportunity for healing the deeper wounds that are expressed in fights about money.

When you finally do, the refrain "welcome to the family business" takes on a whole new meaning.

Chapter 18

Financial Gerontology

The Good, the Bad, and the Phony

Laughter always was the best medicine in my family because we couldn't afford health insurance. So when someone would get hurt, we'd just laugh and laugh.

—Tom Cotter

With your "business plan for aging" in place and some clear goals and values articulated, you're now in a position to delve into some of the minutiae that can make this journey a successful one. I've urged you to adopt an evidence-based strategy in evaluating health-care and lifestyle practices. Similarly, there are tried-and-true financial strategies that can have an important impact on your financial (and therefore physical and emotional) health as you age. Just as researchers at academic medical centers regularly discover or invent new medications or surgical techniques, their colleagues over at the business school are doing some research of their own, trying to cut through the marketing hype of the financial-services industry to give you some sound (and generally free) advice on what to do with your money.

Look, I'm a doctor, not a financial planner or investment guru, and worlds of money and health might seem very disparate at first glance. But I'm just stunned at some of the powerful similarities between evidence-based strategies for maintaining health and those for helping us build wealth. I'm even more struck by how our best-laid plans for health and wealth so often seem to go awry in similar ways—I've seen both in my practice over and over. The truth is, good financial and health practices are never adopted by the vast majority of Americans, or if they are, they tend to be abandoned shortly thereafter. "Why is that?" you might reasonably ask. Because similar internal and external forces are working against your attempts to know about and maintain them. Here are some of those forces and how they operate.

- **The processes are rarely sexy or expeditious.** By and large, proven techniques for maintaining health are much like the ones proven to keep you wealthy—there are no quick fixes. Both involve work and discipline. Adherence to a program of diet and exercise is about as sexy as disciplined monthly savings for retirement or a child's college education. Maybe it's just me, but the commercials for supplements that promise twenty pounds of weight loss in one month sound a heck of a lot like the ones that promise a 100 percent investment return over the same period. Believe me, there's no free lunch in either undertaking, no matter what the infomercial says.

- **The best advice is generally free but ignored.** Many proven interventions often fall upon deaf ears because people believe that something they get for little or nothing is of no value and probably won't work. In the health-care world, good examples are quitting smoking, exercising regularly, or keeping weight off. Mountains of data demonstrate the health benefits of these simple interventions, and hundreds of free pamphlets, Web sites, and publicly funded programs are available to assist anyone who wants to get with the program, yet I still see patients who spend tons on unproven supplements but never bother to exercise—and still smoke!

An analogous evidence-based financial example would be the proven value of index-mutual-fund investing over the long haul. Hundreds of academic studies have demonstrated the inability of the great majority of investment advisors, mutual-fund managers, and even hedge-fund gurus to beat, over the long haul, a "monkey-could-do-it" approach like buying and holding an inexpensive, unmanaged index mutual fund.[1] Some believe that this is not true during times of recession or economic duress, but the last American bear market also proved that idea wrong.[2] Yet many investors still fall for slick marketers' promises of sensational returns. (Did someone say "ten-minute abs"?)

- **They don't want you to see the real data.** There are exceptions, but most people who try to sell you financial products—stock and insurance brokers, mutual-fund companies, financial-services corporations—would prefer that you didn't know about inexpensive and uncomplicated products like index-fund investing, term life insurance, and competing financial planners who charge by the hour rather than commission (see below). They want to keep you in the dark for the same reason drug companies don't want you to know about generic alternatives when their expensive medication goes off patent: There's little or no money in it for them. But over the long haul, products like index mutual funds that generate smaller commissions and fees usually produce returns equal or superior to those of highly paid money managers, just as generic drugs are usually just as effective as their much pricier brand-name counterparts. And both industries "sex up" their products to hide the real data and confuse you (for example, putting two generic drugs in the same pill to get a new patent, or selling annuities or financial instruments that have some novel but inscrutable bells and whistles to get you to bite).

- **Snake oil comes in two flavors: health and wealth.** The tactics employed by charlatans to sell you dubious financial products are incredibly similar to the ones used to sell dubious health-care products. The claims are equally outrageous, gurus are in abundance, and fear and desperation—financial or medical—can drive vulnerable people to make irrational decisions.

- **Both outrageous health claims and outrageous investment claims can produce temporary insanity in even the most rational people.** If you're an aficionado of harebrained get-rich-quick schemes or dubious health care advice, I'm sorry if I've offended you. But here's something to make you feel better: You have a lot of intelligent company. I've seen some of the most hard-nosed, data-driven financial people submit to dangerous and unproven medical procedures that would make your skin crawl. I've seen scientists and physicians who in their own work insist on evidence-based medicine and hard data before making any decision adopt some of the nuttiest health-care practices imaginable. And I've seen both doctors (lots of doctors, actually) and financial people throw every last principle of evidence-based reasoning out the window to invest in crazy financial ventures, from commodities to real estate speculation. The returns Bernie Madoff promised his "investors" were a near statistical impossibility over the time frame he proposed to deliver them, yet he duped some very sophisticated businesspeople with his scheme (some of whom I care for or know and were wiped out). Quite a few Madoff investors had strong quantitative backgrounds and were highly familiar with the economic and investing precepts.

What's to be learned here? Fear of poverty and fear of disease both seem to create an emotional short circuit in the brain of otherwise intelligent people, causing them to respond in a way that reminds me of an audience member under the influence of a hypnotist's suggestive powers.

Immunizing Yourself Against Bad Health and Financial Decisions

Once you see the eerie similarities in the way your brain approaches health and money and you understand how a good proportion of the entrepreneurial world is trying to exploit your vulnerability, you can begin to create a sensible strategy for responding. Before we get to specific strategies for savings, insurance, and health-care spending, there's one big-picture element to consider: emotion.

Many financial advisors contend that the best decisions are made without it. "Create a plan for the long haul and stick with it," they might say. While I certainly believe that better decisions about both health and money are made when emotion is taken out of the equation, I don't see how it's possible to do so completely. These are, by their very nature, emotional issues for everyone to some degree, and the stakes rise exponentially as we age and test the physiologic and economic margins of reserve. How could it be otherwise? Implicit in your search for health-enhancing and life-extending concoctions is your knowledge that you're going to leave this earth someday. How do you stay emotionless for existential decisions like this?

In the case of money, the Wall Street guys say that the primal emotions of "fear" and "greed" drive bear and bull markets, respectively. I don't know a soul who hasn't experienced appropriate angst over at least a few financial decisions—overextending for the mortgage on that house you love that's just out of your price range (assuming you actually qualify for it, unlike some of those subprime victims), deciding to bite on a stock tip a friend gave you, or choosing to sit at the blackjack table while on vacation, even though you don't generally gamble and are well aware that the odds are stacked hopelessly against you. In cases like this, I don't believe that everyone can (and should) throw emotion completely to the wind.

All this notwithstanding, there are things you can do to minimize emotion or its impact when it seems to be taking over health and money decisions.

- **First, recognize when it's happening.** Think about when you've made rash financial or health-care decisions, especially ones you've regretted. It could be something as small as responding to an infomercial for hair-loss products or as significant as buying a life-insurance policy that, in retrospect, didn't really make sense for you. What were the circumstances? How did you feel beforehand? Were you tired? Were you "pitched" by someone you trust? Was it at an especially vulnerable moment in your life? The first step to averting a hasty or bad decision is to know when you're susceptible to making one. Salespeople in any field are taught to recognize and create situations in which the potential buyer is most vulnerable. They do this by managing how you're contacted, by whom, with what pitch, and when. (Example: There's a reason that automobile promotions are launched around the time people are due to get their tax refunds.) My point here is that if you have a general sense about when you're likely to be solicited (and are able to recognize that it's actually happening), it's easier to have your defenses up so you can avoid rash choices.

- **Next, stop or slow the clock.** When you've identified yourself as at risk for making an impulsive health or wealth decision, call a "time-out" on yourself. Whatever you're being pitched will still be available tomorrow (despite what the salesperson is telling you). I'm a big fan of sleeping on any decision that can wait. Slowing the clock also gives you time to consult with other sources that might have valuable knowledge on the subject at hand.

- **Make decisions when you're at your best.** Most people think more clearly at the beginning of the day. That's a good time to tackle big decisions, as opposed to when you're tired or irritable. Similarly, when you're worried, anxious, or under the weather, it's no time to be making investment or health decisions. Unfortunately, during illness is often the precise time when many such decisions get made.

- **Finally, build on your rational strengths.** If your left (rational) brain is tending to things in either the medical or the financial sphere calmly, responsibly, and with data, the goal is to try to put the same approach to work in the sphere that is being unmanaged, ignored, or overdriven by emotion. If both your financial and health-care decisions are being made in this haphazard way, I won't sugarcoat it: You've got trouble, and you need some good professional advice to help you straighten things out. I've told you how to find a "gero-friendly" doctor. Read on about how to find a credible gerontological financial planner.

Financial Gerontology 101

While an extensive discussion about taxes, insurance, savings, and *longevity planning* (the term preferred to *retirement planning* by gerontologists who work in this area) is certainly beyond the purview of a medical book about aging, I can point out the kinds of financial difficulties or disasters that I see again and again in my practice. Sometimes these result from harebrained financial decisions by patients and families. But often the culprit is a predatory scam from the financial-services community, which I find out about when a patient has stopped buying medicines or is not eating well and meekly tells me he has fallen prey to such a scheme. Or I hear about a problem in my capacity as an elder-abuse expert, for which I'm called to testify or opine in a criminal court or before a state or federal legislature considering laws to protect older people from financial exploitation. Whether someone is the victim of financial exploitation by a stranger's scam or an unscrupulous family member's efforts to separate her from her money, she's likely to feel a devastating sense of loss and shame over having been suckered. And by the time it becomes clear that the economic assault has occurred, the horse has left the barn: All the assets that could have been used to assist her in her day-to-day needs are now stolen, gone, and spent, with little or no chance of recovery.

For all these reasons, you need to arm yourself and/or your loved one with financial advice to avoid these kinds of mistakes. There are significant lessons to be learned from the rapidly growing field of *financial gerontology*. Here are recommendations from some of its experts to get you started.[3]

Begin a family dialogue about money sooner rather than later. One of my first bosses used to say, "It's easier for many people to talk about sex than to talk about money." He underestimated the phenomenon; I think it's true for *most* people. But it's time to expand your comfort zone. Discussing finances is best done when everyone's able to think calmly and clearly, before a health or financial crisis has you frantically trying to understand where a parent's assets are stashed and how you're going to pay for any number of unexpected and unpredictable needs that could arrive like a tsunami. I don't care who goes first. If you're the parent and you have a bashful adult kid, by all means, take the bull by the horns. If you're the kid and Mom or Dad won't speak up about these issues, you're just going to have to find a way to start the conversation. Sometimes recent life experiences can offer a useful hook. Perhaps a friend or neighbor was hospitalized suddenly or died, leaving an estate in financial disarray (and a surviving spouse in double bereavement); this would be a good jumping-off point. Or if the word *money* is not an acceptable icebreaker in your house, start by beating around the bush, perhaps using "housing" as the conversation starter. "Mom, where would you like to live if you couldn't stay here? Have you saved enough money for that?" Discussions about money and dwelling and health invariably coalesce when these issues are broached properly.

The time to start understanding Medicare and Medicaid is now. If you're fifty-five or younger, these probably seem like far-off things you'll worry about when you get older. In fact, many younger people I speak to confuse the two programs. But ignoring them is a huge mistake, for many reasons. Not knowing what Medicare does and doesn't pay for can get you into trouble at any age when it comes to making decisions to extend or keep private health insurance. Understanding how the programs reimburse for various expenses, such as rehabilitation or a nursing-home stay, can influence your decision to buy long-term-care insurance (more on that shortly); and it can help you help a parent wade through the issues they are facing in the here and now. If these pragmatic reasons to school yourself in the basics of Medicare and Medicaid don't compel you, how about the fact that so many upcoming political debates and decisions about these programs will have profound influence on you, your children, and the financial stability of this country? You'd be wise to understand them simply as a responsible voting citizen.

I could dedicate an entire book to Medicare and Medicaid; instead I've included a quick reference table (see the next page) as a cheat sheet. My favorite unbiased Web source for information on the programs is the Kaiser Family Foundation's sites: www.kff .org/medicaid and www.kff.org/medicare.

Become your own health and financial guru. If you're looking for a new hobby and have the time, inclination, and patience, getting a handle on your finances and investments is a terrific way to marry avocation and need. No one is going to manage them in a way that better represents your interests than you. The resources for getting a good do-it-yourself financial education are limitless, but make sure you get your information from someone who's not trying to sell you anything. My favorite starting point: Eric Tyson's *Personal Finance for Dummies* and any of his subsequent books on mutual funds, investing, real estate, and other money matters. In the best tradition of evidence-based practice, Eric provides sound advice on almost every aspect of financial planning and has nothing to sell. He began his career counseling people of modest means on how to handle money; stunned by the lack of financial literacy in America, he's made it his mission to educate people of all ages about money in prose that's easy to read, sensible, and straightforward. Another great resource is his Web site, www.erictyson .com, which offers no-nonsense approaches to money and shows you how to identify the people who are trying to get at yours for the wrong reasons.

Or find someone knowledgeable about financial gerontology. So you've decided that your "thing" is raising orchids, not working the stock market. Fine! But that means you'll need to get sound financial help from an expert. Be careful, though, it's a hornet's nest out there. And though your old family stockbroker may be the most familiar option, he might not be the best big-picture guy. There are several criteria for choosing a "longevity planner." First, be sure whoever you choose is a certified financial planner; while

A Geriatrician's Ten-Minute Guide to Medicare and Medicaid

	MEDICAID	MEDICARE
What it was supposed to do when enacted into law in 1965	Pay for medical care for poor people of all ages.	Fund medical care for the last few years of remaining life expectancy after retirement at 65, because health insurance is tied to employment (a distinctly American phenomenon). Prior to this, when you retired, you lost your insurance. At the time, little expensive technology was available to sustain life. My, how times have changed.
What it's become	That and more. It's the way most nursing-home care gets paid for in the United States, which was never the original intent of the program.	Infinite and unmanageable financial risk to the federal government. America continues to age. Expensive technologies continue to evolve that can extend life. The program is therefore unsustainable over the long haul without major surgery.
How it's funded	Through a combination of federal and state dollars. As a result, what's covered varies considerably from state to state.	Exclusively a federally funded program, through a specific payroll tax. Benefits, therefore, are much more uniform across states.
How and when you get it	When you meet certain low-income requirements. With long-term care, this usually happens after you've been in a nursing home for some time and are "medically indigent" because paying for it has depleted your life savings. You have to apply. Social workers in various health-care settings are very familiar with the process (because it's how their facility gets paid) and can help.	When you turn 65, after having contributed (through payroll taxes) to the system over time. You'll get a notice in the mail as the time draws near. Younger patients with some forms of disability can receive Medicare. Dialysis for some younger people is also paid for by the program.

What it covers medically	Basic physician and hospital services and some medications, though coverage varies from state to state because the program is partially state funded.	Hospital services and tests (Part A), physician services and certain therapies (Part B). Most recently some medications (Part D). Hospice.
What it covers in long-term care	The major payer for chronic (long-stay) nursing-home care, as any extended time in a nursing home will typically deplete the finances of most Americans. Medicaid may also pay for some long-term care services at home (such as home attendants) as well as other community long-term care services (such as adult day care), but this varies considerably from state to state.	Not a long-term payer but will pay briefly for services after a hospitalization for an acute illness. Examples include short-stay subacute rehabilitation in a nursing home after a hip fracture, or a visiting nurse to see you at home after you've been hospitalized for pneumonia.
What else you should know	Medicaid is bankrupting state governments, and the culprit is long-term care, not just poor and uninsured people. Federal and state governments are also constantly trying to shift the costs of elder care to each other.	The Medicare Trust Fund will be bankrupt soon, and all kinds of solutions are being proposed, including higher copayments for patients, the use of "managed-care" strategies to keep costs down, and delaying enrollment to later ages.

this doesn't guarantee that you won't wind up with a scammer, it greatly decreases the probability. Be cautious about other designations (such as "senior advisor") that suggest skill or expertise in this area; often these can be obtained through mail-order degrees. News outlets like the *New York Times* have done lengthy exposés on some of the unsavory folks who have bilked older Americans out of their life savings using phony titles like these.[4] A highly credible organization that certifies investment advisors in financial gerontology is the American Institute of Financial Gerontology; their Web site (www.aifg.org) provides links on how to find a registered financial gerontologist or RFG.

The Securities and Exchange Commission keeps a list of fraudulent financial "advisors" on its Web site: www.sec.gov. The Financial Industry Regulatory Authority has a similar tool for brokers and firms: www.finra.org/Investors/ToolsCalculators/BrokerCheck/index.htm. The federal government also has an excellent Web site that gives general advice on selecting a financial advisor: www.pueblo.gsa.gov/cic_text/money/financial-planner/10questions.html.

Pay for financial advice by the clock, not by commission. This is an extension of the conflict-of-interest dogma I've been preaching. When a financial planner makes money from investments, insurance policies, annuities, stocks, or other products he sells you, he's incentivized to point you in the direction of his most lucrative products. Not so for someone who is simply charging by the hour or year.

If you encounter an investment proposal from a commissioned financial advisor that seems both reasonable and enticing (in all fairness, this does happen), how about seeking a second opinion? Get the advice of a financial advisor who doesn't work on commission; this way you're not trading one conflict of interest for another. You'd make the extra effort for a medical problem, and financial decisions can have consequences that last just as long and can be nearly as serious.

Understand that your risk tolerance has changed with age. (If it hasn't, you're either very rich or very obtuse.) Nearly every financial-planning exercise for a new client involves an assessment of his "risk tolerance" (that is, how much can you stomach the vicissitudes of a fluctuating stock market to earn a potentially higher return instead of putting your money into safer CDs or a money-market account). But rarely are these exercises repeated as we age, and that's really unfortunate. Why? Because risk tolerance usually changes as we get older, and it can move in either direction. The stereotype of the older person wanting absolute security and guarantee of principal is not always true. Yes, many people become more risk-averse as they get older, especially if they must rely on a fixed-income investing strategy in retirement to meet monthly expenses. But some older people become less risk-averse, perhaps because they've accumulated enough money to allow them to "speculate" responsibly or because major expenses they shouldered in younger life (such as children's educational costs) have been dispatched and they're a bit freer now to chase higher returns. The point here: Risk tolerance is not a static feature of human beings like eye color or blood type. It changes and should be reassessed periodically.

And while we're on the subject, the changing nature of risk tolerance as we age occurs with regard to health-care decisions, too. Just as I have many patients who refuse safe and clearly indicated surgical procedures, such as repair of a potentially problematic hernia ("Not at my age!" they often say), I have others who are more willing to "take a shot" on slightly riskier procedures that could improve quality of life. They've done the calculation in their heads and decided that being happy and independent for their remaining time on the planet is worth the risk of serious complications, and in some cases even death.

Rethink everything you've ever thought about life insurance. This becomes a far more complex issue as we get older, in that we may need more of it or we may not need it at all. It's pretty straightforward when you're thirty with a new family: Your death would be financially devastating to your survivors, and you simply must have life insurance to protect them from that unlikely event. But what if you've reached boomer age or beyond with good savings and health, and major expenses like the kids' college educations are behind you and your mortgage is paid off? If your retirement nest egg is large enough for you and a spouse to retire on, it may very well be big enough for your spouse to live on alone. That's a case where you might not need life insurance; after all, it's another financial product that gets very expensive as you get older. The money you save from canceling your policy could be invested elsewhere or simply enjoyed.

That said, there are many instances when more life insurance is necessary as we get older. Some examples: A surviving adult child or spouse will have ongoing and/or expensive care needs from acquired or developmental disability; you yourself have ongoing medical problems that could bankrupt your estate and wipe out your spouse's inheritance; or you're part of a complex business arrangement or partnership in which insurance is used to "buy out" a partner who predeceases the other.

The bottom line: Life insurance is not necessarily a "buy and hold" proposition as we get older. It should be revisited.[5]

Long-term-care insurance: not "if" but "when." This, on the other hand, is a kind of insurance you may not have thought about much when you were younger that you could very well make use of as you get older. It pays for nursing-home care or care at your home should you need it. It usually goes into effect when you develop two or more impairments in activities of daily living (you remember ADLs—tasks like bathing and eating). And just like any other health-related coverage, long-term-care insurance gets more and more expensive as you get older, especially if you develop chronic diseases that are likely to worsen and be associated with disability in their later course (the "insuring a burning house" metaphor applies here). I generally urge people to buy long-term-care insurance in their forties, certainly by their fifties.

But be careful: This area, too, is filled with reputable and disreputable companies and characters. The horror stories range from insurance companies that have simply gone bankrupt after you've paid into a policy for years to ridiculous fine-print clauses like exclusions for dementia—the reason more than 50 percent of people ultimately come to need long-term-care insurance. Then there are the companies that simply won't pay when the policy is supposed to go into effect.

As a geriatrician I have done battle with several companies that refused to pay for care for my patients when they legitimately deserved it. I find these fights kind of therapeutic because, after all, I'm on the side of the angels, and I just about always win. (The phone calls are fun: Usually an agent on the end of the line tells me he's going to educate me about activities of daily living and other geriatric principles.)

Don't count on your regular health insurer to pay for long-term-care expenses, because they won't. And Uncle Sam? As we talked about in the discussion of Medicare and Medicaid, state governments are being bankrupted by Medicaid's exposure to long-term-care expenses. So it's probably not a good idea to look there, either.

Other things you may not know about long-term-care insurance that should increase its appeal: Many states offer tax benefits to purchasers. Federal employees have access to an unusually good program. And some states have partnership programs with private insurance companies, at preferred rates, with special features if you buy specific policies (such as the opportunity to legally shelter your assets from Medicaid for a spouse so you get care and he or she keeps the fruits of your retirement savings). These incentives make perfect sense for states trying to protect both their budget and their citizens.

My favorite resource for researching long-term-care insurance is the National Clearinghouse for Long-Term Care Information's Web site, which includes an excellent, unbiased discussion on the topic: www.longtermcare.gov/LTC/Main_Site/Paying_LTC/Private _Programs/LTC_Insurance/index.aspx.

Consider supplemental health insurance. Many people are delighted when they reach sixty-five and can trade in their employment-based insurance (or the mandatory health insurance the government will now require under health-care reform) for Medicare. But Medicare doesn't pay for a ton of stuff, and I'll bet dollars to doughnuts that as boomers move through the belly of the snake, the list of uncovered needs is only going to get longer. Besides out-of-pocket expenses like co-pays, deductibles, and drugs not covered by the Part D Medicare benefit (the list is long), you'd probably be surprised at some of the things Medicare doesn't cover that your current insurance probably does. For example, did you know that it won't pay for medical care anywhere outside the United States, you globe-trotting retiree? Nor does it pay for the first three units of blood you need in an accident or emergency.

Rather than keep blood in your freezer or apply for dual citizenship for each country you're planning to visit, you can sign up for "Medigap" insurance; as the name suggests, it pays for many of the things Medicare won't. Gap policies are available for commercial health insurance as well. All my comments on long-term-care policies apply to gap policies: There are good and bad policies, good and bad purveyors, and they differ substantially with respect to what's covered and what's not. But the basic features of Medigap policies are highly prescribed by the government so you can compare apples to apples. In fact, the government has decreed that there be specific plan types (lettered A through L), and each company selling plan A, say, has to offer exactly the same benefits. That makes it easier to comparison shop, because mostly what you're comparing is cost.

Two very important points on Medicare supplemental policies: First, since the advent of Medicare Part D (the Medicare drug benefit), they no longer cover prescription drugs. Gap policies for drugs, known as Medicare supplemental prescription plans, can be purchased separately. Second, the best time to buy a Medigap policy is in the open-enrollment period (the first six months after you turn sixty-five and become eligible for Medicare), because you can't be refused coverage, don't have a waiting period before coverage starts, and can't have your premiums increased because of new or worsening health problems.

As you might expect, the best information on Medigap policies comes straight from the horse's mouth. The federal government's Medicare site is at www.medicare.gov/medigap/Default.asp. Be sure to download the associated guide, "Choosing a Medigap Policy," which is indispensable and superb (and perhaps the only effective tool in trying to understand this complicated topic): www .medicare.gov/Publications/Pubs/pdf/02110.pdf. (Be sure to put up a huge pot of coffee before proceeding, or take a printout to the coffee shop.)

Also be aware that gap policies are not only for patients on Medicare. If you're still commercially insured it's worth scrutinizing your employer-sponsored insurance plan to see what's covered and what's not in order to see if a gap policy makes sense. In this context however, you find there's considerably less regulation than for the gap policies meant to augment Medicare.

Estate planning becomes increasingly important as we age. Estate plans are your instructions as to how you want your surviving assets used, how they will be taxed, and where they will be directed. These need to be reviewed at regular intervals—most professionals suggest every two years—or when something changes dramatically in your life (a financial windfall or loss, the arrival of a new grandchild, the loss of a spouse) or in the environment (including congressional changes to tax laws that affect estate planning—this happens fairly frequently these days as Republicans and Democrats cycle through control of the White House and legislative bodies every few years).

Additionally, estate planning should include provisions about end-of-life care and advance directives (chapter 19 talks about these in great detail), as well as tackling some of the legal aspects of aging that you may not have thought about (such as avoiding the need for guardianship).

A Few Choice Words about Retirement

Ending a chapter about money with a discussion of retirement makes sense, right? This is, after all, a chapter about money, and working is how most people get their hands on it. So when you retire, the implications are primarily financial, true?

Au contraire, mon ami!

Let me share a geriatrician's secret with you: For some folks—a minority, thankfully—retirement is one of the most stressful events life can foist upon them. That stress often has little or nothing to do with the loss of a paycheck and everything to do with damage to one's sense of self.

I believe that in American culture we are overdefined by our occupations. Just go to any cocktail party these days; the icebreaker you'll hear most often is no longer "What's your sign?" but more likely "What do you do for a living?" Note the verb "do" and the object it's directed at: "living." The implication is clear: When you're retired, you do nothing for a living.

My coy grammar lesson is not meant to be abstract. Some of the darkest depressions and worst stress-related illnesses I have ever encountered in medical practice have occurred in patients following their retirement. I have several theories about why: existential crises over looming mortality, newfound time to reflect on the fact that you may have just wasted forty years in a profession you disliked, or more time to spend in relationships that are much harder to navigate when you're at home instead of at work. One of my female patients has this favorite lament about retirement: "Twice the man, half the money!"

But the theory I think fits best is this one: Since we're overdefined by our occupations, retirement can produce a profound loss of meaning for some people, especially with the simultaneous severance of work relationships that have been important for years, perhaps decades. Again and again I see new retirees in a kind of rudderless state. And their sadness and disillusionment is only magnified by familial and societal expectations that retirement is supposed to be some kind of nirvana. Well, maybe for most it is, but not for everyone.

The worst retirement crises I encounter usually result from forced retirement, whether through some mandatory corporate policy (less common these days) or through downsizing or buyout. For most people, the best coping strategy is to dive back in rather than test-drive retirement. Find other employment if you can, even if the situation cannot entirely match the work or compensation you previously enjoyed. Volunteer opportunities should be included in the potential mix, too. If the new gig doesn't meet your expectations, at least you'll be entering retirement from a position that holds less allure and nostalgia for you.

Most of my patients, however, have just had it with work and are counting every bloody minute until they get the gold watch. (One guy sent me countdown e-mails daily starting with day "T minus 100.") If that's your take on it, congratulations; I'm delighted for you. But be aware that retirement may not be all it's cracked up to be, and venture carefully. I'm a big fan of the "toe-in-the-water" approach to retirement whenever possible, perhaps incrementally phasing out long hours over a year or two, or taking on consulting projects before going cold turkey. The goal here is to wind down in such a way that nobody notices. Not even you.

It's a bit like my favorite *Seinfeld* episode, in which Kramer announces to the gang that he's retiring. His friend Jerry pauses thoughtfully for a second and asks, "From what?"

Chapter 19

It Ain't Over Till It's Over
(and Sometimes Not Even Then)

A Geriatrician Talks about Death and Dying

Man plans, God laughs
—Yiddish proverb

I considered a variety of titles for this chapter before settling on this one; it was the "death and dying" part that gave me pause. Euphemisms, I thought, might be less jolting to readers, whether flippant ("kickin' the bucket," "buying the farm"), literary ("shuffling off this mortal coil"), or religious ("meeting your maker"). But as I began writing this chapter I learned of the death of comedian George Carlin, who marveled at the many euphemisms we use to avoid talking about death. I thought he would despise any manipulation of the English language that served to sugarcoat, conceal, or otherwise distract the reader from what I really want to talk about: our limited time here on the planet and what to make of it from cradle to grave. Shame on me as a geriatrician—no, as a physician—for even briefly contemplating the easy way out, because it's one of the most profound disservices a doctor can do to a patient or family.

I believe that geriatricians have a unique view of this topic, and not just because we're often called to assist people at the very end of life in so many ways. We also frequently have ongoing relationships with families after bereavement (such as when we care for surviving spouses or adult children) and therefore get to see the

294

aftermath of losing a loved one in a way many people and even many physicians don't. How we live and die can have a long-lasting influence on surviving loved ones in the form of guilt, peace, anger, family feuding or bonding, and any number of other legacies we leave through these choices. So "It Ain't Over Till It's Over" is actually inaccurate in these circumstances: It can go on, in fact, long after it's over. This is especially true when a loved one experiences a protracted end-of-life journey during which family members disagree on the course of action; there's no worse time for a family feud than when you're just trying to hold yourself together amid enormous anguish and grief.

What's so frustrating about the majority of the toxic legacies that result from bad end-of-life experiences is that most are completely avoidable. They result from two highly addressable problems. The first is abysmal physician training in the field of palliative medicine (more about that later). I'm in the health professions, so I'm willing to take some of the heat for that. Where I won't let you off the hook, though, is for failing to communicate your preferences on this critical subject to the people who matter to you. That's entirely within patient and family control. The other major reason that bad choices (or no choices) get made at or near the end of life is that the conversation simply never gets started in the first place. I'll talk about how to steer clear of this and other major barriers to a "good death" shortly.

These problems are part of the reason I'm so fascinated with the words we use to talk about death (or, more accurately, avoid talking about it). Hard discussions are easy to put off or avoid, and code words or euphemisms are vehicles and tools in service of that exercise; if you don't talk about it, then maybe it won't happen. This is an idea that is pervasive in our culture, and especially in American medicine. Furthermore, the accelerating pace of life makes it even more convenient to put off just about any discussion until tomorrow—about money, sex, anger, frustration, you name it. And death is a particularly tempting one to avoid, because the topic is so, well, consequential.

Don't think you're the only one trying to avoid this conversation. Odds are, you've got a medical facilitator. First, even if your doc is inclined to raise the issue, there's the problem of the "incredible shrinking office visit." When your doctor has to cover everything from seatbelt use to safe-sex practices to cholesterol counseling in a fifteen-minute "drive-by" (and, oh yes, there's a physical exam in there somewhere), where do you suggest we squeeze in a ninety-second mortality discussion?

There can also be powerful cultural factors at work here that can be as difficult for some physicians as it is for patients. Earlier in this book I lamented the overpromising of medicine, a dream world in which everyone is cured (without problems finding a place to park) and goes home happy. Of course, this is utter balderdash. Yes, we've got great treatments for lots of chronic illnesses that can improve symptoms and extend life, but ultimately every person has his day. Physicians, too, are caught up in the world of medical progress and hype, and I've come to believe that many view a patient's poor prognosis as a personal failure. The notion that death is a conquerable enemy seems to have been institutionalized at our medical palaces. So should we be surprised when some doctors have issues with discussions about the end of life?

If you stick your head in the sand on this issue, you risk losing the chance to make the absolute most of your life while you're here. You'll also be in danger of getting treated for a grave illness in ways that you wouldn't want, of forcing your family and friends to make decisions about your health without your guidance, and of blowing whatever small or large fortune you may have accumulated on medical tests and procedures that have little or no chance of improving your quality of life.

My advice: Suck it up and read on. You might wince at first, but as we doctors like to say: It won't hurt a bit. And while it won't save your life, it may just "save your death" in a way that affords dignity, control, and compassion to you and those who care about you most.

A Dummy's Guide to the Documents, Terms, and Forms You've Heard About

Without doubt, you've heard an endless number of confusing terms and been told about just as many documents with names like "advance directive," "health-care proxy," "living will"—the list is long. That's unfortunate, because the confusion obfuscates a very straightforward process. It also intimidates people to the extent that they simply throw their hands up and just avoid the whole thing— something they were probably eager to do anyway. This is a huge mistake. The good news: I'm here to boil it all down for you. Just take five minutes to read and understand the basic vocabulary, and we'll build on that.

- **Advanced directive:** A generic umbrella term for the over-arching process and the stack of documents you can use to express what you would like doctors and other health-care providers to do for you should you become temporarily or permanently unable to express those wishes. A very nonspecific phrase used far too loosely, in my opinion, but acceptable.
- **Health-care proxy (aka health-care agent):** The person you entrust with making your health-care decisions should you be unable to make them for yourself. The process of assigning this role is simple and straightforward and does not require an attorney, but it should involve (1) very serious thought as to who you pick and (2) a frank and open discussion with that person as to what your preferences are (more on that shortly). Ideally you should have an alternate proxy as well, in case something happens to your first choice.
- **Durable power of attorney for health care:** This legally binding document is the most formal way in which you can designate a health-care proxy, and in most cases it's probably overkill, if you'll pardon the expression. In most cases a health-care proxy can be designated right in your doctor's

office using simple forms that are available there or online
and typically require only a witness. My favorite Web site
on this topic is run by the National Hospice and Palliative
Care Organization, which has a state-by-state list of preferred
forms (there are some differences in what various states will
accept) right on the home page (www.caringinfo.org/statead
download). And if you'd like an advanced degree in being a
health-care proxy or assigning one, download the organization's wonderful pamphlet on the topic at www.caringinfo
.org/UserFiles/File/PDFs/AdvanceDirectives/QAHealthCare
AgentsBooklet.pdf.

- **Living will:** A document that describes (sometimes in jarring detail) what you'd like done to you regarding things like
dialysis and feeding tubes under very specific circumstances.
A living will is no substitute for a health-care proxy! More typically, this is a companion document to the proxy designation
that provides more specificity and should reinforce the wishes
you've conveyed to your proxy in discussions. In my opinion,
there are some limitations to living wills (which you should
understand but which shouldn't dissuade you from having
one). The biggest concern is that they can foster misconcep-
tions about the way medical emergencies actually play out. No
two medical circumstances are exactly alike with regard to
end-of-life care, and rarely does one encounter a situation in
which a generally rigid and formulaic document can provide
airtight advice on how to proceed. Bottom line: You need a
health proxy whose decisions can be informed by a living
will, but there's no way to plan for every eventuality.

- **Do-not-resuscitate (DNR) order:** A very specific kind of
advance directive that speaks to what you'd like done in the
event of an "arrest" (your heart stops beating or your lungs stop
breathing or both). In this case, without aggressive (and dare
I say heroic and dramatic) treatment, you would perish immediately. We're talking the last ten or fifteen minutes of the
ball game here, with paddles, defibrillators, ventilators—all

the stuff you see on TV. DNR orders typically come into play in health-care facilities (hospitals, nursing homes) because the technology to "resuscitate" is so readily available here, should you suffer a cardiopulmonary arrest, and because in the United States the default posture is to "do everything" in this situation for anyone of any age. Increasingly, "out-of-hospital DNR orders" are coming into prominence. This makes perfect sense; while your hospital medical chart may be clearly marked "DNR," as soon as you walk out the door there's a city full of paramedics who are unaware of your preference and ready to resuscitate you when someone dials 911. I tell my patients to keep a copy of their "out-of-hospital DNR order" taped to the fridge and another at their bedside. (One ninety-one-year-old patient of mine, vehement in her wish not to have life-sustaining treatment in the case of such an event, asked me what I thought about her getting a DNR tattoo. I'm pretty sure she wasn't kidding.)

The Six Major Barriers to Going Out on a High Note

Now that you know the lingo and some of the basic issues, I'm going to share with you one of the greatest lessons this book has to offer: a brief catalogue of the most common barriers in end-of-life care that cause unnecessary pain and suffering for both patients and families—and more important, how to get around them.

Barrier One:
Failure to Discuss Specific Preferences

There is perhaps no area of medicine that is more individualized as we age than end-of-life care, where patients express the most deeply held preferences of all. Many patients assume that once they've designated a health-care proxy, their work is done. That's certainly better than nothing, but it's no guarantee that your wishes will be honored; you still haven't expressed them.

There's some fascinating research on this issue, in which patients are asked what's important to them with regard to end-of-life care.[1] Guess what: People are different. There are very few universal preferences when it comes to how we'd like to exit the planet. It's a highly personal choice, and understandably so. One example of an "end-of-life issue" with substantial variation: the notion that all patients want to die at home. Sure, some do. But others find the prospect downright spooky, worrying perhaps about the impact it might have on a co-residing spouse or child. Either way, it's an important decision, but if you've lost the ability to express this preference before you told anyone about it, your family and/or doctor might have to make that choice for you.

Add doctors to this mix and it gets even more interesting. A popular folk belief among some docs: Most patients don't want to be awake and alert at the very end of life. Yet in one study, 90 percent of patients asked about their preference in this circumstance said just the opposite, while only 66 percent of physicians were on board with the idea for the same patient. If pain and other symptoms are controlled, many patients would indeed prefer to be alert. Perhaps we shouldn't be sedating people in this situation; maybe we should be controlling their distressing symptoms so as not to deny them this "once-in-a-lifetime" experience so they can spend the last drops of their lives and the last minutes of their existence with their loved ones—but only if that's what they want. And the only way we'll know is if you tell or we ask.

As if this whole area weren't complicated enough, there's another confounding factor: the ever-growing cultural diversity of the United States. This country boasts many different ethnic, religious, and other kinds of constituencies. Each brings unique ideas about death and dying to the mix—in some cases, including ideas that are alien to the way medicine is taught and practiced in the United States. This reality was brutally conveyed to me when, as an intern, I was excoriated by the family of a Native American patient for completely relieving his cancer pain with morphine. An acculturated daughter later explained to me that in their belief system, at least some suffering during dying is required for a peaceful afterlife.

In applying standard Western medical dogma, I had potentially robbed her father of that opportunity. Medical schools call this attribute "cultural competence." Apparently, I had very little in this context.

Don't assume that your medical care will be appropriate, sensible, or humane at the end of your life, especially if you haven't communicated your wishes. Communicate them as soon as possible, because you probably won't have the opportunity to do so when the need arises (see Barrier Two). Do it specifically and thoroughly with someone you know very, very well and who knows you very, very well (see Barrier Four). How specifically and how thoroughly? There's no such thing as too specific or too thorough. However, recognize that patients change their preferences and that medicine is an imprecise undertaking; no amount of planning can cover every contingency (see Barrier Five).

Barrier Two:
Counting on an Epiphany

Many people delay articulating their wishes because they believe they can simply do it "when the time comes"—a big miscalculation but an understandable one, given the way this time of life is depicted in popular culture.

To watch people die on television or in the movies, you'd think that meaningful last words were a dime a dozen. Maybe that's because when you buy the farm in prime time, the mode of exit tends to be dramatic, traumatic, or both—gunshot wound, asteroid mishap, germ-warfare slipup. As these television characters are generally the picture of health up to the very second prior to death, they bring complete intellectual faculties (and occasionally some acting skills) to the big "Rosebud" moment.

The truth is, deathbed confessions of screenplay quality are few and far between in the real world, because this is rarely the way we die anymore in the United States. I have attended the deaths of hundreds of people in the course of my medical career, and I can recall perhaps two or three instances when a dying patient partook in meaningful conversation in the moments immediately prior to death. Why? Because we're living longer: Over the past few centuries this has fundamentally changed both the causes of death and the ways in which we die. Rare are rapid deaths at young ages from acute infectious diseases like typhoid or perilous childbirths or operations without anesthesia in which we have time to say good-bye. That's a good thing. Instead, many of us have prolonged hospital courses (often without advance directives) and diseases like cancer, in which death is more likely to be preceded by a period of incapacity or the inability to communicate. That's not such a good thing.

Don't put off making your wishes known regarding end-of-life care (or any other important preference, for that matter) because you believe you'll have time to articulate them later. It's more likely that you won't. And in that case, someone will be making the choices for you. Or, more ominously, no one will know exactly what you want, and the care providers will default to "doing everything."

Barrier Three:
Insisting on Pomp and Circumstance in Creating Documents

Think you need an expensive lawyer to designate a health-care agent, create a living will, or draw up other legally admissible documents that pertain to end-of-life care? Great if you can afford one, but it's not a prerequisite, as many seem to believe; it's a perceived barrier rather than a real one. I call this the "pomp-and-circumstance" myth about advance directives. Here's the myth buster: Expensive lawyers are not needed to draft lengthy treatises on long legal paper to "make it official." Sure, there are formal documents that are recognized by each state, and these should be used whenever possible and ideally reviewed and executed by attorneys. (Again, see www.caringinfo.org/stateaddownload to get your state's documents and learn about its laws.) But just as you don't need a lawyer to create a last will and testament (just a witness), the same holds true for the legal document that specifies who you'd like making medical decisions for you. Yet many patients and families with limited financial resources tell me the expense of a lawyer is why they're putting off designating a health-care proxy. My response? I listen politely and then pull out a New York State form to complete the process right then and there. How's that for one-stop shopping? Let me be clear: I'm not advocating a particular position on care here. I don't care if a patient wants no aggressive treatment at the end of her life or the whole nine yards. My job is to make sure those wishes, whatever they are, get honored.

So when it comes to advance directives, "Do I need an attorney?" is not as good a question as "How well do you know that person across the breakfast table from you?"

Barrier Four:
Not Letting Your Health-Care Proxy Know
She's Been Elected

While more and more people are choosing to designate a health-care proxy these days, the overall proportion of people who have one is still way too low—for example, about 20 percent in the state of New York where I practice medicine. A substantial proportion of those other 80 percent without one will be dying someday, and no one will know what it is they want done when that happens. If you haven't designated a heath-care proxy, get to it! But even if you've done this, you're not finished yet. A substantial number of people have designated a proxy but haven't told the proxy that he or she has been selected.

When people draw up a will, the lawyers presiding will frequently include "boilerplate" health-care proxies, living wills, and related documents as a convenience. But because the focus is on the will (and money), the health-care planning may be an afterthought. A husband will very likely designate a wife, whether she is present or not. A widow may designate an adult child. A young person may designate a parent. Imagine being summoned to an intensive-care unit to learn that your parent or child has been critically injured and may need to have life support instituted or withdrawn. Now imagine learning at the same time that you have been designated to make that decision for him or her. To put a friend or loved one in this position is unconscionable.

You wouldn't designate someone to be your child's guardian in the event of your death without asking him first, would you? The gravity of this responsibility is similar. Make sure your health-care proxy knows he's been tapped for this role, then explain your preferences to him.

Barrier Five:
Not Updating Your Proxy as Your Values and/or
Prognosis Change

In another of my favorite *Seinfeld* episodes, Kramer decides to designate a health-care proxy and complete a living will. He's motivated by a cheesy movie he's just seen called *The Other Side of Darkness*, in which a lady falls into an irreversible coma. Kramer is adamant about not wanting "heroic measures" in the event of a devastating illness, but people change as their understanding and experience of medical illness evolve:

> *Kramer:* Jerry, listen. I just saw the rest of that movie *The Other Side of Darkness*. Do you know what? The coma lady wakes up at the end! . . . I didn't know it was possible to come out of a coma!
> *Jerry:* I didn't know it was possible not to know that. . . .
> *Kramer:* I gotta find Elaine. Y'know, she's gonna pull my plug!
> *[Kramer exits hurriedly and finds Elaine in the video store. . . .]*
> *Kramer:* Listen, Elaine, I've changed my mind about the whole coma thing. Yeah, I decided I'm up for it.

This little vignette highlights an important point rarely discussed in advance directives: End-of-life preferences often change. For example, a number of studies demonstrate that when patients are asked in two separate interviews conducted years apart about their preferences for aggressive treatment near the end of life, a substantial proportion change their wishes, in both directions.[2] The reasons? There are probably several, but human beings seem to respond differently to disability in the abstract than to disability for real. For example, as a new medical student I recall having to place one of the patients I was following on oxygen at home. As I saw her leave the hospital I remember thinking that a life tethered to a tank was an unfathomable one. But as I've put in the years, I can now envision a worthwhile life in which I can no longer run a four-minute mile. That's just me. Many patients have strong feelings in the opposite direction: If and when disability becomes part of their lives, their appetite for aggressive treatment wanes.

People and their preferences change all the time. You probably restructure your financial portfolio as markets change or update your estate plan as adult children become either more endearing or more insufferable. Why wouldn't the same be true of your feelings on advance directives if some medical event or simply the passage of time changes your worldview on the topic?

Barrier Six:
Being Squeamish about Prognosis

That Kramer's "coma lady" could emerge from her unconscious state helps make my point about the last barrier to good end-of-life care: the failure to seek prognostic information on your own situation. I alluded to this problem in the chapter on money when I asked you to create an aging business plan, but it's relevant to this discussion, too.

On the one hand, emerging from a coma is a bit of a movie cliché. On the other hand, it does occasionally happen. Whether we're talking about a medical event as dramatic and acute as a coma or a condition that produces disability slowly over many years, like arthritis, physicians cannot make guarantees; they can only speak in terms of probability. Ultimately you will have to arrive at some level of comfort for yourself (if you are the patient) or for someone else (if you are the health-care proxy) regarding the degree of certainty with which a physician renders a diagnosis and conveys the prognosis associated with it. My suggestion is that you do this

with data—the info medical science can provide about the "typical" illness or condition you're dealing with. Without data, you're
left only with hunches and anecdotes. The New Testament parable of Lazarus, the beggar who dies but is resurrected, comes to
mind and is frequently cited to me by families in situations such
as a deep coma wherein recovery is highly unlikely, but rare cases
of reemergence are on the record books.

The process of "prognosticating" certainly has improved in recent
years. The familiar query "Doc, how long do I got?" is now addressed
with *longitudinal cohort studies* and *randomized clinical trials.* In this
kind of research, people who are newly diagnosed (with something
like lung cancer) or who have just entered some life-threatening
state (such as coma from a brain injury) are "assembled" into a
group. Researchers then make "baseline" measures of every possible factor they can think of that might tell them who will be alive
versus dead (or still comatose versus awake) in, say, three months.
The variables may be medical (such as the size of the lung tumor or
injured area of brain on a CAT scan), demographic (such as income,
which as we discussed is a good prognosticator for just about anything health-related), and even psychological (such as the quality
of social support, also shown to predict outcomes in many health
conditions). The patients are followed and the outcomes recorded.
Researchers then determine which factors that were measured at
the beginning of the research are best correlated with the more
positive outcome at the end. Sounds like a great way to explain to
patients and proxies what to expect if they find themselves in an
acute situation and have to make decisions, right?

Well, not exactly. These studies tell you only what to expect on
average. In every such study of reasonable size, there will always be a
patient with "poor prognostic features" who outlives the researchers
and another with "great prognostic features" who goes unexpectedly sour in a hurry. Furthermore, these kinds of aberrations tend
to be more common in studies of older people. Why is this? Sorry
to sound like a broken record: If you've seen one eighty-year-old,
you've seen one eighty-year-old. The number of candles on the

cake is an immensely poor indicator of the well-being of older people; it can hide enormous variability in strength and frailty in all health categories—physical, emotional, and mental. Many of those strengths and weaknesses are also hidden from investigators in studies of prognosis and are summarized simply as "age." An extremely "hot" area of gerontological research is the refinement of how we measure health. Doing a better job at this would not only permit better identification of who will do well (or poorly) with a newly diagnosed disease but also which older person is likely to better tolerate (or suffer complications from) a surgical procedure or other potential treatments. One of these days we might actually be able to make sure that our treatments are not worse than the diseases we're treating.

So families of patients in these dire medical straits frequently recall stories they've heard where patients close to death somehow rallied and were back at work the next week. The danger of these Lazarus stories, unfortunately, is that "comebacks" are really quite uncommon; popular culture has deceived us into thinking that they occur all the time. Devastated families understandably cling to the possibility of recovery and use this as the basis for "not letting go" and even to press for more intervention. If you're doing this to honor the wishes of a patient who previously expressed these kinds of preferences for end-of-life care, then you are my hero (especially if you are getting pressure from a dissenting family member or health-care providers to withdraw care). If you are doing this in disregard of an advance directive explicitly requesting noninitiation or withdrawal of life support, your behavior can be construed as not only unethical but illegal. In some cases hospital administrations and physicians have been accused of assault and battery for placing patients on life support when the patient had a living will expressly prohibiting these treatments.

Much of this can be avoided if you do your job properly: Ask your physician *in quantitative terms* how likely recovery is not only in terms of survival but also in terms of meaningful quality of life (that is, living independently again). Most patients and families accept the doctor's prognostication at face value. I'm suggesting that you dig a bit deeper. "Unlikely" and "survive" are not good enough. You would make your physician estimate the probability of a complication if you were undergoing an operation. Why would you not require at least some specificity around prognosis in the face of illness? Implicit in this question is a deeper question that I believe is at the root of patient temerity: *What is the chance you could be wrong, Doctor?*

There is no substitute for discussion of these matters, in the most exacting detail that you can tolerate, with your physician and your family. I say this because the very act of talking these issues out—even if you can't come to a definitive resolution about all of them—provides more and more insight for your health-care proxy into the way you think about them. That's priceless.

And when and if you do find yourself in the uncomfortable position of having to make decisions for someone who has entrusted this monumental task to you (or vice versa), remember this: It's not what you want and it's not what the physician wants; it's what the patient would have wanted. These kinds of discussions afford a health-care proxy the best opportunity to exercise what ethicists call substituted judgment. With this information, you can begin to implement the wishes of the person who entrusted you with these deeply personal decisions. In these situations I often say to families, "Although your father cannot communicate now, imagine for a minute that the man you knew a few years ago could hover over us in this room and take in all the details—his physical condition, your anguish over the decision to be made. How would he react?"

Now that we've discussed the major barriers to getting good end-of-life care, let's talk about the antidote to the rotten kind: palliative care.

Palliative Care

Over the past decade or two, a growing movement, driven equally by families and health-care professionals, has gained enormous steam in the United States, and it may just be the remedy to the overpromising of medicine that I've railed against throughout this book. I'm talking about the growing call to improve care for patients with chronic disease who may or may not be cured but still have suffering that needs to be addressed. This area of medicine is called palliative care, or palliative medicine. Here, too, geriatricians have been at the vanguard; in many hospitals and medical centers (including mine) palliative care falls under the jurisdiction of geriatrics, even though the patients served by palliative-care physicians and palliative-care teams can be of any age.

Beautifully derived from the Latin *palliare* (to "cloak" or "protect"), *palliation* refers to the process of treating symptoms that cause suffering, such as pain from a cancer that has spread to bone, anxiety or depression about leaving family members in need, or breathlessness due to emphysema. We're talking about *addressing people's symptoms* with treatments that need not be directed at the actual cause of the disease. This is completely antithetical to the tenets of modern medicine, which holds that every disease should be addressed aggressively and relentlessly at its source. Holistic healers (and physicians) will often speak disparagingly of "Band-Aiding" the symptoms of a disease without getting to its origins. Well, guess what: Sometimes when people have unaddressed wounds, you need Band-Aids.

There are several myths about palliative care that I'd like to dispel:

Myth 1: It's just for the dying. Palliative care is about helping people live with chronic disease, and once we reach seventy, this includes just about everybody. Sure, palliative-care physicians see many patients close to the end of life, but anyone with chronic disease who is suffering could benefit from the expertise of a palliative-care physician.

Myth 2: It's just for patients with cancer. While cancer is the most common reason people seek palliative-care consultation, palliative-care physicians can be enormously helpful in easing suffering of every type. I have referred patients with just about any chronic disease you can think of—Alzheimer's, multiple sclerosis, arthritis, ulcerative colitis—to palliative-care docs. But this is yet another persistent myth that creates a barrier to getting palliative-care services.

Myth 3: It's the same as hospice. Hospice is a service provided to patients at or near the end of life (the official Medicare definition is someone with an estimated life expectancy of six months or less), and certainly palliative care is provided to hospice patients as part of an overarching plan of care. But you need not be a hospice patient (nor have a "terminal" diagnosis) to receive it. This misconception often prevents patients from seeking palliative-care consultations; they sometimes believe that once a palliative-care physician appears in the doorway, they've been "given up" on. Quite the opposite! I tell families that this care can be aggressive, too, as in "I'm going to use every tool at my disposal to treat your father's pain." I'll talk more about hospice in a moment.

Myth 4: It's all about pain relief. Palliative-care physicians are certainly expert in treating the pain associated with cancer and many other diseases. But that's only a small part of the job. Besides addressing other symptoms that can cause distress (such as breathlessness, nausea, and depression), one of the major goals of palliative-care physicians and teams is to *clarify goals of care*. Often physicians involved in the day-to-day management of patients are too close to see "the big picture." They may be focused on lab tests rather than symptoms. They may not be able to see that a patient is doing poorly or is becoming depressed. They may be in "cure mode" even after cure is not possible, or they may not be able to hear patients' desires to change gears. Families may have different expectations than patients and physicians. The prognosis and plan may not have been well-communicated to patients and families, leading to expectations going unmet. Or, alternatively, goals of care may have been communicated by physicians but not "heard" or "processed" by patients and families who are overwhelmed by grief, sadness, or denial.

What's the Difference Between Hospice and Palliative Care?

Used liberally, the words *hospice* or *hospice care* generally refer to a philosophy of care rendered to people with limited life expectancy. It, too, focuses on symptom relief and providing comfort to patients and families during those difficult times; hospice care also philosophically accepts the dying process as a natural part of life. Accordingly, much of the work of hospice involves palliative care but for patients with a limited prognosis.

In the United States, *hospice care* can have an even more specific meaning: It refers to a Part A Medicare benefit to which beneficiaries are entitled (most private insurers have adopted similar policies and benefits). And just as palliative care isn't only for cancer patients, you need not have cancer to be enrolled in a hospice program. In fact, hospice is underused for many clinical conditions, including Alzheimer's and other illnesses.

Hospice care can be delivered in many places: in health-care buildings specifically designated as a hospice, at home, in nursing homes, and sometimes in the hospital. Hospice patients are always followed by a physician; in some cases this is a physician who works for the hospice, but many physicians (and especially geriatricians) follow their patients into hospice. In order for someone to be enrolled, a physician must certify that the patient has a prognosis of less than six months (sounds ironclad, but fret not; it rarely is—many patients in hospice outlive their six-month certification, in which case they can be recertified or even taken off hospice if their condition or prognosis improves). Enrollment brings a variety of services to the patient that would not normally be covered by Medicare: visiting nurses, social workers, family support, and so on. In general, patients who choose the Medicare hospice benefit forgo subsequent hospitalization, although if circumstances warrant (such as a hip fracture), this can be overridden.

When to Call for Palliative Care

As someone leading a division that is responsible for palliative-care service in our hospital, I've gotten to see up close when this care is done well. However, some common errors in how palliative care is delivered occur repeatedly throughout the United States. The most common: Consultation is requested too late, after a ton of aggressive treatment has already been rendered. Now that the patient is doing poorly or experiencing some kind of distress palliative care is called for, but by this point it may have less to offer than it might have earlier. Suffering that has been ongoing could have been treated days sooner.

There are many reasons for these delays in consultation: the misconception that accepting palliative care means you're "giving up," a belief among physicians that they can handle pain management as well as anyone (many can, but palliative care is not simply about pain), a physician's lack of time to participate in lengthy patient and family discussions, and even doctors' lack of awareness that a palliative-care team exists at their hospital. And then there's the other physician phenomenon I've already described, wherein patients who are dying are not recognized as such by their doctors because they are too close to the hour-to-hour changes in tests and isolated symptoms as opposed to the big picture.

What can you do to avoid this problem? If you or a loved one are hospitalized with a serious illness, with or without symptoms that are being poorly controlled (such as pain or shortness of breath), you should adopt an active posture around palliative care that is consistent with your wishes, including the following:

- **Ask staff at your institution whether palliative care is available.** The first step, whether you think you might need it or not, is to determine whether anything resembling palliative care exists there. Increasingly, this is an important part of the modern hospital; I predict that within the next decade or so, it will be mandatory for them to offer such services.

If de facto palliative care is not offered, it may be hidden in the form of other services that are doing this "without portfolio," such as in geriatrics or a pain-management program (see below).

- **Get your physician's thoughts on palliative care.** At any point during your hospitalization (ideally as early as possible), ask your physician about it. His response (whether it's appropriate or utterly unreasonable) will be telling. As I always say, be wary of closed-minded men bearing stethoscopes. What physician would not entertain assistance in relieving patient suffering?

- **Know that doctors haven't cornered the market on palliative care.** There's no need to limit your discussion to your doc; speak to nurses and social workers, too. While the "party line" on medical consultation is that it needs to be ordered by a physician (in the same way medications or other interventions are ordered), the truth is that nurses and social workers are often well positioned (dare I say, even better positioned than physicians) to make the assessment as to when a palliative-care consultation is reasonable. After all, they are involved in the minute-to-minute assessment of symptoms (unlike the docs, who roll by once or twice a day at most to make their proclamations). In some enlightened institutions, nurses and/or social workers can make palliative-care consultations directly, which totally turns the militaristic model of medical care (doctor in charge orders everything) on its head. I for one just love this idea. Why shouldn't the clinicians (nurses) who know you best have a substantial (if not definitive) voice in determining how you get cared for?

- **See what assistance pain-management services may provide.** Many hospitals also have these services, which can be inpatient, outpatient, or both. As the name suggests, the focus tends to be exclusively on pain; accordingly, these services are often run by anesthesiologists and/or neurologists (although geriatricians and palliative-care specialists may participate).

In general, these folks can be superb adjuncts when the issue is primarily pain. But the larger issues of psychological distress and goals of care are probably best addressed by a palliative-care team.

A Man on a Mission

One of the heroes of the palliative-care movement in the United States is my colleague Sean Morrison at the Mount Sinai School of Medicine in New York City. Born in Canada (where the populace tends to have a more reasonable view of what medicine can actually deliver), Sean is yet another Beeson scholar and a former medical resident at my institution (I've always thought of him as "the one who got away").

Sean has devoted his career not only to helping those who are suffering, in the form of direct practice, but also to the study of palliative care at a variety of institutional and community levels. Some of his most compelling work has been in the area of "spreading the palliative-care gospel." He believes, as I do, that everyone in an American hospital should have access to this service.

Often the biggest perceived barrier to palliative care is cost. Hospitals are in an ever-worsening economic tailspin. Why should they fund yet another service that does not cover its costs? (As with geriatrics, direct physician reimbursement for seeing palliative-care patients in the hospital, talking with them and their families at length, and doing a "good job" does not nearly cover that doctor's salary, not to mention the other members of a team that might include social workers, nurses, and chaplains.) And palliative care is not a terribly "marketable" service, the way gastric bypass for obesity or Lasik surgery for nearsightedness is. Understandably, I know of few hospitals that would want to advertise the fact that there are patients behind their walls in many different forms of duress.

Sean's recent work has demonstrated quite convincingly that palliative care actually pays for itself many times over.[3] How? When these services help to clarify goals of care, patients are often moved to other areas of the hospital, other facilities, or home (for rehabilitation, hospice, and so on)—locations that are more goal-appropriate and, as it turns out, less expensive. This frees up beds and resources for patients who really need the services of an acute-care hospital (and whose care tends to be more remunerative). For patients who remain in the hospital to receive palliative care, the number of costly (as well as unpleasant and potentially dangerous) tests and procedures that may have little benefit are decreased. More to the point, these are interventions that the patients often don't want, or would not want if someone bothered to pose the question to them! I've seen it again and again at great institutions throughout the United States: ICU patients getting stuck over and over for blood tests unlikely to change their course; oncology patients receiving nauseating chemotherapy, unaware that there are other palliative options; heart-failure patients receiving powerful drugs in a cardiac unit to make their hearts beat harder or rid their bodies of fluid, all because they feel that taking a less-aggressive tack will disappoint their families. When these patients learn that there are other honorable options that are not synonymous with giving up, patient and family anxiety goes down and quality of life improves. But let me be clear: This is not about providing less care to save money; it's about providing the care that patients and families want and need, which just happens to be less expensive—more "high-touch" than "high-tech." When practiced correctly, palliative care aligns the goals of good doctors and of good administrators in a way that is rather unusual in modern medicine.

Sean and his colleagues have gone so far as to develop specific business plans that will help a hospital understand how much this care will cost and how the program will pay for itself (and then some).

In my opinion, palliative care is now viewed in the way geriatrics was in the 1980s. There were few formal training programs. Physicians and patients did not see the need. A medical student or resident declaring an interest in geriatrics drew quizzical looks from colleagues and professors. There was only marginal recognition by the august bodies that certify medical professionals and subspecialists. Fast-forward three decades and geriatrics is a fully recognized board certification; it has growing acceptance in medical schools and hospitals, in Congress, and at the National Institutes of Health. There are trainees who profess interest in geriatrics early in their careers and stick with it (although never enough, in my opinion).

Palliative care is now undergoing a similar cultural sea change in the United States. Americans are demanding it, and good for them. A growing number of medical students and residents have seen this type of medicine practiced "up close" and are choosing to make it their life's work. In the future, hospitals will be unable to get accredited without some attention to palliative care. And a new board certification in palliative medicine is being created, with specific training programs sprouting up throughout the United States. I believe that one of the most egregious oversights in modern American hospitals is the lack of widespread availability of palliative care, but a revolution is in the air, and you can join it. If you're in a position of influence in your community or local hospital, advocate for a palliative-care service. (Visit the Center to Advance Palliative Care's Web site to learn how to introduce the idea to the powers-that-be: www.capc.org/support-from-capc/capc_publications/the-guide/.)

Death and Taxes:
Still Compulsory, Despite What They Tell You

In this chapter, I've tried to get you to recognize an increasingly pervasive and widely held Western belief about death that is especially prevalent in the United States: that it may actually be completely preventable. This belief has been stoked by many forces, including irresponsible factions of the anti-aging movement and a steady diet of miraculous made-for-TV recoveries in which patients seem to bounce back after just about any medical misadventure, however serious. And my profession is to blame, too; we've promoted the misguided idea that medical science can fix just about anything.

These beliefs have become ingrained in our system of care in subtle ways you may not realize. If you are over the age of sixty and arrive unconscious at an emergency room in Europe and things look grim after an initial evaluation, you are far less likely to make it to that hospital's intensive-care unit than you would if you were in the United States. In the absence of advance directives to the contrary, American medicine presupposes that you want everything. And like it or not, you'll probably get everything. Physicians in many other societies (even many Western ones) find these "default settings" unfathomable.

I'm assuming you're way too smart to believe that death will be eradicated from the planet anytime soon, and therefore I refuse to insult your intelligence. By now you've probably figured out that the temptation to temporize or procrastinate on end-of-life discussions is just another form of ageism. In fact, ageism in all its various incarnations—youth worship, the anti-aging complementary medicine brigade, books about never getting old, TV shows with nary a sixty-year-old to be found, age discrimination in the workplace— really stem from a single powerful force in the collective human psyche: fear of death. If you don't get old, you won't die.

It's one thing to feel superstitious about death or to water it down with metaphors like "passing" or "at peace" as a salve against an understandable human fear. But it's another thing altogether to avoid discussing end-of-life issues with your family and doctor (or for your doc to avoid discussing it with you). I'm not just talking about people who are at the end of life and facing "terminal" diseases. No, this is an ongoing discussion that I have with patients of every age. (I was an internist before I was a geriatrician and still care for younger patients.) And here's a surprise: Almost without exception, every patient I have raised this issue with has been grateful rather than spooked after I've done it.

The ultimate irony: A discussion about death with a geriatrician is really much more a conversation about living than dying! It's about making sure that you, your family, and your doctor understand what your values and preferences are should you be alive but unable (even temporarily) to express them. If you suffer from chronic illness, it's about understanding the likely trajectory of that illness so you can make intelligent decisions about accomplishing all you'd like to in the proper time frame (could be months, could be decades); that way, you don't find yourself frustrated and disappointed by a long list of unfinished projects or unreached goals when and if disability restricts you. And it's about making sure that the people you love and who love you aren't saddled with more emotional and financial baggage than absolutely necessary when and if things get hairy concerning your health—it's going to be tough enough for them just worrying about you.

How ironic that the greatest gift you can give the people you love during your life is related to the end of your life: Going out on a "high note."

Chapter 20

Staying in Control

Making and Encouraging Good Choices as We Age

This guy goes to a psychiatrist and says,
"Doc, my brother's crazy; he thinks he's a chicken."
The doctor says, "Well, why don't you turn him in?"
The guy says, "I would, but I need the eggs."

This chapter is about making good choices (and avoiding bad ones) as we age. It differs from the ones that have preceded it in two important ways. First, in all my previous diatribes I've portrayed aging as a continuum and, in doing so, tried to speak to boomers and their parents simultaneously. I've made the case that the interventions I described (such as methods of staying safe in the hospital) are equally applicable whether you're fiftysomething or eightysomething. This chapter is about issues and challenges that arise more commonly among older readers. But boomer-aged adult children shouldn't fast-forward too quickly, because these very same issues provoke the most frustration and anxiety when they occur with parents (and other older loved ones). What's more, you may also want to stay tuned because you might recognize some of these early bumps in the road developing in your own path.

The other way that this chapter differs from the preceding ones is in its slightly different take on independence. Throughout this book I've argued for taking matters into your own hands whenever possible, whether researching medications and supplements, under-standing financial gerontology, or communicating with hospital staff.

But in this chapter I will address one of the most difficult decisions we make as we get older: when to accept a carefully titrated amount of assistance so that you can retain your independence along with your dignity. People often misconstrue accepting help as loss of control when nothing could be further from the truth. This chapter is not about losing control but exactly the opposite: retaining it.

Good Decisions Promote Independence

Last year one of my patients fell on a New York City subway and fractured a vertebra. He was left with an unstable but improving stride, and his family worried endlessly about his falling at home, especially the possibility that he might be unable to reach a phone to summon help. Their solution was to hire a twenty-four-hour home attendant to shadow his every move so he would not fall. Some patients love this kind of assistance, but he absolutely hated it. He was an eligible (and active) eighty-eight-year-old bachelor who had lived alone before this, and having a babysitter was the ultimate indignity. It also cramped his style. But as a proper and considerate man, he would not voice his objections to his family. He complained only to me. The situation was really wearing on him.

I suggested that he get an Internet home-monitoring system. "But I don't know a computer from a toaster!" he protested. I explained that he didn't need to. This was no "computer" in the traditional sense. I suggested having a company install a DSL line in his home and place Wi-Fi sensors over key places in his home: near his refrigerator, in the bathroom, in the corridors, by his front door. It would cost only a few hundred dollars. I explained how it worked: Over the first few days a computer that he would never see would learn his movement patterns: how many times he went to the bathroom at night, when he typically got out of bed, how many times he opened the fridge. When he deviated substantially from these patterns, his kids and I would get an e-mail indicating that there might be a problem.

"Too Big Brotherish!" he protested.

"Would you rather have Big Brother or a babysitter?" I responded.

I negotiated this idea with him and his family. They argued that he could still fall; there would be no guarantee of preventing this unless someone was trailing behind him every waking minute. I explained that his gait was improving, and with the device at least someone would get to him more quickly. They reluctantly agreed, and we proceeded.

Now each morning I get a "robot e-mail" telling me when and if he got out of bed, what the temperature in his apartment is, and how many times he opened the fridge in the past twenty-four hours. Everybody's happy. His kids feel a sense of control and vigilance about his well-being (their guilt that they can't be there every day has improved, too), he's got his privacy (the thing doesn't tell me when he's socializing), and he no longer has a live-in babysitter. (There is one wrinkle to this happy ending. Sometimes he stays at a friend's and forgets to turn the damn thing off. Then the monitoring company calls me in the middle of the night, thinking he's had a stroke, when in fact he's having a fine old time.)

Oh, and let me give you the economic punch line. The device, once installed, costs about fifty bucks a month. The cost of his home health attendant? Eleven bucks an hour. You do the math. How's that for health-care savings?

P.S. You want evidence that there's something wrong with our health system? Insurance would not pay for this service, but *was* willing to pay for the home attendant for a few hours a day indefinitely.

If Only It Were That Easy

I've got hundreds of wonderful stories like this, wherein a combination of negotiation with patients and families and good old-fashioned ingenuity created a situation that maintained (and, dare I say, promoted) independence and dignity.

But I also have some misfires—stories about attempts to encourage good decisions that didn't go as smoothly. You need to hear those, too, not because I want to rain on your parade but because I want you to understand the many reasons why people sometimes make poor decisions as they age. You'll see how things go wrong as a consequence of that and learn what you can do to avoid the same quicksand. For the next story you may want to sit down.

As a newly minted physician I rotated through the local VA hospital. This was one of my favorite things; I loved taking care of our nation's veterans (I have done this at several VA hospitals during my training and career), and I especially enjoyed taking care of the older guys who served in World War II.*

One of the patients admitted under my care was a man in his early seventies with diabetes and vascular disease (narrowing of blood vessels in his legs). That made it hard for his body to heal from even the smallest wounds or scrapes. Unfortunately this time he had been admitted with gangrene (a severe skin infection associated with low blood flow). I gave him powerful antibiotics and used every other trick I could think of in the hope of avoiding amputation. I even called a vascular surgeon buddy to see if he would perform a "bypass" surgery on the man's legs ("jumping" the narrowed vessel using a vein from somewhere else); my thought was that greater blood flow would help the legs heal and that more antibiotics would get to the infection. Alas, his vessels were too diffusely narrowed for a bypass to be of any value.

Sadly, I had to break the news to him that he would need amputation of both his legs below the knees. Remarkably, he was more worried about my feelings than he was about himself. "Don't worry, Doc!" he told me. "I've been in far tougher scrapes than this one." He went on: "Amputation is a walk in the park compared to some

---

* By the way, the Department of Veterans Affairs has been at the vanguard of American geriatrics and is responsible for minting some of the best geriatricians in the country. Kudos to it for doing a better job than our private system of health care in investing in the care of older people.

of the things I've had to see and do in my life, especially in the war. Don't you sweat it one bit, Doc. You're a prince!"

His buttering up worked; he played me like a Stradivarius. I know doctors are not supposed to have "favorite patients" (or at least admit to it), but after that he became mine. Although he had no formal education beyond the eighth grade, he had a stunning intellect. Self-educated, as a young man he had developed enormous guilt over his role in the Allied bombings of Europe and had pledged to "rehabilitate both my heart and anyone else I could help along the way." "God let me out of there for a reason," he would often say. And he seemed to believe that I was one someone he could help.

Nor did I complain. He was an intensely philosophical man, and it was a joy to watch his mind work, especially in the face of such medical hardship. He was something of an inspiration to every medical student and resident he came across.

I saw him in the recovery room after his amputation. He was in remarkably good spirits. He sailed through the operation and did just fine. He was not yet ready for prostheses, but I figured with a little bit of rehabilitation at a local subacute facility (which the government was willing to pay for) he might be able to live in some kind of assisted-living environment.

A sound geriatric plan, I thought. It would require some work, certainly, but ultimately he would wind up in the "least restrictive environment"—the goal of all geriatric medicine. When he was medically out of the woods from the surgery a few days later, I eagerly shared my suggested plan of care with him. And that's when it got really interesting.

He politely digested everything I said, studied my face, and then considered my proposal for a second.

"I'm going home tomorrow," he told me.

"But Jim," I reminded him, "you told me you live on the third floor of an apartment building that has no elevator, and you have no friends or family nearby who can assist you. How are you going to get to the bathroom or to the kitchen or into bed, much less out of your apartment to buy groceries?"

"I'll manage," he offered bluntly.

I thought carefully for a moment; I somehow knew that the next volley would probably determine which way this conversation was going to go. I chose to counter with a dazzling display of finely honed physical examination skills and anatomy training that only an Ivy League medical professor could muster:

"Jim, you have no legs," I pointed out.

"My cleaning lady comes once a week." He was formulating a plan in real time. "I'll ask her to come every other day to check up on me, and pick me up some groceries, beer, and cigarettes," he suggested, rather anemically.

"You use the bathroom only every other day?" I queried.

"Yup," he said. "At least for 'number two.' For 'number one' I'll keep one of these bedside urinals on my night table."

You'll need several, I thought to myself. This line of questioning was a dead end, so I adopted a new strategy.

"What if there's a fire?" I hypothesized. I had him!

"Hmmm. . . . Not a bad way to go," he pontificated.

And so it went. He had thought a great deal about this. There was no way he was going anywhere but home. Unfortunately, there was also no way he was going to last more than a day there. *This guy is nuts,* I thought to myself!

But here's the problem: He wasn't nuts, at least in the psychiatric sense. His mind was working just fine, and I knew it—I had debated politics with the guy that morning, and he kicked my butt. But the hospital, appropriately concerned about being at the doling-out end of this "unsafe discharge" from a medico-legal vantage, asked a psychiatrist to weigh in. They were interested in assessing his *decision-making capacity* to return home. Perhaps he had had a stroke or something during the surgery that had impaired his thinking or judgment. After all, diabetes is a risk factor for stroke, and we already knew that the disease had narrowed the blood vessels elsewhere in his body (his legs).

I also knew beforehand what the outcome of this charade would be.

"He's fine," said the psychiatric consultant. "Send him home, he knows exactly what he's doing. I should have so many marbles at that age."

I'll never forget the medical-transport guys picking him up for the ride home and loading him into the ambulance—the same guys who had brought him in a month earlier. They were not happy with him and were even angrier with me. Nor were they happy with the feeble medical-ethics lecture I gave them on "capacity" and "patient autonomy" as the justification for my decision to release him. I'll never forget the scornful look on their faces as they loaded this legless man into the back of the vehicle.

And though I didn't get to see it, as I went to sleep that night, I pictured in my mind these two hulking paramedics schlepping this double amputee on a gurney up three flights of stairs, whereupon they put him into bed and "let themselves out." I was so sick with worry that I promised myself that after doing rounds in the hospital the next morning I would make an unscheduled and unannounced house call.

As it turns out, I didn't need to, because he came back to *my* house. On my way into the hospital the following morning, I passed him in the emergency room with a fractured hip. He had fallen from bed trying to get himself to the bathroom. He looked at me, frightened and tearful for the first time since I had known him. In refusing to accept a little bit of help to remain independent, he had put himself at an even greater risk of losing it.

Why Do We Sometimes Make Poor Choices as We Age?

Why have I decided to share this lighthearted little chestnut with you? Because it's an extreme example of one of the most common and frustrating scenarios I encounter in my practice: people who have increasing care needs of one type or another but are unable or unwilling to request, access, or recognize the need for more services that could keep them in the best shape possible. It's one of the most maddening things for everyone involved. Adult children who are worried sick about a parent and can't understand why, even when they have adequate resources, simple "fixes" are not employed to make things better. The needed services and things people inexplicably deny themselves? The list is long: household help (even if it doesn't involve personal assistance). Someone to do errands, cleaning, or chores that are now simply too demanding, such as cleaning gutters or mowing the lawn. Better doctoring (or health care in general) that is more responsive to the kinds of difficulties you are experiencing. The need for home improvements (some inexpensive and simple, such as better lighting) that could save you some serious grief down the road. And, if things get hairier, choices that get undeniably tougher, such as accepting live-in help, a new dwelling, restrictions on driving, or any number of significant changes to one's life that preclude the need for yet more restrictive changes.

You might even recognize "milder" behaviors in yourself or a loved one that serve as less severe forms of my patient's poor self-care and safety choices. These might include not taking medications regularly, not keeping doctor appointments, or not sticking with a diabetic or low-cholesterol diet when the potentially dire consequences seem to be well understood. On the lifestyle side, these behaviors could involve partaking in a variety of potentially dangerous activities, from driving with visual or cognitive problems to using a ladder at home despite having arthritic hips and knees. The most extreme cases of "self-neglect" involve ignoring obvious medical or environmental problems (such as skin breakdown, shortness of breath, or hoarding of newspapers to the extent that you cannot walk in your home) that would cause any "reasonable" person to seek medical or other attention much earlier in the game. I view these kinds of behaviors as I would any other medical symptom, as existing on a spectrum that runs from mild to moderate to severe. Just as there are some stroke patients who recover and go to work every day while others become eternally bed-bound, so it is with low self-care states, which can worsen over time if not attended to.

The "Differential Diagnosis" of Bad Decision Making

While refusing care or deciding to live in a hopelessly unsafe environment can be purely a personality issue ("He's been stubborn and independent his whole life" is the kind of family editorial I often get), that's not the place to start when you're trying to fix the problem. If you do, you've adopted a fatalistic viewpoint that subliminally says you've given up any hope of turning things around. As I said, I prefer to think about bad decision making as a *symptom*. This is a useful medical exercise, because when physicians encounter symptoms, their brains are trained to look for all the potential causes. We have a medical name for this top-ten list of possibilities: We call it the "differential diagnosis." And the differential diagnosis of bad decision making has a few top contenders, some of which are purely medical conditions and some of which are not. Furthermore, there are easy solutions for a few of the causes of poor decision making, tougher solutions for others, and sadly, absolutely nothing you can do for the rest. This is unfortunate but good to know, because if the problem is truly unfixable, it's better to know what you're looking at than to toil in utter frustration.

Medical Causes of Bad Decision Making

Before you jump to the immediate conclusion that your relative is simply being obstinate, you need to exclude medical causes as the basis for his laissez-faire attitude. What are some of the medical reasons that can explain why people act this way? Well, this book is not big enough to cover in any meaningful detail the many potential causes of altered mental status, how to evaluate them, and what to do about them if they're responsible for the erratic behavior and poor judgment. So rather than make you do a neurology residency, I'll focus on the causes that are the most common, or the most treatable, or both.

Dementia. Leading the list of medical conditions most likely to produce these kinds of problems are illnesses like Alzheimer's disease (although there are hundreds of causes of dementia, in this part of the world the most common is Alzheimer's). How and why do patients with these problems neglect their care needs? While it's tempting to simply invoke memory loss as the basis ("I forgot my doctor appointment"), it's actually far more complicated than that. Many patients with dementia (and with Alzheimer's particularly) *have very poor insight* into their deficits, often to the point of denial. This finding is so common that neurologists have a fancy medical name for it—anosognosia—and some even postulate that the disease affects the part of the brain that is responsible for insight and self-awareness (the way memory is affected).

There are two reasons that it's incredibly important to figure out whether this kind of cognitive impairment is playing a role in refusal or self-neglecting behavior. First, depending on the kind of dementia that's causing the problem, there might be a specific intervention that could restore some cognitive performance and perhaps insight; the best example would be an untreated thyroid problem or some other biochemical imbalance. Second, if the dementia that's responsible is truly untreatable, you're heading down an entirely different road that may involve psychiatrically assessing the older person's decision-making capacity (as was done for my patient). Furthermore, some of the worst family dynamics I've seen around this issue are when families misconstrue "refusal behavior" as a willful choice when brain disease is the cause. A variety of ill-picked battles invariably ensue, in which the older person is told to "cut it out" or "pick themselves up by their bootstraps" or, even worse, is accused of neglecting his or her own needs as a way of vindictively getting back at a child or spouse. This kind of confrontation is always a very bad idea and only escalates an already incendiary situation. You wouldn't yell at diabetic Dad because his pancreas isn't making enough insulin; why are you blaming his struggling brain cells for his obstreperous behavior?

Depression. Mounting evidence speaks to the role depression plays in patients' inability to accept or keep up with a variety of medically recommended treatments—diets, exercise regimens, and medications, to name just a few.[1] (By the way, *nonadherence* is the newer, politically correct term we're now supposed to use for patients' not following our instructions. It replaces the older, paternalistic *noncompliance*, which suggested that the problem always stems from ungovernable patients who were behaving badly, meaning not subserviently following our health advice to the letter.)

There is no doubt in my mind that depression in persons of any age can produce profound inattention to health and hygiene. Furthermore, when doctors and lay people look for the usual "young person's" picture of depression in trying to diagnose the problem in older people—crying, staying in bed all day with the sheets over your head, loss of sexual desire—they get burned. Many older people with clinical depression have no sadness at all; sometimes the only symptoms are things like a decline in self-care, odd beliefs, memory loss, or a variety of bodily complaints (so-called somatization) that lead to their getting endlessly scanned, poked, and prodded by eager subspecialists (particularly when they have health insurance—it's called Medicare).

There are three reasons you should keep your antennae receptive to the possibility of depression as a cause or contributor to refusing help. First, it's incredibly common, especially in people who are experiencing the kind of advancing health problems that raised concern about needing help in the first place. Second, it's one of the more treatable causes of these behaviors, far more so than dementia. There are highly effective treatments for depression in people of all ages; medicines are especially helpful when used in conjunction with some form of supportive psychotherapy. Third, many primary care doctors are not trained to recognize the unusual "face" of geriatric depression, and even if they happen to, they may have little experience or training when it comes to treating it with medications.

And there's one more barrier to add to the identification and treatment of depression: embarrassment. Many older patients believe that accepting any psychiatric diagnosis or medication means you've got one foot in the funny farm. In fact, much of my time spent in treating older patients with depression is spent getting them to understand that this is a "brain problem" and not a lack of moral fiber. In other words, I'm actually treating two problems: depression and stigma. The good news here: As we boomers move into that age range, we're arriving with far more exposure to and experience with mental health services (usually starting with a Psychology 101 course in college), and I hope we will be much more accepting of treatment.

Medications. Changes in mental status can be caused by a medication or a combination of medications. If a decline in self-care seems to coincide with the start of a new medicine or a change in the dose of an existing one, tell your doctor or your parent's doctor, and consider a drug holiday as I described in chapter 15 (but again, always in consultation and collaboration with your personal physician).

Other causes. After dealing with the biggies I've already discussed, the list of contributors to a decline in self-care is nearly infinite and includes many medical conditions that are associated with behavioral changes. They include endocrine abnormalities (such as overactive or underactive thyroid or adrenal gland), psychiatric illnesses other than dementia or depression (bipolar disorder, forms of mania), and acute infections (pneumonia, urinary tract infection) that can provoke some of the worst mental-status changes. I can't cover all of them here, but suffice it to say that you're going to have to work with a primary care physician to figure it out or find a geriatric-medicine program. But here's a tip: Changes in behavior of any type that occur abruptly usually portend some unusual medical cause as the basis. A patient who has fastidiously attended to health and similar matters all his life who quickly becomes disheveled is more likely to have an underlying medical diagnosis as the basis for declining self-care ability. Slowly worsening patterns of refusing help that have persisted over decades are less likely to have such a treatable basis.

Nonmedical Causes

Okay, you've excluded some medical "eureka" as the basis for the problem. What are we left with if Dr. House isn't going to pull a rabbit out of his hat?

You don't have to be demented, depressed, or medically ill to refuse services and neglect yourself. There are plenty of physically healthy and robust older people without major medical problems who just want to be left alone. They've got all their marbles and some very good reasons as to why they should be spared an intensive medical evaluation; this would be a perfectly valid life decision for a younger person who does not want to deal with doctors. So what exactly is this all about?

It's about many things: Loss of control. Avoiding the first step on a slippery slope of being yanked from your home and placed into an assisted-living facility. Losing other "human" activities and connections like driving. Not wanting to be a burden on your family. And, yes, fear of death.

When you as a concerned adult child, parent, friend, or spouse really begin to understand this, it provides a gateway into what I believe is the most important tool you have to address the problem: empathy. If there ever was a place for empathy in family relationships, this is it. I'm asking you to truly picture living in the same home for fifty years without anyone meddling in your business. Then suddenly you lose a spouse or suffer a medical setback, and almost overnight you have your kids insisting you need a home attendant watching your every move. Or think about what it must be like to get a driver's license at sixteen or seventeen, use it for sixty years, and then be told you no longer can. Or what about living privately in your own home for a lifetime, and then being sent to a facility where you not only will have to prune down your most prized possessions to those that will fit on a night table, and then get a roommate for the first time since you were a college freshman or in the army?

That's tough stuff, my friend. Earnestly trying to put yourself in those shoes provides a window into why many people simply don't want to begin thinking about heading down that road. And if you honestly think that you're going to make constructive headway by simply "talking some sense" into Mom or Dad, you're being intellectually dishonest with yourself (and not terribly empathetic to boot).

When you start to take a step back to understand the underpinnings of care refusal, you can begin to adopt solution strategies that are more likely to be successful.

Getting Someone to Accept Help: A Twelve-Step Program

Here are the steps that I suggest families use to get a parent, a spouse, or someone else you care about to accept assistance when they've been refusing. This process is derived from practical advice gleaned from more than twenty-five years of doctoring and includes tips from families, social workers, and professional care managers who contend with this issue every day.

1. Exclude medical causes. As I said before, if there's a treatable (or untreatable) underlying medical problem that's causing someone to refuse care or services, that's really important to know from the get-go. You'll be spinning your wheels indefinitely if you try to implement any of the strategies below with someone who has altered mental status from thyroid disease, bipolar disorder, advanced dementia, or any other medical problem that influences thinking. Debate skills do not hold sway over brain biochemistry.

2. Identify sensory problems that may be contributing. Sometimes lack of awareness of declining self-care skills can be attributed to sensory disturbances that are more common as people get older. This was never more apparent to me than when I sent such a patient for cataract extraction; when I saw her a month after the procedure she said she had no awareness that the clothes she had been wearing for a year were stained, that her apartment was in dire need of a painting, and from recent photographs she could now appreciate that her makeup had been "harlequin" (her word). She was delighted to have her vision restored, but she was also mortified. I've seen similar circumstances wherein older people were unaware of body odor because of declining olfactory function (sense of smell) or unaware of wounds, rashes, or skin cancers because of decreased skin sensation due to diabetes or other disorders. And while we're on the subject of visual impairment, it's very easy to take medications improperly if you can't read the prescription bottle or draw up insulin correctly; in that case you might get accused of neglecting your health when the issue is more medical than willful.

3. Start the conversation. How you broach this topic may very well determine whether it gets shut down or you make some headway. The best advice I can offer is to start with the most sympathetic tone you can muster and combine it with your understanding of your loved one and the kind of overtures that he or she will likely respond to. Some examples: If vanity is a personality trait previously exhibited, then you might go there first: "Mom, you are still one of the most beautiful women I know, and with some assistance and some new dresses you'd look and feel better. How about getting someone in periodically to help with your hair and wardrobe?" Other family members respond to sincere and heartfelt concern when expressed honestly: "Dad, I'm sorry, but I'm worried about your health. I need you around for a long time. Your grandchildren need you, too. How can I get you to be more interested and involved in getting your diabetes under control?"

4. Listen, and understand the issues. If you do this right, your overture might just open a window into what's going on, and you might be very surprised at what you hear. Familiar refrains certainly include fear of losing one's home and autonomy, but in many of these situations interesting stuff comes to light that no one could have ever predicted. Some families have learned that a proud mom or dad had financial losses they didn't know about. Some find out about elder abuse by a sibling or spouse; the refusal of household assistance was based on shame—patients did not want others to learn of the situation. Other personal curveballs I've encountered have included marital affairs being concealed, drug or alcohol habits no one suspected, and understandable fears of loss of privacy. In several cases the major barrier to seeking care was a simple transportation problem, unbeknownst to anyone other than the patient.

Whatever the specifics, once you've identified the driving concern, you can begin to reassure your loved one with a carefully crafted plan that acknowledges his or her position.

5. Evaluate resources. All right, you've gotten a foot in the door, as unobtrusively as possible. You're now going to have to figure out which resources can be brought to bear on the situation. What good is getting a parent to accept help if there's no money to pay for it? In many communities, social workers associated with geriatric-medicine programs or area agencies on aging (find them through www.eldercare.gov/Eldercare.NET/Public/Home.aspx) can often come to the home and make you aware of what resources are available, even which ones the patient might be entitled to. These can be based on anything from income to military service to simply being a resident of that community.

But to be clear, I'm not just talking about money. Equally valuable resources in this context include family, friends, and neighbors who can assist; social-service agencies that offer older people in the community free friendly visitation programs or any number of services (such as medical escort); and churches or synagogues that can serve as an important social network for older people, who may become increasingly isolated.

6. Ask trusted others to assist in the campaign. Sometimes people need to hear concern from more than one individual in their social network, lest they perceive your involvement as meddling. Are there people you trust in your loved one's orbit that share your concerns? Peers are especially useful here; when concerns about the need for assistance come from someone in the same age group, it may make your mom or dad sit up and take notice.

7. Get everybody on the same page. Let's say you've gotten everything in place: The older person has agreed to accept some assistance, see the doctor, seek psychological counseling, or drive a bit less at night. Just as you're giving yourself a well-deserved pat on the back, you get beaned by an undermining curveball: A sibling, friend, or other interested party (often with little recent contact with Mom or Dad) swoops in and declares that you and the other family members who have painstakingly put together this plan have overreacted or misconstrued your parent's wishes. (Some geriatricians call this the "Daughter from California" syndrome, based on a famous paper describing a dissenting sibling, unknown to anyone over weeks of providing care, who mysteriously appears and declares a mutually agreed-upon plan of care to be inconsistent with the parent's wishes.)[2]

You can avoid this jarring complication by keeping everyone in the loop to the greatest extent possible so that there are no last-minute surprises. Although I recoil at the use of e-mail to negotiate difficult emotional terrain, this is an area where I think it can be valuable when used as a kind of "blog" to keep the other natives from getting restless.

8. Pick the low-hanging fruit first. If you've finally gotten a loved one to accept assistance, you'd be well advised to make your first intervention one that brings immediate tangible benefit (and perhaps even joy) to the recipient. It's very much like when I see a new patient, reluctantly schlepped to my office by a spouse, who has ten new medical problems that need attention. If none are immediately life-threatening, I always first address the ones that quickly improve quality of life in the eyes of the patient (for example, back pain, incontinence, erectile dysfunction) rather than the ones that are "just another pill" without any perceived benefit (cholesterol-lowering medication, colonoscopy). An immediately happy patient gives me more "cred" (as my teenage daughter would say) when I begin to address those very important issues in the second visit. Here are some concrete nonmedical examples of this that you can use to grease the wheels: If Dad needs some supervision at home while Mom is in rehabilitation, how about a helper who is a super cook to fill that void? If there are architectural changes Mom's house needs for her to remain mobile there, how about integrating some fashionable redecorating into the mix (like new chairs or sofas of appropriate height that she won't sink into). One of the more creative solutions I've seen was one a woman arranged for her mother, who was recovering from hip surgery: a "gift certificate" booklet for a chauffeured car so she could get to her weekly bridge game until she could drive herself again. ("She arrived in style, and her friends were green with envy," the daughter later told me.)

9. **Small steps first—they add up.** If you go from zero to sixty in attempting to get your loved one to accept assistance, you may lose the passenger altogether. Having identified an area of difficulty where she is willing to consider assistance, you should propose interventions that are minimalist and nonthreatening and that preserve her dignity to the greatest extent possible. Examples? If someone needs some basic housekeeping assistance a few hours a week, hiring a full-time home attendant is not going to make you popular. For patients whose driving appears to be safe but is still of some concern, yanking car keys can be draconian; how about convincing them to limit driving to shorter distances or just daytime trips? And rather than taking away the checkbook when arithmetic ability begins to wane, offer them one of the bookkeeping or accounting services that are growing to fill this niche. The goal is to take charge by providing some assistance, not by taking over.

10. **If help is required at home, you'll need to do some matchmaking.** Perhaps the most difficult form of help to accept is someone in the home as either a housekeeper or a personal attendant, especially when the presence is 24/7. And why not? If you've ever had someone live in and assist you—as a nanny, housekeeper, au pair, you name it—you know that it can be an unnerving violation of privacy (and that's when the help is caring for your kids, *not you*). I get about a call a week from frustrated adult children of one of my patients telling me that Mom or Dad has fired yet

another live-in companion or similar in-house employee. And I have several patients who have fired dozens, including many who never even made it in the door.

While there are some people who will not accept home help under any circumstances, my experience has been that a common error underlies why this goes wrong so often: failure to carefully think about the match between the client (note I did not say patient— this is your home, not my hospital) and the person coming in to assist. The mismatches I have seen have ranged from silly to idiotic: Spanish-speaking client with Chinese-speaking housekeeper, racist stroke victim (we're all God's children, and everyone deserves care) with Swahili physical therapist, bed-bound Hasidic rabbi (can't touch women other than the missus) and Muslim female home attendant (she was to do the bathing). When you're not thrilled about help in the first place, even less dramatic fix-ups typically result in a short first date and certainly not a second.

The remedy: Do your homework and make sure the agency hiring the person for you has done theirs. For example, if your dad has a hobby or interest, then having someone come who can share that interest is just awesome. My favorite example: A newly bereaved male patient of mine was just useless—depressed, couldn't shop, couldn't cook, couldn't clean, had no friends (his wife had done all those chores as well as maintained the social calendar). Fred had good long-term-care insurance and the agencies that tried to help him sent a parade of home health attendants, all women (because that seemed to be what he was missing): young ones, old ones, attractive ones, demure ones, quiet ones, "take-charge" ones. I don't think a single attendant made it more than twenty-four hours before Fred gave them their walking papers, along with some choice words that are not fit to print here.

When I made a home visit to scope out the situation, I found the patient sitting animatedly in front of the TV, booing at the Boston Red Sox as they trampled the New York Yankees in one of their traditional summer brouhahas. I had no idea that Fred (the nerdiest-looking accountant I'd ever seen) had any interest in baseball.

When he took me to his bedroom so I could examine him, there was Yankee paraphernalia everywhere. It looked like my ten-year-old's bedroom, not that of an eighty-one-year-old guy. He told me he had been a Yankee fan since he was five, when his Dad took him to the stadium, and the saddest part of his immobility was not being able to go to the games; when his wife was alive, they had gone together (he proposed at Yankee Stadium).

As soon as I got back to the office I called a patient whose son had just come to live with her here in New York. He was a superb baseball player who had been recruited to play minor-league ball but wasn't quite good enough to make the big leagues. He was going to school part-time and was looking for work: Here was a match made in heaven.

And indeed, the personal and professional relationship that evolved between these two persisted long after the companion's "tour of duty" with my patient was over. The most heartwarming moment came when he wheeled Fred into Yankee Stadium for the first time in a decade, and they both sat in some killer "handi-capped" seats. ("I could never get seats like this any other way," the younger man confessed. "Fred gets to Yankee Stadium; I get to enjoy his company and wave to my buddies in the bleachers—if they can see me from back there. A couple of them asked me if Fred needed extra help!")

Pick caregivers for your loved one carefully or you'll be replacing them on a regular basis.

11. The role of ethical deception. It's a bit Machiavellian, I know, but I believe that for patients who are refusing help on the basis of cognitive and behavioral impairment as a result of diseases like Alzheimer's, there's some ethical wiggle room for a few "white lies." When patients lack capacity and can't understand their need for assistance (and how quickly they'll wind up leaving the environment they're trying to protect), I view it as my duty to protect them by almost any means possible, as long as it comports with the wishes that were articulated before they lost the ability to weigh in. What do I mean? Dr. Rick Moody, ethicist and director of academic programs at AARP, tells the story of the patient with dementia who lost his spouse and became tearful and agitated every time his nursing assistant responded to his question "Where's my wife?" with the answer "She died." In a geriatric version of the movie 50 *First Dates*, it was as if she died anew every single time the aide reminded him. What I would regard as the ethical and proper though untrue answer ("She's away visiting your kids, I'm here until she gets back, what would you like for dinner?") put an immediate end to that perpetual wake. In a case of mine, a woman was firing aide after aide until I introduced the next one as her "personal assistant and secretary." Now the woman is safe, she believes she's the CEO of a Fortune 500 company, and both her son and I sleep a heck of a lot better.

You got a problem with that?

12. Good old guilt. And speaking of Machiavelli, there's always the good old-fashioned guilt card. I'd certainly play this one last, but if you're out of options, consider it, even if it's not your style. If your investment in trying to keep a loved one safe—whether it's time, money, worry, anxiety, neglect of your own job or family, mental health—is becoming overwhelming, then you should find a kind way of telling him or her that. You'll need to adjust the volume on this based on your understanding of Mom or Dad ("I'm going to lose my job because of your refusal to accept services" might better be brokered as "My coworkers are upset that I'm out so frequently"). You don't want to provoke a major depression here, just get the message across.

When It Just Won't Work

If you've followed my instructions scrupulously and are still unable to make any headway in terms of getting Mom or Dad to accept more assistance and live more safely, you're far from alone. As I said, it's one of the most common and frustrating things in every geriatric practice, so don't beat yourself up. But there still is one more thing you can try. Before getting into what could be some very uncomfortable territory, you've got to ask yourself two questions about the demeanor of the parent or loved one who's driving you nuts: (1) Does the behavior actually pose a danger to the person or others (and if so, what exactly is that danger?) and (2) Does the person actually understand the poor choice that he or she is making and its likely consequences? These questions are pretty complex, so let me break them down for you.

Is the Behavior Actually Dangerous?

Before you try to have Mom committed for missing a dose of insulin or a doctor's appointment, you'd do well to take a step back and ask yourself: Is this a truly dangerous situation? Just because someone doesn't want to live the way you do doesn't necessarily make them a personal or public health threat. People have a right to be messy or clean, bathe or not, and just generally be ornery even though you may not like it. In fact, there's a whole segment of society who make irrational, frustrating, and infuriating decisions— they're called teenagers. But unless these behaviors actually violate the law, harm others, or harm themselves, it's Mom or Dad's job to reel them in.

In evaluating patients who are allegedly unsafe or not caring for themselves, and before I get to the issue of their mental capacity, I first take a good look at whether the behavior is indeed unsafe or merely anxiety-provoking to the spouse or adult child hauling them into my office. I then ask myself, How would this behavior be construed in a thirty-five-year-old? What if a man brought his wife to see me, complaining that she misses several doses of blood-pressure medicine a month? What if his wife counters that he sneaks ice cream when no one's watching, even though he's overweight and has high cholesterol?

Would I be happy about these situations in patients of any age? Of course not. On the other hand, who among us has taken every single dose of their medication correctly or never cheated on a diet? And what about the huge human range of variation in (as well as variable opinion on) what constitutes "normal" hygiene? No patient in his fifties would be hauled into my "Doctor's Court" by his spouse with the expectation that I could issue some kind of medical restraining order to make him adhere. In fact, it would be a profound violation of his personal rights and liberties unless the behaviors seriously jeopardized him or others.

So what constitutes real danger? Geriatricians have a few hot-button items here, and they're the ones that typically endanger both the individual and the public. Driving is a good example. Taking away car keys is one of the most unpleasant things we do in geriatrics; it does rob people of independence (and often ends relationships with patients). But when others are placed at risk, we err on the side of curtailing activities, whereas in other domains we might allow more "room to fail" (see below). Smoking habits that could cause fires and endanger both the individual and other inhabitants of a dwelling is another example, as is a patient who forgets to turn off the stove, causing a fire. In such circumstances, I tend to be less forgiving in insisting on interventions that are aimed at curtailing the behaviors.

Does the Person Have the Cognitive Ability to Make the Decision?

Okay, let's say we've established that a bad choice—in the form either of not accessing medical care or of living in a precarious environment—is causing harm or the potential for harm. Now the issue is whether the person has the mental ability to make that decision (because, as I said, people have a right to make bad decisions). We're talking about something physicians call decision-making capacity, and it's one of the thorniest issues in providing care for older people (or for people of any age, for that matter).

If the patient neglecting himself or displaying other undesirable lifestyle behaviors does have the mental ability to make that decision (and no one else is harmed), free will is supposed to prevail in this part of the world, no matter what you or I think about it. Conversely, if he has no understanding of the potential impact of his actions on himself or others, we may be heading down a legal path toward *guardianship*. (I'll talk a little bit about that later.)

The proper assessment of decision-making capacity may seem subjective, but when it's done correctly, most physicians skilled in this area come to the same conclusion about a particular patient, and that's reassuring. But it's still a far more complicated process than other, tidier problems docs deal with, such as the interpretation of EKGs and chest X-rays. No, the evaluation of decision-making capacity is far more nuanced than drawing a tube of blood or running someone through a scanner.

Specifically, the assessment is focused on determining whether the person really understands the significance, ramifications, and likely outcome of his or her behaviors and choices. When I assess decision-making capacity, besides administering some formal mental-status testing, I try to solicit what the person's understanding of his or her predicament is. I find posing hypothetical questions extremely useful. "Mary, I know you want to live alone, but tell me what you would do if, god forbid, you fell in the middle of the room and broke your hip?" Answers like "I plan to get an electronic pendant that would summon help" suggest more decision-making capacity than "I would wait until it heals" or "I might still be able to walk to the bus to go to the doctor's office."

Central to decision-making capacity is the ability to understand the implications and likely manifestations or consequences of one's actions. I'll never forget an assessment recounted to me by a hospital lawyer. A developmentally disabled young woman who had the intelligence of a five-year-old had just given birth and wished to care for her infant at home. The psychiatrist kindly asked her a series of questions about how she would care for the child, to get a sense of whether she had the capacity to do this.

"What would you feed the baby, Sarah?"

"Hamburgers," she replied.

That interaction provided insight into her capacity to provide care for a newborn.

The critical point: *Decision-making capacity cannot be assessed outside the context of the actual decision that needs to be made, because different decisions require different degrees of mental ability.* A patient may be perfectly capable of consenting to a surgery when the choices and ramifications are clear and the decision is simple and straightforward ("You have appendicitis. If you do not have surgery now, your appendix will burst and you will become very sick and likely die. What would you like us to do?"). Many very impaired patients can participate reasonably in such a discussion. But that same patient might not have the cognitive ability to parcel out a sprawling multinational corporation to eleven heirs, or make a complex decision between radiation therapy, chemotherapy, or surgery for newly diagnosed lung cancer (each treatment having its own statistical chance of success or failure, as well as side effects—complicated even for an oncologist to wrap her brain around). Formal assessments of decision-making capacity are usually performed by psychiatrists, but many geriatricians and other generalists are very comfortable making these determinations. (Certain states may or may not require psychiatrists for the purpose of formal proceedings like guardianship; see page 346.)

Room to Fail: When to Get Aggressive about Frustrating Behaviors and When to "Lay Off"

One last point before we take it to the next (and rather draconian) level of interventions for people who exhibit poor decision making. You've heard me talk about finding the "least-restrictive alternative" as we age; it's the balance between safety and independence that we all strive for. How do you make sure that people you love are reasonably safe without driving them nuts (not to mention stoking an understandable paranoia that you are meddling in their life and trying to undermine their independence)?

The answer: with some space. Many of us have had at least one aging parent, family member, or friend who just worried us sick. We knew that someday there would probably come a time when they would be unable to function independently. Believe it or not, they often know this, too. Still, we may wind up putting off doing anything for as long as possible, even though we'd feel just rotten if our procrastination allowed something horrible to happen.

I know throughout this book I've advocated for an aggressive, proactive stance around planning for our own aging and that of our loved ones, but we have another saying in geriatrics: "Sometimes things have to get a little worse before they can get better." If a person has dwindling mental or physical abilities and a definitive loss of independence is somewhere on the horizon, sometimes the only way to make that transition is to let it happen, as safely as possible. If your parent is unable to handle finances, for example, perhaps the only way to get him to recognize this is to let him write out a check that is incorrect or have a utility threaten to end service for failure to pay a bill. If he's prone to frequent respiratory infections and refuses to see the physician, get flu shots, or take other appropriate preventative measures, sometimes an avoidable hospitalization for mild pneumonia is the only way to get him to recognize the vulnerability you've been angsting over. Let me be clear: I'd never put a patient at risk of losing his or her life savings or jeopardizing life and limb from neglected medical problems. But if the downside of giving room to fail is getting scammed out of $300 and the upside is many more months of independence because the patient accepted intervention, that's a risk I might consider taking. Patients in situations like this should always be stealthily monitored (for example, that checking account shouldn't have $100,000 in it, and the patient with a history of respiratory infections should be visited on a regular basis). Furthermore, permitting behaviors that risk the health and safety of others (like driving) are absolutely verboten, but what's the problem with affording some prolonged dignity to people if their poor decisions are unlikely to cause significant harm? Besides, if the person has the decision-making capacity to make those poor choices, there are really very few options (or at least no legal option) other than the twelve-step strategy I've outlined for you. The goal here is the "soft landing." Often medical or social crises (especially when they involve hospitalization) serve as important transition points for families (and patients themselves) to understand that the previous situation was simply not working anymore.

Guardianship

So now you have a gerontological framework to help you think about less-than-ideal decision making in someone you care about, and even some concrete advice on how to gently intervene (with the assistance of experienced health-care professionals). If you're creative and lucky, perhaps you've been able to improve the situation, if only partially. If so, congratulations, you're a hero. But what if things don't go so smoothly? The thorniest circumstance you or your loved one may find themselves in is what I call the trifecta of impaired decision making: (1) The person is indeed repeatedly making poor decisions that are dangerous to them, (2) the person refuses assistance despite your best attempts to provide or arrange it, and (3) the person lacks the ability to understand the implications of his or her actions. We might then be heading for the ugliest end point of these common scenarios: a *guardianship proceeding.* (In some states, guardianship is also referred to as *conservatorship.*) Guardianship is an increasingly common occurrence these days in American life, not only because people fail to specify their wishes in advance but also because there is an epidemic of incapacity as America ages and mobility patterns disperse potentially helpful relatives or friends far from home (and also because there are some unscrupulous people who would like to get ahold of older people's resources, particularly by taking advantage of deteriorating mental status).

I wish the public were more aware of guardianship. Most law and crime shows on television would probably find the topic profoundly "unsexy," especially when compared to topics like "murder one," the "insanity defense," and the death penalty. But guardianship in real legal settings is considered to be one of the most serious matters in American jurisprudence. Why? Because it rescinds one of the most basic human rights guaranteed by the Constitution: the freedom to make decisions for oneself. Until age eighteen, minors are considered to have no rights in this regard; decisions are ultimately in the hands of their parents (their legal guardians). At eighteen, children arbitrarily attain the right to self-determination (including the right to make bad and potentially self-injurious decisions). What's more, that right stays with them until death, or until someone believes that they have lost the capacity to exert the right safely. This was probably a reasonable posture when some tenets of the Magna Carta were imported to create an American system of laws and average life expectancy was the ripe old age of thirty-two. Just about everyone who died did so with most of their marbles, even if you did not agree with their choices.

The details of guardianship vary a bit from state to state, but the basic elements are the same. A petitioner approaches the court and alleges that a person has impaired capacity. At a formal proceeding, a physician certifies this to be the case. Should the allegation be confirmed, a guardian is appointed, typically to assist the incapacitated person in areas of his or her life in a way that is the least restrictive as possible (there are those buzzwords again). For example, some patients are incapacitated in such a way that they need help with managing finances, but they remain able to make decisions about where they want to live; in that case, the guardianship order might stipulate that the guardian assist only with financial issues. The guardian must make regular reports to the court that include how monies were spent, what health-care decisions were made, and whether the individual still needs a guardian. Being a guardian is a tough job when done properly, and in my opinion there's a critical and growing shortage of well-trained, judicious, and ethical guardians.

How to Avoid Medico-Legal Hornets' Nests Like Guardianship for You or Your Loved Ones

The news these days is filled with stories of older people who allegedly have been exploited by guardians or other folks to whom they have entrusted their care and/or finances. Most of the stories that make the news are about wealthy types (the Brooke Astor situation is a good example), but people with modest or few resources find themselves in these situations, too, and in some ways it is even more tragic. Losing $100,000 stinks if you're loaded, but if it's your entire nest egg, it is devastating, particularly if it happens at a time when your resources are needed most. Then there are the lawyers' fees, which can consume all or most of your savings if these proceedings drag on.

And money is only one part: People may find themselves in care situations that they never would have agreed to earlier in life as adult children squabble endlessly over what Mom or Dad "would have wanted."

How can you avoid guardianship or similar kinds of hot water for you or a loved one? With regard to health-care decisions, I've already told you: Designate a proxy ASAP, and let that person know about it. Then go buy your proxy a fancy dinner, over the course of which you lay out all your preferences. Do this right and when you become incapacitated, your proxy will meet your doctor with a plan reflecting your wishes, rather than a dumbfounded blank stare.

That will go a long way toward inoculating you from health-care monkey business, but it won't do much to fix the next problem: handling your money and finances when you no longer have the ability to do it. Ask yourself this: If you were laid up in the hospital for a month (or indefinitely) to the extent that you could not think or communicate clearly, what would happen to your financial world? I suspect your landlord would still want the rent, the car-leasing company would still want its payment, and the electric company would still want its bill paid. How will money from your checking account get to your mortgage holder? And let's not forget the stuff only you can do that's not directly related to money but in the same neighborhood. This could be anything from paying your taxes to getting into your safe-deposit box to picking up a certified letter at the post office. In fact, just about anything for which your signature and/or identification is required (and that's a growing number of places in a security-minded world) will be inaccessible when you can't get out of your hospital bed. And should you be lucky enough to do that at some point, you may find you've come home to utter financial turmoil, ranging from repossession of your car to foreclosure to a ruined credit rating. What's a poor boomer to do?

Enter the *power of attorney*, a document that gives someone you've designated (as you did when you designated a health-care proxy) the ability to transact financial and other business as if they were you. A power of attorney comes into play in a very specific circumstance: when you lose decision-making capacity to handle finances, temporarily or permanently. If you've picked your power of attorney carefully, she will have a good general sense about what you want to happen in your financial world should you be unable to run it. She should also have a good sense of what you've got and where you've got it. For this reason, I often suggest to all patients (of every age) that they have a *document locator*, which summarizes all bank accounts (location, number, approximate amount), retirement accounts (same), life-insurance policies, and all other documents one would need to keep your financial house in order. Certain software and some Web-based programs can help you organize this relatively quickly and painlessly. A great and easy-to-use free program is offered by TIAA-CREF at http://www.tiaa-cref .org/pubs/pdf/financial_organizer.pdf.

All Bases Covered

Between your health-care proxy and your power of attorney (if you've done it correctly), you're pretty much set. Once these decisions are put into effect, the person who holds power of attorney can make sure your financial and related matters are correctly executed, and your health-care proxy can make sure your health-care wishes are honored. Sometimes the same person assumes both these roles; sometimes not. For example, if an adult child is especially gifted with finances, he might serve as the power of attorney and cede the proxy role to a sibling who is more familiar with those matters (for example, if she is in the health-care profession). The most important points—whether we're talking power of attorney or health-care proxy—are to make sure that (a) the person you've selected knows you've tapped them for this role and (b) this person knows what you'd like him to do should he have to assume it.

One last point: Many attorneys these days will suggest that you also complete a HIPAA-designation form. HIPAA (the Health Insurance Portability and Accountability Act) does many things; in this context, its most important function is to make sure your medical records are kept confidential. If anyone wants to see them, you need to give the okay—a perfectly reasonable safety feature in the era of the information superhighway. But what if you don't have the ability to give your assent (for example, if you're incapacitated and a physician is in need of understanding your medical history to provide emergency treatment)? Well, we've got a process and forms for that, too. See http://www.hhs.gov/ocr/privacy/index.html for information about the health insurance Privacy Rule or about HIPAA.

In the Eye of the Beholder

Bad decisions are a bit like beauty—they're in the eye of the beholder. Everyone makes them from time to time, and some of us do so habitually. Ironically, many of us would even look favorably upon some of our worst decisions, for any number of reasons—denial, stupidity, foolish pride, and even strong convictions.

Whether the topic is health-care heroics or money, when you pick people who know you and your opinions and permit them to express these on your behalf when you no longer can, you get to have your wishes honored indefinitely, even when you can't articulate them. How's that for staying in control?

Chapter 21

It's Never Too Late . . .

Had I known I'd live this long,
I would have taken better care of myself.
—Eubie Blake, 1883–1983, or Mickey Mantle, 1932–1996

Depending upon whom you believe, the quotation I chose for the epigraph of this chapter came from one of two giant figures in twentieth-century popular culture: the piano impresario Eubie Blake or the baseball legend Mickey Mantle. Conveniently for us, a side-by-side examination of their lives in the context of expectations about aging is as useful as it is profound. It speaks volumes about the control we have over our destinies as we get older, even in the face of what we often misperceive as insurmountable genetics, environment, or life's random misfortunes. Both men's stories also rebut the ridiculous and overused refrain that you can't teach an old dog new tricks. Take it from a hardened geriatrician: You absolutely can, often with surprising results.

Mantle was described as having been born with "gifts from God"—not only his athleticism but also his astonishing physique, his good looks, and his rapport with fans and the public (at least before he started drinking heavily). Certainly some of those gifts were genetic, but he also cultivated them as a child and teenager. Driven by a dedicated but often disapproving father, he nurtured these talents with a work ethic that would make any parent proud. He also inherited some gifts that were not as enviable; the Mantle lineage was rife with Hodgkin's disease. Mantle watched his grandfather, uncle, and father die of the cancer while relatively young. He also lived to see one of his sons contract the same disease and perish at age thirty-six, although not from the illness itself. Talk about life's curveballs. My patients who have experienced the loss of a child tell me it's the most unfathomable card fate can deal out.

Mantle's response to this combination of physical gifts, personal tragedy, and guarded prognosis? By all accounts, a death wish. He thought he would die early, as had the Mantle men before him, and he was determined to suck every drop of life from what he was sure would be a short run on the planet. "I won't be cheated," he would say of his calculated excesses. But as I've described in this book, the aging profit-and-loss ledger begins when you're young and is scrupulously maintained throughout every subsequent decade. Predictably, Mantle's ledger went deep into the red from the poor choices he made in nearly every aspect of his life—medical, psychological, financial, lifestyle, and interpersonal. These were bound to come back and bite him in the ass.

He burned through many of those god-given gifts and his physiologic reserve quickly. Rather than take time to heal, he played through an astonishing number of injuries: some thirty-six different fractures, sprains, and other orthopedic nightmares. He was my childhood hero, and one of my earliest baseball memories is of watching from the stands with my grandfather at Yankee Stadium as he rounded the bases after hitting a home run. After that season he would retire, at the ripe old age of thirty-six, no less. In what could have been an advertisement for accelerated aging, his late-career stride around the bases was so hobbled, it might have belonged to one of my geriatric patients.

I've taught you that aging bodies, minds, friends, and bank accounts interact in some remarkable ways, and unfortunately Mantle's aging miscalculations weren't limited to the ball field. He had no business plan for aging to help him avoid many common missteps, so he made just about all of them. The most poignant: During his life Hodgkin's disease stopped being a uniformly fatal disease and became a curable one. How ironic that he never developed the disease he feared most; if he had, yet the odds were overwhelming that he would have been cured of it. It was his fear of this illness that served as the rationale for his "live hard, die young" strategy.

Finances? Here, too, the Mick was a case study in unsuccessful aging, at least in the years immediately after he left baseball. It's one thing to play injured if you've got a plan, like stashing away your paycheck for a rainy day. Many thoughtful modern players do that all the time, mindful that their high-earning years will be brief and that a nest egg will probably need to last for at least a forty-year retirement. Either they've done the math or someone has done it for them. Although Mantle was one of the highest-paid players of his era, he left the game with little to show for it and then embarked on a series of business ventures that were far from home runs. These, in turn, put him on the publicity circuit, where he found himself at banquets, golf tournaments, and other gigs that created more than a few opportunities to indulge his well-documented drinking problems. And this impacted the other essential ingredients needed for successful aging, such as pursuing meaningful or fulfilling interpersonal relationships. If you think you have to be eighty to experience a geriatric cascade, look no further than Mantle for proof that boomer-aged folks are vulnerable, too. His other family problems and infidelities have been described in great detail, and I refuse to impugn my childhood hero any further.

But the story has a happier (if bittersweet) ending: Mantle ultimately resurrected himself in one of the greatest Lazarus stories ever. (I'll get to that shortly.) Nonetheless, we boys of a certain generation thought that he was immortal, and his passing at any age would have been tough to stomach. I've come to believe that wise statement of my childhood icon. I think that, had he been able to self-prognosticate a bit more accurately, he certainly would have taken better care of himself.

But on the subject of imprecise prognostication, let me tell you about another miscalculation—one that was substantially bigger and in the opposite direction. If any physician or scientist had been asked to predict the life expectancy of the other author of the quotation, they probably would have been even more wildly off the mark.

If circumstance and family history are any harbinger of life expectancy, Eubie Blake should not have survived his first year. He was born to former slaves (Blake was the name given to his parents by their owner); eight other Blake infants died before reaching two months of age. Later Eubie would ascribe this to his mother's lack of prenatal care, but the cards were stacked high against him in many other ways, at least at the outset. In his biography *Eubie Blake*, Al Rose wrote: "Actuarial tables of Baltimore Life (in 1886) would have pegged his life expectancy at about fifty-one, but given his in some ways insalubrious environment, his wispy physique, and the family history of mortality, that would have seemed to be too optimistic a forecast."[1]

Blake ultimately lived a long and rich life, reaching one hundred years of age.* Did all the choices he made over his lifetime that enabled him to prevail over genetics, environment, and decades devoid of penicillin and modern medicine reflect an orthodox interpretation of all the aging strategies I've outlined in this book? Not even close, but that's what makes his story so much more inspiring for readers of any age who want a better and longer life but don't want to spend the rest of it in some kind of gerontological boot camp. Eubie's story speaks to the impact of making even modest changes at any point in life and stopping to smell the roses along the way whenever possible.

He adopted some strategies for successful aging as a youngster, probably by chance or some unidentifiable force (the term *geriatrics* had not even been introduced yet). Some strategies he never adopted. Others he adopted much later in life, even after the onset of modest disability. Eubie was no healthy-aging zealot, but the

---

* Blake's date of birth has been disputed. Some scholars assert that he lived to the age of ninety-six, not one hundred.

impact of his strategy on longevity, quality of life, and legacy were undeniable.

Blake detested sports ("I couldn't care less who won or lost," he would say), and later he said he chose music in childhood to escape after-school athletic requirements. By age fifteen he was playing piano in Baltimore brothels, and he had his first swig of booze well before that. He had a sweet tooth that persisted into his nineties and had him consuming generous quantities of doughnuts and 7-Up (even as his later-life handlers tried to insist on better nutrition). The cover of Rose's 1979 biography shows him with a cigarette in his mouth.

But as he got older and life hurled all kinds of difficulties at him, he adapted. His response to physical, financial, emotional, and even existential curveballs—at every age—is a study in preservation of physiologic and emotional reserve. This guy had a plan for getting older, and as the years passed he began to talk about it with greater and greater specificity.

Personal losses were met with adaptive competence rather than Mantle's scorched-earth approach. He lost his first wife to tuberculosis while in his fifties (they'd met in grade school), as well as many friends (extraordinary longevity invariably brings these losses). With each loss he mourned appropriately but ultimately moved forward, choosing to take a philosophical approach to life's twists and turns. In his eighties he offered his worldview:

"I just decided right there that I wasn't going to be an old man. God! If I could be 56 again, I'd feel like a kid. I had plenty going for me that other people don't. I had my health and a way of makin' a livin' doin' what was more important to me than anything else, and not only that, I knew how to live, and that's somethin' a lot of people older than me never learned."

Blake was a pragmatist who could roll with the punches, even tough ones. I'm doubtful that he could have predicted his unusual longevity as a young man, but from early on he was a shrewd planner, a trait he would carry all his life. As a teenager he squirreled away his bordello tips, quickly realizing that he could make more money in an evening than his father, a Baltimore dockworker, could make in a month. In his nineties he founded his own record label (a dream usually harbored by teenagers these days, not nonagenarians). As he aged he stayed astute in business affairs, never falling into the stereotype of old, destitute jazz musician.

But he enjoyed his bounty, too, and was never thrifty to the point of self-deprivation in matters of lifestyle or medical care. When he was in his nineties, his physician commented that he saw Eubie regularly at his home and as often as necessary, often on very short notice. The rationale: Medical problems should be attended to when minor, rather than after they've had a chance to escalate. Blake's doctor described his care as "highly personalized," adding that "preventative care assumed the highest priority." Sounds like geriatric medicine to me, and a good way to avoid colliding with health-care institutions.

I'm sure he would never have articulated it this way, but Blake seemed to understand physiologic reserve in a way that those of us who are already older (or have established impairments or disability) should pay special attention to, a testimony that you *can* teach an old dog new tricks and that it's never too late to start. Blake was never a big drinker, but he decided to stop drinking and gambling in early adult life because he did not want it to interfere with his music and travel schedule. In his eighties, when arthritis began to threaten his piano playing, he shifted his disability curve (chapter 3) in a way only a gerontologist could love:

"I know I got to practice on the piano every day for two or three hours, because I can't let my fingers get stiff," he would say. "At my age you let 'em get stiff and that's it!"

And how did Eubie Blake handle the search for meaning, legacy, and the other potential existential crises I've talked about? After his "retirement" in his sixties, he felt unfulfilled. The new trick he taught himself? He decided to go to college for the first time in his life to earn a degree in music theory from NYU. This was in the 1950s, long before it was fashionable for older students to share the classroom with pierced and tattooed younger classmates. The degree he earned would ultimately share a wall with honorary ones from Dartmouth, Rutgers, and the New England Conservatory of Music, institutions at which he delighted in meeting and mentoring the next generation of musicians.

And on the subject of slowing down or checking out altogether, Blake had this to say:

"Ninety-six ain't too old to start doin' new things. . . . I'll keep performing until, one day while I'm on stage, the man upstairs says 'eight, nine, ten, you're out!' "

At this point you might be asking: Why would a guy who had such an extraordinary ride assert that he should have taken better care of himself? Didn't Mantle have a much more reasonable claim to that gripe? How could you be anything but delighted and grateful for a run like Eubie's?

———

As I work in gerontology longer and longer and care for more and more older people with varying longevity and quality of life, I think I'm beginning to understand. To believe that simply because you've lived a long and good life (or even a shortened and medically beleaguered one) means that you're not allowed to want or have more is just downright ageist. Sure, Eubie Blake had a long life, and a high-quality one at that. But as he got to the margins of physiologic reserve, with lots of unfinished business and much more to accomplish, he began to see and appreciate the benefits of many of the interventions I've described in this book—even when he adopted them later in life. And maybe he started to believe—as do I—that there's always more quality and quantity to be squeezed from any aging body and mind. Even without cramping the inimitable style of someone like Eubie Blake.

I am not a Pollyanna. I am an expert in aging, and I am here to tell you that there are profound benefits to getting older that are substantial, real, and supported by a growing body of biological and social science. I'm not talking about those inane "ten good things about getting old" lists that try to put a funny spin on aging to relieve your anxiety (one example, "Your secrets are safe because your friends can't remember them"). Those are as ageist as some of the provocative jokes I've used to begin many chapters in this book.

No, I'm talking about bona fide and reproducible findings from real scientists that should convince you that there's some great stuff to look forward to as we age. You want examples? No problem. I can give them to you in any sphere of human endeavor you'd like.

Work and retirement? Despite my rant about the stresses of retirement for some people, study after well-conducted study demonstrates that for the majority of retirees, retirement is all its cracked up to be—a downright great phase of life. Relationships? Spouses in marriages that endure into late life report some of the highest levels of marital satisfaction at any time in the life course and the lowest rates of divorce. Meaning? As we age, the constraints that made us nuts when we were younger—dealing with a crappy boss, putting up with obnoxious acquaintances, buttoning your lip when you'd rather express your political views or other sentiments—can give rise to a newfound freedom. You can speak your mind. Pick your friends. Tell the other numbskulls to go take a hike. How's that for emancipation?

Biology? At the extremes of age, *rates of death actually begin to fall*. Are you with me? Sure, as we get older the risk of shoving off increases on average (that's why life insurance goes up). But as we reach the oldest decades, mortality rates actually fall. This fascinating finding has been demonstrated in everything from worms to primates. And in one of my favorite scientific papers,[2] the authors found this same phenomenon in a nonhuman lineage that blew my mind: automobiles. But you knew that. Hondas or Volvos that make it to 200,000 miles run like a dream, long after their siblings have been junked. Why not try to coddle your body to make it past that threshold?

You want to talk quality? A mountain of studies clearly indicates that not only is life expectancy improving, but so is disability-free survival. The percentage of people spending the last years of their lives in relative immobility is actually falling. The bottom line is that we're going to live longer, and I expect every one of these inspiring trends to continue over our lifetimes.

Don't get me wrong, I am well aware of the challenges that an aging society can create. But in this book I've given you a bunch of tools to deal with many of them. That should free you up to make getting older anything you like. Who wouldn't look forward to that? It's your ride; use it however you like! After all, we're the generation of Americans that redefined youth. It's time to redefine getting older. My vote: The only rule should be that there are no rules.

———

For readers who are not baseball historians, the Mantle story ends with what many regard as his finest hour, even after a lifetime of excess and miscalculation. In the end the Mick did try to take better care of himself, and while it didn't afford him as much time as he or his fans would have liked, it was enough time for him to get it right.

Newly sober for the first time in decades, he reconciled with family, friends, and the fans he thought he may have disrespected, and courageously told his story to millions. The baseball-memorabilia craze that started in the 1980s put money back in his pocket, and he took better care of that, too. He created a foundation to support organ transplantation, raised money for victims of the Oklahoma City bombings, and dedicated himself to helping retired ballplayers who were down on their luck. Organ donations and organ donors increased dramatically in the months after his heroic and forthright public declarations about his mistakes as a younger man. "I feel more important as Mickey Mantle now than when I played for the Yankees," he said.

When Mantle died, President Clinton observed that he would be remembered not only for his heroics on the ball field but also for "the honor and redemption he brought to the end of his life." And in his eulogy, Bob Costas commented on how Mantle finally got it right and was able to receive "love for what he had been, love for what he made us feel, and love for the humanity and sweetness that was always there mixed in with the flaws."

The missteps of his youth would not rob the older Mantle of legacy or meaning. Sure, as a young man the Mick could have taken better care of himself. But the point is that he got around to it, and in time to look back on his life and take it all in. Now when I think of my ageless childhood hero, I don't think of someone who squandered God's gifts. For me, Mantle's swan song invokes Will Rogers's timeless observation about aging; it's the most compelling reason to approach getting older with the knowledge, honesty, and wonder that it truly deserves:

"One must wait until evening to see how splendid the day has been."

Appendix

Lay Interpretations
(*Summaries for Patients*)
of CAM trials from
The Annals of Internal Medicine

I. Comparison of Yoga, Exercise, and Education for the
   Treatment of Chronic Low Back Pain
II. Glucosamine Sulfate to Treat Hip Osteoarthritis
III. The Relationship between Green Tea Intake and Type 2 Diabetes
   in Japanese Adults
IV. Adding Acupuncture to Physical Therapy and Anti-Inflammatory
   Drugs in the Treatment of Knee Osteoarthritis

Summaries for Patients are a service provided by *Annals* to help patients
better understand the complicated and often mystifying language of
modern medicine.

Summaries for Patients are presented for informational purposes only.
These summaries are not a substitute for advice from your own medical
provider. If you have questions about this material, or need medical advice
about your own health or situation, please contact your physician.

I.   Comparison of Yoga, Exercise, and Education for the Treatment of Chronic Low Back Pain

What is the problem and what is known about it so far?

Low back pain is a common problem that often goes away after several days or weeks but can also be chronic, lasting for months or years. Treatment goals include decreasing pain and improving function so that patients can do their normal activities. Treatment options include educating patients about ways to prevent back injury and to deal with back pain, drugs (pain killers, anti-inflammatory drugs, and muscle relaxants), and exercise. We do not know which particular types of exercise will best improve outcomes for patients with low back pain. Yoga is an activity that combines physical exercise with relaxation techniques. Although many people with chronic low back pain use yoga, little is known about its effectiveness for this condition.

Why did the researchers do this particular study?

To compare the effectiveness of yoga, traditional exercise, and an educational book for people with chronic low back pain.

Who was studied?

101 patients between 20 and 64 years of age who visited a primary care doctor in the past 3 to 15 months for chronic low back pain. All patients were members of the insurance plan Group Health in Seattle, Washington. To be in the study, patients had to rate their pain as being at least 3 on a scale of 0 (no pain) to 10 (worst pain). Patients who had major illnesses or conditions (cancer, pregnancy, bone fractures, previous back surgery) that could explain the back pain could not participate in the study.

How was the study done?

The researchers assigned patients at random to receive: (1) 12 weekly 75-minute yoga classes designed for patients with back pain and instructions to practice daily at home; (2) 12 weekly 75-minute sessions of aerobic, strengthening, and stretching exercises, which were developed by a physical therapist, and instructions to practice daily at home; or (3) a personal copy of *The Back Pain Helpbook* by Jim Moore and colleagues (Reading, MA: Perseus Books; 1999). Study patients could use drugs, such as anti-inflammatory agents or acetaminophen, as needed. Interviewers, who did not know which treatment each patient received, called patients after 6, 12, and 26 weeks and used standard questions to collect information on pain and dysfunction.

What did the researchers find?

After 12 weeks, patients in the yoga group had better back-related function than patients in the exercise or education groups. Reports of pain were similar in all 3 groups. At 26 weeks, patients in the yoga group reported better back-related function and less pain.

What were the limitations of the study?

The study followed patients for about 6 months, so this study does not tell us about the effectiveness of yoga over longer periods. The study involved only 1 yoga instructor and 1 exercise instructor. Other instructors might have achieved different results. The study was too small to come to firm conclusions about the safety of yoga for patients with low back pain.

What are the implications of the study?

Over 3 to 6 months, yoga appears to be more effective than traditional exercise or an educational book for improving function and pain in patients with chronic low back pain.

ARTICLE AND AUTHOR INFORMATION

This summary is from the full report titled "Comparing Yoga, Exercise, and a Self-Care Book for Chronic Low Back Pain. A Randomized, Controlled Trial." It is in the December 20, 2005, issue of *Annals of Internal Medicine* (vol. 143, pages 849–856). The authors are K.J. Sherman, D.C. Cherkin, J. Erro, D.L. Miglioretti, and R.A. Deyo.

II. Glucosamine Sulfate to Treat Hip Osteoarthritis

What is the problem and what is known about it so far?

Osteoarthritis is the most common type of arthritis in middle-aged and older people. It often occurs in large joints, such as the knees and hips. The pain may limit a person's ability to get up from a chair, stand, walk, or climb stairs and tends to get worse with activity. Treatment aims to decrease pain and other symptoms and to keep people active. Treatments include drugs to decrease pain and inflammation; weight loss, if needed; physical therapy; and exercise. Unfortunately, these treatments do not always help, and some have side effects. Many people with knee osteoarthritis seek alternative treatments, such as glucosamine sulfate. Glucosamine sulfate is a natural substance that is found in healthy joint cartilage. Some studies suggest that glucosamine sulfate helps osteoarthritis, particularly that of the knee. Others studies have not shown a benefit. It is also not known whether glucosamine sulfate helps patients with hip osteoarthritis.

Why did the researchers do this particular study?

To see whether glucosamine sulfate is effective in treating hip osteoarthritis.

Who was studied?

222 patients from the Netherlands who had hip osteoarthritis.

How was the study done?

The researchers assigned patients to receive either 1500 mg of glucosamine sulfate or a placebo pill daily for 2 years. The placebo pill looked and tasted like the glucosamine pill, but it contained no active ingredients. The researchers reported patient outcomes at 3, 12, and 24 months after starting treatment. They collected information on patients' pain and their ability to do their usual activities. They also did x-rays to measure the joint space in the hip, because as osteoarthritis gets worse, the joint space becomes narrower.

What did the researchers find?

Pain, ability to do normal activities, and joint space narrowing did not differ between patients who received glucosamine and those who received a placebo.

What were the limitations of the study?

Twenty of the patients had hip replacement surgery during the study, which interfered with the researchers' ability to measure patient outcomes.

What are the implications of the study?

Receiving 1500 mg of glucosamine sulfate daily for 2 years seems to offer no benefit in relieving pain, increasing the ability to do normal activities, or reducing joint space narrowing in patients with hip osteoarthritis.

ARTICLE AND AUTHOR INFORMATION

This summary is from the full report titled "Effect of Glucosamine Sulfate on Hip Osteoarthritis. A Randomized Trial." It is in the February 19, 2008, issue of *Annals of Internal Medicine* (vol. 148, pages 268–277). The authors are R.M. Rozendaal, B.W. Koes, G.J.V.M. van Osch, E.J. Uitterlinden, E.H. Garling, S.P. Willemsen, A.Z. Ginai, J.A.N. Verhaar, H. Weinans, and S.M.A. Bierma-Zeinstra.

III. The Relationship between Green Tea Intake and Type 2 Diabetes in Japanese Adults

What is the problem and what is known about it so far?

Type 2 diabetes mellitus is a common disease that interferes with the body's ability to store energy from food. The pancreas makes insulin, a substance that helps store energy from food. In people with type 2 diabetes mellitus, the body makes enough insulin but cannot use it normally. The result is high blood sugar levels, which can lead to blindness, kidney failure, nerve damage, and heart disease over time. Risk factors for type 2 diabetes mellitus include being overweight, lack of exercise, and family history of the disease. Because type 2 diabetes mellitus is common and has serious complications, it is important to understand factors associated with the disease. It is known that caffeine influences the way the body handles sugar. Recent studies show that people with higher coffee intake are less likely to develop type 2 diabetes mellitus than are people with lower intake. However, these studies have largely been done in western populations and have not evaluated whether tea intake is also related to type 2 diabetes.

Why did the researchers do this particular study?

To examine the relationship between type 2 diabetes mellitus and drinking green, black, and oolong teas.

Who was studied?

6,277 men and 10,686 women from 25 communities in Japan who were participating in a study of cancer risk factors. To be included in the study, people needed to be 40 to 65 years of age and free of diabetes, stroke, heart disease, or cancer when the study began.

How was the study done?

At the start of the study and again 5 years later, the study participants completed surveys that asked about health issues, including whether they had been diagnosed with diabetes. The survey also asked about how much coffee and tea (green, black, and oolong teas) participants drank. The researchers looked for associations between participants' intakes of the various beverages and the development of diabetes over the 5 years of the study. The analyses examined other diabetes risk factors, such as body size, exercise, family history, and age.

What did the researchers find?

People who were frequent drinkers of green tea (>6 cups per day) or coffee (>3 cups per day) were less likely to develop diabetes than those who drank less than 1 cup of these beverages per week. Higher total caffeine intake was also associated with lower risk for diabetes. These relationships were strongest in women and in overweight men. No association was found between black and oolong teas and reduced risk for diabetes.

What were the limitations of the study?

The design of this study did not permit the researchers to be certain that green tea, coffee, and caffeine protect against type 2 diabetes. There may be another factor about people who drink these beverages frequently that protects them from diabetes.

What are the implications of the study?

People who drink more green tea, coffee, or total caffeinated beverages are less likely to develop type 2 diabetes than people who drink none or very little of these beverages.

ARTICLE AND AUTHOR INFORMATION

This summary is from the full report titled "The Relationship between Green Tea and Total Caffeine Intake and Risk for Self-Reported Type 2 Diabetes among Japanese Adults." It is in the April 18, 2006, issue of *Annals of Internal Medicine* (volume 144, pages 554-562). The authors are H. Iso, C. Date, K. Wakai, M. Fukui, A. Tamakoshi, and the JACC Study Group.

IV. Adding Acupuncture to Physical Therapy and Anti-Inflammatory Drugs in the Treatment of Knee Osteoarthritis

What is the problem and what is known about it so far?

Knee osteoarthritis is a common condition in which changes in the knee joints lead to pain. Treatments include drugs to decrease pain and inflammation; weight loss, if needed; physical therapy; and exercise. Unfortunately, these treatments do not always help and some have side effects. Consequently, many people with knee osteoarthritis seek alternative treatments, such as acupuncture. Acupuncture is an ancient Chinese treatment that involves putting special needles into specific points on the body to treat medical conditions. Mainstream medicine is increasingly recognizing acupuncture as an effective treatment for some disorders. Past studies about acupuncture for osteoarthritis have had inconsistent results.

Why did the researchers do this particular study?

To find out whether acupuncture is an effective treatment for knee osteoarthritis.

Who was studied?

1,007 patients with osteoarthritis knee pain for at least 6 months.

How was the study done?

The researchers assigned patients to receive either 10 sessions of traditional Chinese acupuncture (TCA), 10 sessions of sham acupuncture, or

10 doctor visits without acupuncture over 6 weeks. Traditional Chinese acupuncture was "real" acupuncture according to Chinese protocols that specify the location and depth of needle placement in the treatment of knee pain. Sham acupuncture was "fake" acupuncture in which the acupuncturist placed the needles at a shallow depth in places other than the TCA points. Patients in all 3 groups could receive 6 physical therapy treatments and could take anti-inflammatory medications as needed up to a certain amount. The researchers compared changes in patients' pain after 26 weeks.

What did the researchers find?

After 26 weeks, patients in the TCA and sham acupuncture groups had greater improvement in pain than those in the no acupuncture group. Surprisingly, the changes in pain were not different in the TCA and sham acupuncture groups. However, patients in the TCA group reported higher satisfaction with treatment than those in the sham acupuncture group, but both acupuncture groups reported higher satisfaction than the no acupuncture group. Of note, patients in both acupuncture groups had more contact with health care providers during the study than did those in the no acupuncture group.

What were the limitations of the study?

Patients knew whether they were getting acupuncture. The researchers did not monitor whether the acupuncturists were following the TCA and sham protocols exactly as the study plan specified.

What are the implications of the study?

Compared with patients with knee osteoarthritis treated with physical therapy and anti-inflammatory drugs alone, patients who also received TCA or sham acupuncture had improvements in pain at 26 weeks. Surprisingly, the researchers found no difference in pain reduction between real and fake acupuncture. Several potential explanations are possible. First, because of psychological effects, patients who know they are getting special types of treatment report feeling better regardless of whether the treatment really works. Second, patients who received acupuncture had more intense contact with health care providers, which could explain why they felt better. Third, sticking needles into the body may have a physical effect on pain, regardless of whether the needles are placed according to TCA principles.

ARTICLE AND AUTHOR INFORMATION

This summary is from the full report titled "Acupuncture and Knee Osteoarthritis. A Three-Armed Randomized Trial." It is in the July 4, 2006, issue of *Annals of Internal Medicine* (vol. 145, pages 12–20). The authors are H.-P. Scharf, U. Mansmann, K. Streitberger, S. Witte, J. Krämer, C. Maier, H.-J. Trampisch, and N. Victor.

Reprinted with permission of *The Annals of Internal Medicine*.

NOTES

Chapter 2: You're a What?

1. http://www.presidency.ucsb.edu/ws/index.php?pid=9572.
2. J. Kaprio, M. Koskenvuo, and H. Rita, "Mortality after Bereavement: A Prospective Study of 95,647 Widowed Persons," *American Journal of Public Health* 77, no. 3 (March 1987): 283–87, http://www.pubmedcentral.nih.gov/articlerender.fcgi?artid= 1646890.
3. Lisa F. Berkman, Linda Leo-Summers, and Ralph I. Horwitz, "Emotional Support and Survival after Myocardial Infarction," *Annals of Internal Medicine* 117, no. 12 (December 15, 1992): 1003–9, http://yalerei.org/intmed/resources/docs/Berkman .pdf.
4. H. G. Koenig et al., "Does Religious Attendance Prolong Survival? A Six-Year Follow-up Study of 3,968 Older Adults," *Journals of Gerontology: Series A, Biological Sciences and Medical Sciences* 54, no. 7 (July 1999): M370–76.
5. L. F. Berkman and S. L. Syme, "Social Networks, Host Resistance, and Mortality: A Nine-Year Follow-up Study of Alameda County Residents," *American Journal of Epidemiology* 109, no. 2 (February 1979): 186–204.
6. M. J. Lenzen et al., "The Additional Value of Patient-Reported Health Status in Predicting 1-Year Mortality after Invasive Coronary Procedures: A Report from the Euro Heart Survey on Coronary Revascularisation," *Heart* 93, no. 3 (March 2007): 339–44, Epub 2006 Sep 15.

7. Candyce H. Kroenke et al., "Social Networks, Social Support, and Survival after Breast Cancer Diagnosis," *Journal of Clinical Oncology* 24, no. 7 (March 1, 2006): 1105–11.

Chapter 3: The Biology of Aging

1. Angus Maddison, *The World Economy in Millennial Perspective* (Paris: OECD, 2001), chart reproduced in "Crude Life Expectancy Estimates," Semi-Daily Journal of Economist Brad DeLong, July 25, 2003, http://econ161.berkeley.edu/movable_type/2003_archives/001846.html.
2. This reference comes from a governmental report that can be found at http://www.healthypeople.gov/Document/tableofcontents.htm.
3. E. F. Binder et al., "Effects of Extended Outpatient Rehabilitation after Hip Fracture: A Randomized Controlled Trial," *JAMA* 292, no. 7 (August 18, 2004): 837–46.
4. J. P. Allegrante et al., "Methodological Challenges of Multiple-Component Intervention: Lessons Learned from a Randomized Controlled Trial of Functional Recovery after Hip Fracture," *HSS Journal* 3, no. 1 (February 2007): 63–70.

Chapter 4: A Geriatrician's Perspective on Ageism

1. http://jhupbooks.press.jhu.edu/ecom/MasterServlet/GetItemDetailsHandler?iN=9780801874253&qty=1&viewMode=3&loggedIN=false&JavaScript=y.

Chapter 5: Do No Harm, but for God's Sake, Do Something!

1. Sanjay Saint et al., "Are Physicians Aware of Which of Their Patients Have Indwelling Urinary Catheters?" *American Journal of Medicine* 109, no. 6: 476–80, http://linkinghub.elsevier.com/retrieve/pii/S0002934300005313.

Chapter 6: Cookbook Medicine

1. Gina Kolata, "Sharp Regional Incongruity Found in Medical Costs and Treatments," *New York Times,* January 30, 1996, http://www.nytimes.com/1996/01/30/science/sharp-regional-incongruity-found-in-medical-costs-and-treatments.html?scp=12&sq=wennberg%20dartmouth%20prostate&st=cse.
2. Jane E. Brody, "Cookbook Medicine Won't Do for Elderly," Personal Health, *New York Times,* December 30, 2008, http://query.nytimes.com/gst/fullpage.html?res=9C02E6D91539F933A05751C1A96E9C8B63.
3. Jane E. Brody, "How Perils Can Await the 'Worried Wealthy,'" Personal Health, *New York Times*, November 12, 2002, http://www.nytimes.com/2002/11/12/health/personal-health-how-perils-can-await-the-worried-wealthy.html?sec=health.

Chapter 7: Bedside Matters

1. P. J. Leigh et al., "Physician Career Satisfaction Across Specialties," *Archives of Internal Medicine* 162 (July 2002): 1577–84.
2. R. D. Adelman, M. G. Greene, and M. G. Ory, "Communication Between Older Patients and Their Physicians," *Clinical Geriatric Medicine* 16, no. 1 (February 2000): 1-24.
3. http://www.americangeriatrics.org/policy/geriatrician_shortage.shtml.

Chapter 8: How Many Specialists Does It Take to Screw in a Lightbulb

1. "The Medical Home: Position Statement," Association of American Medical Colleges, March 2008, http://www.aamc.org/newsroom/pressrel/2008/medicalhome.pdf.

Chapter 9: Care Transitions as We Get Older

1. Institute of Medicine, *To Err Is Human: Building a Safer Health System* (1999), http://www.iom.edu/Reports/1999/To-Err-is-Human-Building-A-Safer-Health-System.aspx.
2. C. Moore, J. Wisnivesky, and J. McGinn, "Medical Errors Related to Continuity of Care from Inpatient to Outpatient Settings," *Journal of General Internal Medicine* 18 (2003): 646–51.
3. E. A. Coleman, J. D. Smith, D. Raha, S. J. Min, "Posthospital Medication Discrepancies: Prevalence and Contributing Factors," *Archives of Internal Medicine* 165, no. 16 (September 12, 2005): 1842-47.
4. C. C. Roy et al., "Patient Safety Concerns Arising from Test Results That Return after Hospital Discharge," *Annals of Internal Medicine* 143 (2005): 121–28.
5. P. L. Cornish et al., "Unintended Medication Discrepancies at the Time of Hospital Admission," *Archives of Internal Medicine* 17, no. 3 (2002): 186–92.

Chapter 10: No Place for Sick People

1. "John Glenn Returns to Space," Glenn Research Center, NASA, http://www.nasa.gov/centers/glenn/about/bios/shuttle_mission.html.
2. S. K. Inouye et al., "A Predictive Model for Delirium in Hospitalized Elderly Medical Patients Based on Admission Characteristics," *Annals of Internal Medicine* 119, no. 6 (September 15, 1993): 474–81, http://www.ncbi.nlm.nih.gov/pubmed/8357112?dopt=Abstract.
3. S. K. Inouye and Charpentier, "Precipitating Factors for Delirium in Hospitalized Elderly Persons. Predictive Model and Interrelationship with Baseline Vulnerability," *JAMA* 275, no. 11 (March 20, 1996): 852–57, http://www.ncbi.nlm.nih.gov/pubmed/8596223?dopt=Abstract.

4. S. K. Inouye et al., "A Multicomponent Intervention to Prevent Delirium in Hospitalized Older Patients," *New England Journal of Medicine* 340, no. 9 (March 4, 1999): 669–76.

5. S. K. Inouye et al., "The Hospital Elder Life Program: A Model of Care to Prevent Cognitive and Functional Decline in Older Hospitalized Patients," *Journal of American Geriatrics Society* 48, no. 12 (December 2000): 1697-706.

6. Adapted from HELP, "Avoid Confusion in the Hospital—10 Tips," http://hospitalelderlifeprogram.org/public/prevention.ph p?pageid=01.01.03&PHPSESSID=fce0f9d2c341a35c9af3cef2fa6 6cfdd.

7. Find out more about delirium. The American Psychiatric Association's "Patient and Family Guide to Understanding and Identifying Delirium" is available online.

Chapter 13: Maybe You're Not the Problem

1. R. Bakker, Y. Iofel, and M. S. Lachs, "Lighting Levels in the Dwellings of Homebound Older Adults," *Journal of Housing for the Elderly* 18, no. 2 (2004): 17–27.

Chapter 14: Homes Away from Home as We Age

1. See Vikram R. Comondore et al., "Quality of Care in For-Profit and Not-For-Profit Nursing Homes: Systematic Review and Meta-analysis," *BMJ*, August 4, 2009, http://www.bmj.com/cgi/content/full/339/aug04_2/b2732. Also see http://www.consumerreports .org/health/doctors-hospitals/nursing-home-guide/0608_nursing-home-guide.htm.

Chapter 16: Complementary and Alternative Medicine, Vitamins, and Supplements

1. Full disclosure: I serve on the board of directors of this foundation.

2. See http://www.annals.org/site/patientinformation/patientinfor mation.xhtml for a listing of all patient summary sheets from

this collection, which is a fabulous resource and available to the public without charge.

3. "The Beta-Blocker Heart Attack Trial," *JAMA* 246, no. 18 (1981): 2072–74; see https://biolincc.nhlbi.nih.gov/studies/bhat.

4. Fabrizio Benedetti et al., "Neurobiological Mechanisms of the Placebo Effect," *Journal of Neuroscience* 25, no. 45 (November 9, 2005): 10390–402, http://www.jneurosci.org/cgi/content/full/25/45/10390.

5. B. R. Levy et al., "Longevity Increased by Positive Self-Perceptions of Aging," *J Pers Soc Psychology* 83, no. 2 (August 2002): 261-70.

6. See American Medical Association, "CEJA Report 1–A-99: Sale of Health-Related Products from Physicians' Offices" (1999; http://www.ama-assn.org/ama1/pub/upload/mm/369/ceja_1a99.pdf), although at around the same time the AMA did manage to get itself into hot water through product and commercial endorsements that were eventually abandoned (see Glenn Collins, "Sunbeam Sues the A.M.A. on Voided Marketing Deal," *New York Times*, September 9, 1997, http://www.nytimes.com/1997/09/09/business/sunbeam-sues-the-ama-on-voided-marketing-deal.html).

7. *Swindlers, Hucksters and Snake Oil Salesmen: Hype and Hope Marketing Anti-Aging Products to Seniors*, report on hearing before the Special Committee on Aging, United States Senate, 107th Cong., 1st sess., September 10, 2001, Serial No. 107-14, http://www.gpo.gov/fdsys/pkg/CHRG-107shrg190/pdf/CHRG-107shrg190.pdf.

Chapter 17: Money and Aging

1. As I discuss in the next chapter, my favorite "conflict of interest–free" financial author on these topics is Eric Tyson (see www.erictyson.com). His *Personal Finance for Dummies,* 4th ed. (New York: Wiley, 2003), is a classic; another superb Tyson book is *Mind Over Money* (New York: CDS Books, 2006).

2. There are many superb books on creating and starting a business plan for anything. Among my easy-to-read favorites is Guy Kawasaki's *The Art of the Start: The Time-Tested, Battle-Hardened Guide for Anyone Starting Anything* (New York: Penguin, 2004).

Chapter 18: Financial Gerontology

1. Mark Hulbert, "The Index Funds Win Again," *New York Times*, February 21, 2009, http://www.nytimes.com/2009/02/22/your-money/stocks-and-bonds/22stra.html.
2. Karen Damato and Diya Gullapalli, "Managed Funds Offer Little Cover from the Bear," *Wall Street Journal*, April 5, 2009, http://online.wsj.com/article/SB123889089021689987.html.
3. More information can be found at the American Institute of Financial Gerontology's Web site (www.aifg.org).
4. Charles Duhigg, "For Elderly Investors, Instant Experts Abound," *New York Times*, July 8, 2007, http://www.nytimes.com/2007/07/08/business/08advisor.html?_r=1&scp=3&sq=gerontology%20financial%20planners&st=cse.
5. New York Life Insurance Company, "What to Do with That Old Life Insurance Policy," http://www.newyorklife.com/cda/0,3254,14579,00.html.

Chapter 19: It Ain't Over Till It's Over

1. Karen E. Steinhauser et al., "Factors Considered Important at the End of Life by Patients, Families, Physicians, and Other Care Providers," *JAMA* 284 (2000): 2476–82.
2. Sara Carmel and Elizabeth J. Mutran, "Stability of Elderly Persons' Expressed Preferences regarding the Use of Life-Sustaining Treatments," *Social Science & Medicine* 49, no. 3 (August 1999): 303–11.

3. R. S. Morrison et al., "Cost Savings Associated with U.S. Hospital Palliative Care Consultation Programs," *Archives of Internal Medicine* 168, no. 16 (September 8, 2008): 1783–90.

Chapter 20: Staying in Control

1. M. R. Dematteo, H. S. Lepper, and T. W. Croghan, "Depression Is a Risk Factor for Non-compliance with Medical Treatment: Meta-analysis of the Effects of Anxiety and Depression on Patient Adherence," *Archives of Internal Medicine* 160 (2000): 2101–7.
2. D. W. Molloy et al., "Decision Making in the Incompetent Elderly: The Daughter from California Syndrome," *Journal of the American Geriatrics Society* 29 (1991): 396–99.

Chapter 21: It's Never Too Late...

1. Al Rose, *Eubie Blake* (New York: Schirmer Press, 1979). All Eubie Blake quotations in this chapter are from this book.
2. James W. Vaupel et al., "Biodemographic Trajectories of Longevity," *Science* 280, no. 5365 (May 8, 1998): 855–60.

INDEX

Page numbers in *italics* refer to illustrations.

AARP, 339
abnormal lab findings, 126
ACL (anterior cruciate ligament), 121
*ACP Evidence-Based Guide to
    Complementary & Alternative
    Medicine, The,* 242n
activities of daily living (ADLs), 205,
    207, 212, 288
actuarial tables, 264–65, 266–67
acupuncture, 241, 243
admitting privileges, 140–41
advance directives, 297, 302, 317
ageism, 34, 42–51, 199, 317
aging:
    alternative housing and, 203–23
    biology of, 26–41
    business plan for, 257–74, 354
    care transitions and, 116–30, 173,
        183–84, 220–21
    complementary and alternative
        medicine (CAM), 235–56
    emergency room care and, 156–72,
        186–88, 189–91
    families and, *see* family
    financial gerontology, 275–93
    geriatricians and, 12–25
    home modification and, 192–202
    hospital care, *see* hospitals
    hospital discharge process and,
        173–91
    medical ageism and, 44–46, 47–48,
        53–57
    medications and, 109, 122–23, 124–25,
        151, 177–78, 224–34, 277
    physiologic reserve and, 24–25,
        26–27, 28, 29–30, 34, 75, 120, 351,
        355, 356

primary care physicians and, *see*
    primary care physicians
role models and, 271, 350–59
social factors and, 22–25
specialists, subspecialists and, 19–21,
    81–82, 105–15
Alameda County Study, 22
alcohol consumption, 227
ALFs, *see* assisted living facilities
alternative housing, 203–23
    assisted living facilities (ALFs), 21,
        206–10, 215–23, 331
    continuing-care retirement
        communities (CCRCs), 211–23
    financial factors and, 206, 212
    independent senior housing, 210–11
    not-for-profit facilities, 215–16
    skilled nursing facilities (SNFs),
        205–6, 207–8
Alzheimer's disease, 21, 33, 187, 195, 205,
    250, 267, 310, 311, 327–28
American Board of Medical Specialties,
    252
American College of Physicians,
    237n, 242n
American Diabetes Association, 71
American Geriatric Society, 90
American Institute of Financial
    Gerontology, 286
American Medical Association, 252
amplified stereo listeners, 201n
angina pectoris, 53–54, 55
Annals of Internal Medicine, 243
anosognosia, 328
anti-aging medicine, 252–56
antidepressants, 232
arthritis, 197, 243, 267, 310

aspirin, 237
assisted living facilities (ALFs), 21,
    206–10, 217, 331
    evaluating, 209–10, 215–23
    financial factors and, 208
    transition from, 221
Association of American Medical
    Colleges (AAMC), 114–15
atrial fibrillation, 234
attending physicians, 140–42, 146, 172

back pain, 238, 243, 335
Bakker, Rosemary, 195–96, 197
Beacon Hill Village, Boston, 211
bed rest, 132, 134
bedside manner, 83, 113–14
bedsores, 138, 152, 208
bereavement, 22, 62, 203, 261, 294
Beta-Blocker Heart Attack Trial
    (BHAT), 246–47, 248
beta-blockers, 247
biology of aging, 26–41
    age-related disability and, 33–38,
        35, 38
    life expectancy and, 29–32, 30, 31, 37
    muscular strength and, 27–29, 27, 32,
        35, 37, 38, 38
    physiologic reserve and, 24–25,
        26–27, 28, 29–30, 34, 75, 120, 351,
        355, 356
    quality-of-life improvement and,
        38–41
bipolar disorder, 106–7, 226, 332
Blake, Eubie, 350, 353–56
Bogdanov, Alexander, 255
breast cancer, 23, 43
bronchitis, 166–68
bronchoscopy, 179
Burns, George, 12
bursitis, 106, 107
Butler, Robert N., 1, 46

CAM, *see* complementary and
    alternative medicine
caraway oil, 236
cardiograms, 125–26
care transitions, 116–30, 173
    avoiding problems in, 124–28
    definition of, 121–22
    from hospital to subacute care, 183
    long-term-care and, 220–21
    medical errors and, 122–24, 130

personal medical records and, 128–30
    readmission to hospital, 183–84,
        185–89
Carlin, George, 294
catheters, 133, 145, 149
CAT (computerized axial tomography)
    scan, 129, 144, 167, 306
CCRCs, *see* continuing-care retirement
    communities
Center to Advance Palliative Care, 316
certified nursing assistants (CNAs), 218
chemotherapy, 137, 232, 238, 241, 315
cognitive impairment, 127–28, 149,
    227–28, 326, 328, 341–43
Coleman, Eric, 122, 124, 175
colonoscopy, 48, 74, 335
comparative effectiveness research,
    68, 238*n*
complementary and alternative
    medicine (CAM), 235–56
    anti-aging medicine and, 252–56
    choosing worthwhile therapies,
        237–39
    do-it-yourself evaluation of evidence,
        240–42, 243–46
    geriatricians and, 235–36, 255–56
    placebo effect and, 238, 246–49
    research studies and, 239–40
    takeout evaluation of evidence,
        240–43
    treatment choice evaluation, 249–52
concierge medicine, 101–4, 164
confusion (delirium), 132–33, 138–39,
    143, 144–45, 149, 151, 154, 187
conservatorship, *see* guardianship, legal
consultants, 146–47
continuing-care retirement
    communities (CCRCs), 211–15, 217
    evaluating, 215–23
    financial factors and, 212–13, 219
    medical services access and, 220
    postacute care patient (case history),
        213–14
    transition to another care, 220–21
convalescence centers, *see* nursing
    homes
cookbook medicine, 65–77
    definition of, 68–69
    practice variation and, 67–68
Coumadin, 225–26, 233–34
Crohn's disease, 111
custodial care, *see* nursing homes

daughter from California syndrome, 335
death and dying, 294–318
   discussing preferences in, 299–301,
      304–5, 317–18, 347
   documents, terms, and forms in,
      297–99
   at home, 300
   hospice care, 14–15, 310, 311
   informing and updating proxies,
      303–5
   palliative care in, 295, 308–10, 312–16
   prognosis and, 305–8
delirium, *see* confusion
dementia, 70–71, 327–28, 329, 332
depression, 62, 117, 238, 292, 309,
      328–30
diabetes, 24, 224, 243
differential diagnosis, 327
disability, age-related, 33–38, 35, 38,
      63–64
   end-of-life care and, 305
   home modifications and, 192–202
   managing at home with, 320–25
   see also specific conditions
discharge instructions, 176
discharge planners, 177, 180, 182
"Discharge Preparation Checklist"
      (Coleman), 175
discharges, 123, 173–91
   from emergency room to home, 189–91
   follow-up doctors and, 175–76
   from hospital to home, 173–79
   from hospital to subacute
      rehabilitation, 179–85
discharge summary, 176–77, 190
diverticulitis, 213
doctor-patient relationships, 79, 82–87, 93
   chronic tardiness and, 97
   complaint articulation and
      prioritization, 87–88
   follow-up plans and, 89
   hospitalists and, 97
   interval events, listing, 88–89
   medications and, 89, 229–32
   after office hours, 96
   physician telephone accessibility, 96
   specialists and, 111–14
   test results and, 95–96
   transparency in, 90
document locators, 348
do no harm, 52–64
do-not-resuscitate (DNR) orders, 298–99

double blind studies, 245
drug-disease interaction, 107
durable power of attorney, 297–98,
      348–49

elder abuse, 208, 281
Eldercare locator, 202, 211
elder law attorneys, 221–22
electroconvulsive therapy, 62
emergency room, 156–72
   discharges, 189–91
   hospital admissions and, 160–62
   how to avoid, 162–64
   medical errors in, 159–60
   older patients in, 157–59, 170, 171–72
   primary care physicians and, 163, 164,
      168–69
empathy, family relationships and,
      331–32
emphysema, 45, 194, 309
endocrine abnormalities, 330
end-of-life care, *see* death and dying
erectile dysfunction, 335
estate planning, 259, 272–74, 291–92
ethical deception, 338–39
Eubie Blake (Rose), 353
excess disability, 63–64, 75, 195, 197
exercise programs, 37, 244
eyeglasses, 144, 151

family:
   dialogues about money, 281–82
   emergency rooms and, 170–71
   empathy and, 331–32
   evaluating care facilities, 209–10
   getting someone to accept help,
      332–39
   hospital care and, 143, 150, 151
   refusal behavior and, 328
   sibling rivalry, 273
   visits to relatives by, 184–85
Ffirth, Stubbins, 255
financial gerontology, 257, 275–93
   emotion and decision-making,
      278–80
   estate planning and, 291–92
   family dialogues and, 281–82
   getting information and advice on,
      283, 286
   life insurance and, 287–88
   long-term-care insurance, 282,
      288–90

financial gerontology (*cont'd*)
  Medicare, Medicaid and, 282–83,
    284–85, 289, 290–91
  need for and benefits of, 275–78
  planning for, 281–92
  retirement and, 292–93
  risk tolerance and, 287
  supplemental health insurance and,
    290–91
Financial Industry Regulatory Authority,
  286
financial planners, 263–64, 277, 280,
  283, 286
financial planning, traditional, 259–61
fish oil, 236
flooring safety, 200
forced retirement, 293
functional longevity, 263, 264, 267, 270
functional prognosis, 216
furnishings, safety and, 200–201

genetics, 28
geriatric assessment programs, 217
geriatric cascade, 144–45, 187, 352
geriatricians, 78–79
  alternative medicine (CAM) and,
    235–36, 255–56
  on death and dying, 14–15, 294,
    309, 317
  emphasis on patient function, 13–14,
    15–19, 40
  functions of, 13–16, 21–25
  as hospitalists, 16–19
  how to find, 90–92
  medications and, 229–31
  patient aftercare and, 99–100
geriatric nurse practitioners, 157–58
gerontological financial planners,
  280, 281
gerontology, 13, 22, 34, 49, 253
glaucoma, 226
Glenn, John, 48–50, 51, 139
glucosamine, 243
Google, 127, 129
Google Scholar (Web site), 243–44
green tea consumption, 243
guardianship, legal, 342, 345–48

Harvard University, Aging Brain Center
  of, 138
health-care proxies, 297, 302, 303–5,
  308, 347, 348, 349

health insurance, 67, 74, 161, 180, 282
  see also long-term-care insurance;
    Medicaid; Medicare
Health Insurance Portability and
  Accountability Act (HIPAA), 349
hearing aids, 151, 201
hearing impairment, 196
heart attacks, 247
HELP, *see* Hospital Elder Life Program
hip fractures, 136–37, 145, 146, 186
Hippocrates, 237
hip replacement, 179
HMOs, *see* managed care
home-care agencies, 214
home environment:
  emergency room discharge to,
    189–91
  modifying of, 195–202
  pre-discharge evaluation of, 174, 177
  recovery and aftercare in, 173–79
  after retirement, 192–95
  when help is required, 336–38
home for the aged, *see* nursing homes
home-monitoring systems, 320–21
hospice care, 14–15, 310, 311
Hospital Elder Life Program (HELP),
  143–44, 149, 150, 151–53
hospital food, 135
hospitalists, 16–19, 123, 147, 169, 175
"hospitalitis," 138–40, 143, 144, 149–52,
  159
hospitals, 16–18, 21–22, 131–55
  admissions, 160–62
  ageism and, 44–46
  attending physicians and, 140–42,
    146, 172
  care structure in, 141–43
  care transitions and, 117–18, 173,
    183–84, 185–89
  common problems in, 132–35
  discharge, *see* discharges
  family, friends, and recovery in,
    135–37, 143–49, 150–52
  geriatric programs and, 92
  HELP interventions in, 143–44,
    152–53
  hospitalists and, 97, 123
  identifying and treating hospitalitis,
    138–40, 149–52, 159
  palliative care in, 309, 312–13
  readmissions to, 183–84, 185–89
  role confusion in, 146–49

tests and test results in, 95–96, 161,
    179, 190
  see also emergency room
Housing and Urban Development
    Department, U.S., 211
Huges, Bart, 254–55
hygiene, personal, 329, 340, 341
hypertension, 231, 246

IADLs, *see* instrumental activities of
    daily living
iatrogenic events, 149
incontinence, 133–34, 197, 226, 335
independent living, *see* staying in
    control
independent senior housing, 210–11
index-mutual-fund investing, 276–77
Inouye, Sharon, 138–40, 143, 144, 149,
    152–53
Institute of Medicine, 119
instrumental activities of daily living
    (IADLs), 207
International Longevity Center, 253
"Is There an 'Anti-Aging' Medicine?"
    (International Longevity Center),
    253

John A. Hartford Foundation, 122
Johnson, Samuel, 250

Kaiser Family Foundation, 283
Kennedy, John F., 15, 49
kitchen utensils, safety and, 201

lawyers, *see* elder law attorneys
least-restrictive alternative, 204
legacies, *see* estate planning
life-care communities, 21, 205
life expectancy, *see* longevity
life insurance, 277, 287–88
lifestyle choices, 34–38
lighting levels, safety and, 196, 200, 326
living will, 298, 302
longevity, 15, 248, 357
    actuarial tables and, 264–65, 266–67
    biology of aging and, 29–32, 30,
        31, 37
    functional, 263, 264, 267, 270
    impact of financial status on, 257–58
    traditional financial plans and,
        260–61
longevity planning, 281, 283, 286

long-term-care facility, *see* nursing
    homes
long-term-care insurance, 205, 257, 282,
    288–90
lung nodules, 74, 75–76

macular degeneration, 196, 263, 267
malnutrition, 138, 149
mammography, 95
managed care, 81–82, 91, 164
Mantle, Mickey, 350–52, 358–59
manual-dexterity issues, 197, 228
massage therapy, 236
Meals on Wheels, 21, 22
Medicaid, 180, 206, 208, 221
medical-equipment providers, 178–79
medical errors, 118–19
    aging and, 119–21
    care transitions and, 122–24, 130
    emergency rooms and, 159–60
medical homes, 114–15
medical records, 109
    electronic, 110, 118, 123–24, 127, 234
    low-tech approach to, 123–24, 127
    viewing personal, 128–30
Medicare, 21, 72, 99, 100, 103, 163,
        180, 206, 222, 260–61, 290–91,
        310, 311, 329
medication, 224–34
    adjusting for specific symptoms,
        232–33
    body changes and, 227–28
    care transitions and, 124–25
    decline in self-care and, 330
    discrepancies, 122–23
    discretionary categories of, 231
    doctor-patient relationships and,
        89, 229–32
    drug-disease interactions, 226
    drug-drug interactions, 225–26
    drug holidays, 230–31
    elimination of drugs, 226–27
    evaluating, 228–33
    generic drugs, 277
    geriatricians and, 229–31
    non-optional categories of, 230–31
    non-prescription, 233–34
    postdischarge reconciliation of,
        177–78
    regimen changes of, 229–30
    restoring sleep with, 151
medication reconciliation, 89

medicine:
    advances in, 32, 74
    ageism in, 47–48, 51, 56, 57, 58–59,
        61, 62, 65–66
    anti-aging, 252–56
    concierge, 101–4
    cookbook, 65–77
    evidence-based, 241
    overselling of, 39, 40, 73–74
    preventive, 74, 115
    reductionist, 19–21
    specialists and subspecialists in,
        19–21, 81–82, 105–15
Medigap insurance, 290–91
meditation, 236, 237, 241, 244
memory loss, 217, 256, 329
men's health, social factors and,
    22–23
midlife crises, 62
missed diagnoses, 57–59
mobility impairment, 35–36, 216–17
money and health, 257–74, 275, 347
    broad planning for old age, 258–59
    chronic illness and, 261, 263, 264, 265,
        267, 288–89
    estate planning, 259, 272–74, 291–92
    functional life expectancy and,
        263–68
    misuse of financial resources and,
        265, 272–74
    personal business plan for aging,
        261–63, 269
    pursuit of interests and, 268–71,
        355–56
    traditional financial plans and, 259–61
    see also financial gerontology
Morrison, Sean, 314–15
Mount Sinai School of Medicine, 314
MRIs (magnetic resonance imaging),
    128–29, 137
multiple sclerosis, 310
muscular strength, 27–29, 27, 32, 35, 37,
    38, 38

National Association of Elder Law
    Attorneys, 222n
National Center for Complementary
    and Alternative Medicine, 242
National Clearinghouse for Long-Term
    Care Information, 290
National Hospice and Palliative Care
    Organization, 298

National Institutes of Health, 242, 316
National Resource Center on
    Supportive Housing and Home
    Modification, 201
Native Americans, 300–301
naturally occurring retirement
    communities (NORCs), 210
New York-Presbyterian Healthcare
    System, 17, 91, 110
nonadherence (noncompliance), 329
NORCs (naturally occurring retirement
    communities), 210
not-for-profit (care) facilities, 215–16
nurse practitioners, 97–98, 99–101,
    157–59
nurses, 147–48, 218, 313
nurses' assistants, 148
nursing homes, 21, 152, 165, 194, 204
    evaluation of, 182–85, 188–89, 215–23
    health insurance and, 282, 288
    postacute- or subacute-care in,
        179–81, 183, 184, 185–86
    transfer agreements and, 184, 188–89
nutritionists, 148

occupational therapists, 148
occupational therapy aides (OTAs), 218
olfactory function (sense of smell), 333
oncology, 60–61, 113–14
orthopedists, 47, 106–7, 136–37
osteoarthritis, 106
osteoporosis, 32, 196
Oz, Mehmet, 267

pain management, 300, 309, 310,
    312–14
palliative care, 15, 295, 308–9
    cost factors and, 314–15
    growing acceptance of, 316
    in hospitals, 309, 312–13
    myths about, 309–10
    when to call for, 312–14
Palmore, Erdman, 65n
Parkinson's disease, 197, 217, 247
patient autonomy, 325
patient guidelines:
    avoiding bad health and financial
        decisions, 278–80
    avoiding care transition problems,
        124–28
    avoiding emergency rooms, 162–64
    avoiding hospitalitis, 150–52, 153–55

avoiding role confusion in hospital, 146–49
for CAM treatments, 249–52
evaluating alternative housing, 209–10
evaluating long-term-care options, 215–23
for home modifications, 197–202
for medications, 228–34
personal medical record viewing, 128–30
for recovery and aftercare at home, 175–79
for subacute care, 181–85
patient-oriented research, 239–40
Paul B. Beeson Physician Faculty Scholars in Aging Research, 122, 314
peppermint, 236
Perls, Tom, 267
Personal Finance for Dummies (Tyson), 283
physical therapists, 148, 178
physical therapy aides (PTAs), 218
physician's assistants, 97–98, 101
Physician's Desk Reference, 226
physiologic reserve, 24–25, 26–27, 28, 29–30, 34, 75, 120, 351, 355, 356
placebo effect, 238, 246–49
pneumonia, 179, 330
political cartoons, 49–50, 49, 51
polypharmacy, 224–26, 256
postacute care, 181, 213–14
power of attorney, 297–98, 348–49
practice variation, 67–68
prednisone, 106–7, 226
preventative medicine, 21, 74, 115, 116
primary care physicians, 14, 78–104
 attention to detail by, 80–82
 complaints dismissed by, 86
 concierge medicine and, 101–4
 emergency care and, 163, 164, 168–69
 end-of-life care and, 296, 307–8
 finding a new, 94–95
 gero-friendly, 90–92, 93
 hospice care and, 311
 palliative care and, 312, 313
 physician extenders and, 97–101, 147*n*
 preparing for appointments with, 87–90
 reasonable expectations and, 95–97
 recovery at home and, 175, 176, 178–79

specialists and, 105, 107–11
 see also doctor-patient relationships
privacy, loss of, 320, 334, 336
prognoses, 305–8
prostate enlargement, 67
Pubmed (Web site), 244

recovery and aftercare, 136–37, 150–55
 at home, 173–79
 postdischarge symptoms, 179
 self-care at home and, 326, 327–30, 332–33
reductionist medicine, 19–21
reflux (heartburn), 228
rehabilitation facilities, 21, 99, 121, 165, 180, 206, 282
research studies, 57–58
 evaluating evidence from, 240–42
 prognosticating and, 306–7
 types of, 239–40
respiratory infections, 344
restraints, hospital use of, 145, 149
retirement, 257, 260, 261
 enjoyment of, 357
 nest eggs for, 260, 272, 273, 274, 288, 352
 and stress, 292–93
rheumatoid arthritis, 111, 194
risk tolerance, 287
Robert Wood Johnson Clinical Scholar program, 240
Rogers, Will, 359
Roizen, Michael, 266–67

safety:
 electronic monitors and, 320–21
 patients at home and, 195–202, 326, 340–41
sanitation, 31
scleroderma, 250
Securities and Exchange Commission, 286
Seinfeld, 293, 304
self-care at home, 326, 327–30, 332–33
senior campus, 205
senior centers, 22
sensory problems, 227–28, 332–33
sibling rivalry, 273
skilled nursing facilities (SNFs), 205–6, 207–8
sleep disruption, 132–33, 139
sleeping medications, 226, 227

smoking habits, 341
social isolation, 210, 256
Social Security Administration, 266
social-service agencies, 334
social workers, 148, 177, 180, 313
somatization, 329
specialty medicine, 19–21, 81,
    105–15, 108*n*
    medical homes, 114–15
    patient information sharing and,
    108, 109
speech therapists, 148
staying in control, 319–49
    avoiding medico-legal problems,
    346–49
    behaving dangerously at home,
    340–41
    cognitive ability and, 341–43
    depression and, 329–30
    diabetic patient (case history),
    322–25
    getting someone to accept help,
    332–39
    guardianship and, 345–48
    increasing care needs and, 325–26
    loss of privacy and, 320, 334, 336
    managing frustrating behaviors,
    343–45
    medical causes of bad decision
    making, 327–30, 332
    nonmedical causes of bad decisions,
    331–32
    refusing help and, 327, 329–30, 331
Stedman's Medical Dictionary, 129
stents, 23, 179, 231
stereotypes, age-related, 270
steroids, 106–7, 232
stroke, 18, 203, 205, 216, 221, 231,
    250, 324
subacute care, 179–85
    evaluating facilities for, 181–85, 188
    hospital readmission and, 185–89
    nursing homes and, 179–81, 205–6
subspecialty medicine, 81–82,
    105–15, 163
    evaluating quality of, 111–14
    follow-up after discharge, 175, 184
supplements, 234, 276

alternative therapies and, 235, 236
surgical procedures list, 125

testicular cancer, 241
tests and test results, 95–96, 126, 161,
    179, 190
thyroid disease, 332
thyroid hormone replacement, 230–31,
    251–52
transfer agreements, 184, 188–89
treatment:
    CAM choices evaluation, 249–52
    cookbook medicine and, 65–77
    do no harm vs. aggressive
    intervention, 52–64
    financial factors of, 75, 103–4
    practice variation and, 67–68
trepanation, 255
triage, emergency room, 168
TURP (trans-urethral resection of the
    prostate), 67
Tyson, Eric, 283

ulcerative colitis, 310
United States, 157
    assisted living in, 206, 208
    death and dying in, 299, 300, 301,
    309, 311, 312, 315, 316, 317
urinary tract infections, 330

VA hospitals, 322
vascular disease, 322
Veterans Affairs Department, U.S., 322*n*
Veterans Health Administration, 91
visual impairment, 333
vitamin K supplements, 233
vitamins, 233, 235

Weill Cornell Medical College, 17, 37,
    84, 91
Wennberg, Jack, 67
Why Survive? (Butler), 46
women's health:
    breast cancer, 23, 43, 59–61
    muscle training and, 36–37
    social factors and, 22–23

yoga, 236, 237–38, 243, 244